Dietary Fructose and Glucose: The Multifacetted Aspects of Their Metabolism and Implication for Human Health

Volume 2

Dietary Fructose and Glucose: The Multifacetted Aspects of Their Metabolism and Implication for Human Health

Volume 2

Special Issue Editor

Luc Tappy

MDPI • Basel • Beijing • Wuhan • Barcelona • Belgrade

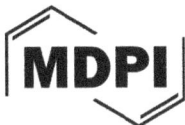

MDPI

Special Issue Editor
Luc Tappy
University of Lausanne
Switzerland

Editorial Office
MDPI
St. Alban-Anlage 66
Basel, Switzerland

This is a reprint of articles from the Special Issue published online in the open access journal *Nutrients* (ISSN 2072-6643) from 2016 to 2018 (available at: http://www.mdpi.com/journal/nutrients/special_issues/dietary_fructose_glucose)

For citation purposes, cite each article independently as indicated on the article page online and as indicated below:

LastName, A.A.; LastName, B.B.; LastName, C.C. Article Title. *Journal Name* **Year**, *Article Number*, Page Range.

Volume 2
ISBN 978-3-03897-083-5 (Pbk)
ISBN 978-3-03897-084-2 (PDF)

Volume 1–2
ISBN 978-3-03897-085-9 (Pbk)
ISBN 978-3-03897-086-6 (PDF)

Contents

About the Special Issue Editor

Luc Tappy obtained his MD degree at the University of Lausanne in 1981, and was trained in the Department of Internal Medicine and the Service of Endocrinology, Centre Hospitalier Universitaire Vaudois (CHUV) and in the Diabetes section, Temple University Hospital, Philadelphia, PA. In 2002, he was appointed full professor of physiology and associate physician at the Division of Endocrinology and Metabolism at the CHUV. He was an invited professor at the Centre Hospitalier Sart Tilman in Liège, Belgium (1998–2001), and in the Department of Nutrition at the University of California at Berkeley (1995). His research has essentially focussed on the environmental factors involved in the pathogenesis of obesity and type 2 diabetes. He has conducted a number of studies to evaluate the role of dietary sugars in the development of obesity and insulin resistance, and others aimed at assessing and evaluating the role of sport and physical activity in the prevention of fructose-induced metabolic disorders. He has published more than 200 original articles and review papers in international scientific journals.

Preface to "Dietary Fructose and Glucose: The Multifacetted Aspects of Their Metabolism and Implication for Human Health"

Fructose was identified by the French chemist, Augustin-Pierre Dubrunfaut, in 1847, and its stereochemical properties, together with those of its stereoisomers glucose and galactose, were elucidated in the 1990s by the German chemist, Emil Fisher (REF https://www.acs.org/content/acs/en/molecule-of-the-week/archive/f/fructose.html). This monosaccharide is a product of plant photosynthesis, and hence is a precursor of most dietary macronutrients. Fructose is naturally present in many fruits, vegetables, honey and natural syrups, either under its free, monosaccharide form, or as a constituent of sucrose, a disaccharide made of one molecule of glucose linked to one molecule of fructose. As such, it has always been present in the human diet, but its consumption increased tremendously during the 19th and 20th century due to the colonial trade of sugars and developments of industrial food products (REF Sweetness and power).

Over the past 50 years, fructose metabolism and fructose health effects have attracted considerable attention from biomedical researchers. It started with the elucidation of specific metabolic pathways used for fructose metabolism and the identification of inborn errors of fructose metabolism in humans (REF). Due to the fact that the initial steps of fructose metabolism are not dependent on insulin, and that fructose ingestion does not increase glycaemia to any great extent, there was a renewed interest in fructose as a sugar substitute for subjects with diabetes mellitus in the 1980s. Much of the specific effects of fructose on glucose and lipids homeostasis was acquired from small clinical trials performed during this period. At the turn of the millennium, several investigators raised concern that excess fructose intake may be closely associated with the pathogenesis of obesity and of several non-communicable diseases, such as diabetes, cardio-vascular diseases, non-alcoholic fatty liver diseases, or even cancers and neurodegenerative disorders. This has led to a large increase in the number of studies and publications on fructose and dietary sugars. Knowledge in this field has advanced at a quick pace, yet many issues remain controversial and many novel questions have emerged. The reviews and original articles included in this book encompass a broad range of open questions in the field. It is commonly proposed that dietary fructose causes insulin resistance and dyslipidemia, which may in the long term lead to the development of insulin resistance, diabetes mellitus, and contribute to atherogenesis. The mechanisms underlying these effects however remain controversial. Several reviews and original articles address the relationships between fructose intake and human diseases and discuss possible mechanisms. Novel research perspectives, such as the role of uric acid as a mediator of fructose toxicity, the link between dietary fructose and gut microbiota, or novel molecular targets mediating fructose's adverse effects are proposed in this Special Issue (include here all references 1–15).

When consumed in high amounts, a large proportion of ingested fructose is metabolized in the liver and exerts stress on this organ. There is ever growing evidence that fructose may be instrumental in the development and progression of non-alcoholic fatty liver disease. This has particular relevance for public health since this condition is highly prevalent and is closely associated with insulin resistance in the population. Several articles address potential mechanisms underlying fructose's effects on hepatic de novo lipogenesis, fat accumulation, and liver inflammation. One clinical study asserts that reducing sugar ingestion can decrease intrahepatic fat content in overweight subjects within 12 weeks. One review proposes that plant polyphenols may offer protective effects on fructose-induced NAFLD (include refs of 16–20).

Prospective cohort studies clearly indicate that a high sugar intake is associated with obesity, and support the hypothesis that sugar intake may play a causal role in body fat gain. Body weight gain is clearly secondary to an excess energy intake, but the reason why dietary sugar drives overfeeding remains hypothetical. It has been proposed that sugar fails to elicit normal satiety signals due to fructose-induced leptin resistance in the brain. It has also been hypothesized that fructose fails to stimulate the release of gut satietogenic factors. Neurosensorial effects of sugars, involving stimulation of sweet taste receptors and activation of mesolimbic dopaminergic reward pathways have also been postulated (include here references of 21–25).

It has long been known that childhood obesity is associated, not only with a high risk of obesity, but also with a high risk of diabetes and cardiovascular diseases during adulthood. Over the past two decades, it has even been robustly documented that maternal nutrition during pregnancy (fetal nutrition) and neonatal nutrition may be strong determinants of metabolic health during adulthood. Several reports address the effects of dietary fructose during pregnancy and early neonatal life on glucose homeostasis and cardiometabolic risk factors (Refs section 26–30).

Finally, fructose may have deleterious effects when consumed in excess in sedentary subjects, but may be a convenient energy substrate for some birds which rely on fructose to build up fat stores before migration, and for athletes for example. Furthermore, physical activity may prevent many of the adverse metabolic effects of a high fructose diet (references of 31–36).

The articles in this book provide a nice overview of fructose science. They illustrate recent scientific knowledge which may link fructose intake to the pathogenesis of obesity and non-communicable diseases. However, they also illustrate that many of the present allegations often presented in the lay press as scientific facts, remain mere hypotheses at this stage, and that still much remains to be discovered about this sugar.

Luc Tappy
Special Issue Editor

nutrients

MDPI

Article

The Acute Effects of Simple Sugar Ingestion on Appetite, Gut-Derived Hormone Response, and Metabolic Markers in Men

Adora M. W. Yau [1], John McLaughlin [2], William Gilmore [1,3], Ronald J. Maughan [4] and Gethin H. Evans [1,*]

[1] School of Healthcare Science, Manchester Metropolitan University, Manchester,
    Greater Manchester M1 5GD, UK; a.yau@mmu.ac.uk (A.M.W.Y.);
    b.gilmore@mmu.ac.uk or ws.gilmore@ulster.ac.uk (W.G.)
[2] Institute of Inflammation and Repair, Faculty of Medical and Human Sciences, University of Manchester,
    Manchester, Greater Manchester M13 9PT, UK; john.mclaughlin@manchester.ac.uk
[3] School of Biomedical Sciences, Ulster University, Cromore Road, Coleraine, Co Londonderry BT52 1SA, UK
[4] School of Sport, Exercise and Health Sciences, Loughborough University, Loughborough,
    Leicestershire LE11 3TU, UK; R.J.Maughan@lboro.ac.uk
* Correspondence: gethin.evans@mmu.ac.uk; Tel.: +44-161-247-1208

Received: 15 December 2016; Accepted: 8 February 2017; Published: 13 February 2017

Abstract: This pilot study aimed to investigate the effect of simple sugar ingestion, in amounts typical of common ingestion, on appetite and the gut-derived hormone response. Seven healthy men ingested water (W) and equicaloric solutions containing 39.6 g glucose monohydrate (G), 36 g fructose (F), 36 g sucrose (S), and 19.8 g glucose monohydrate + 18 g fructose (C), in a randomised order. Serum concentrations of ghrelin, glucose dependent insulinotropic polypeptide (GIP), glucagon like peptide-1 (GLP-1), insulin, lactate, triglycerides, non-esterified fatty acids (NEFA), and D-3 hydroxybutyrate, were measured for 60 min. Appetite was measured using visual analogue scales (VAS). The ingestion of F and S resulted in a lower GIP incremental area under the curve (iAUC) compared to the ingestion of G ($p < 0.05$). No differences in the iAUC for GLP-1 or ghrelin were present between the trials, nor for insulin between the sugars. No differences in appetite ratings or hepatic metabolism measures were found, except for lactate, which was greater following the ingestion of F, S, and C, when compared to W and G ($p < 0.05$). The acute ingestion of typical amounts of fructose, in a variety of forms, results in marked differences in circulating GIP and lactate concentration, but no differences in appetite ratings, triglyceride concentration, indicative lipolysis, or NEFA metabolism, when compared to glucose.

Keywords: glucose; fructose; sucrose; sugar ingestion; appetite; gut hormones; ghrelin; GLP-1; hepatic metabolism

1. Introduction

The ingestion of simple sugars has been the subject of much recent interest. In particular, the proportion of the daily energy intake from the ingestion of added fructose has rapidly increased, and this has been suggested to play a role in the development of metabolic syndrome and obesity [1,2]. Besides the ingestion of the fructose found naturally in fruits, fructose is typically ingested either as its component in sucrose or as high fructose corn syrup (commonly 55% fructose and 45% glucose). Fructose ingestion has been suggested to differentially alter feeding patterns to other simple sugars, leading to a resultant increase in body mass. One potential mechanism for the effect of fructose on feeding patterns is the effect that its ingestion may have on incretin and gut-derived hormones, which are known to influence subjective feelings of hunger.

Previous studies have shown that the acute ingestion of fructose increases blood glucose concentration [3], as well as the concentration of circulating insulin [3–5], though to a lesser extent than the ingestion of glucose. In addition, acute fructose ingestion has also been shown to increase circulating glucagon like peptide-1 (GLP-1) concentration [3] and to stimulate the secretion of leptin [5], though to a lesser extent than the ingestion of glucose. Furthermore, circulating levels of ghrelin following the ingestion of fructose are reported to be suppressed to a lesser extent than following the ingestion of glucose [6]. The effects of fructose ingestion on these circulating hormones, which are known to influence appetite, may therefore explain some of the reported relationships between the rise in dietary fructose ingestion and the increase in the prevalence of obesity.

While investigations in this area have demonstrated the effects of the acute ingestion of fructose on incretin and gut-derived hormone responses, a number of questions remain unanswered. Firstly, the majority of dietary fructose is ingested via sucrose or high fructose corn syrup. However, studies in this area have consistently investigated the effects of fructose alone. To date, and to the best of one's knowledge, no studies have compared the effects of glucose, fructose, sucrose, and a combined glucose/fructose solution on incretin and gut-derived hormone responses. Secondly, according to the National Health and Nutrition Examination Survey (NHANES) data [7], the reported average daily fructose intake in the US is approximately 49 g. In the UK, the reported average daily intake of fructose is 39 g, with the recommended intake of free sugars being no more than 5% of the total energy intake [8]. For an adult aged between 19 and 74 years, this equates to approximately 24–35 g of free sugar, based on estimated average energy requirements [9]. However, many studies that have investigated the acute effects of fructose ingestion have used much higher quantities than this.

The ingestion of large amounts of fructose in the diet is also being increasingly linked to non-alcoholic fatty liver disease (NAFLD), due to its differential and unfavourable metabolism in the liver, where it is considered to favour lipogenesis to a greater extent than glucose [10–12]. Studies indicate that short to moderate-term overfeeding with large amounts of fructose increases fasting and postprandial plasma triglyceride concentrations to a greater extent than glucose [5,6,13–16]. Studies have also shown that short to moderate term increases in fructose ingestion appears to favour the storage of fat to a greater extent than glucose as ingestion has been demonstrated to result in decreased lipolysis and metabolism of fatty acids, indicated by suppressed non-esterified fatty acid (NEFA) [6] and β-hydroxybutyrate [16] concentrations.

The effect of ingestion of an acute bolus of fructose and other simple sugars has also been documented with some conflicting findings. A mixed glucose and fructose solution with 45:55 g composition has been reported to elicit greater blood lactate and NEFA responses but no difference in triglyceride responses when compared to equivalent amounts of glucose alone [17]. On the other hand, serum triglyceride concentrations have been shown to be greater with mixed solutions of glucose and fructose of differing ratios compared to 85 g of glucose alone [18]. As with the studies investigating the effect of fructose ingestion on gut-derived appetite hormones, these acute ingestion studies on the hepatic processing of fructose have involved the ingestion of very high doses of sugars and the effect of a smaller quantity more reflective of a typical serving is unknown. The aim of this study was to examine the effect of simple sugar ingestion in more commonly ingested amounts on appetite, circulating gut hormone responses, and markers of hepatic metabolism.

2. Materials and Methods

2.1. Participants

Seven healthy men (mean ± standard deviation, age 25 ± 4 year, height 179 ± 8 cm, body mass 81.5 ± 12.3 kg, body mass index 25.5 ± 3.8 kg/m^2, and body fat 21.0% ± 7.0%) volunteered to take part in this investigation. All participants were non-smokers and had no history of chronic gastrointestinal disease as determined via completion of a medical screening questionnaire. The participants provided written informed consent prior to participation and ethical approval was provided via the Institutional Ethical Advisory Committee (Reference Number: FAETC/10-11/67).

2.2. Experimental Procedure

Each participant completed five experimental trials with at least six days between trials. Experimental trials were completed in a single-blind randomised order and began at the same time each morning following the completion of pre-trial standardisation. Prior to the first experimental trial, participants were asked to record their dietary intake and physical activity but to refrain from the ingestion of alcohol and the participation of strenuous exercise. Participants were asked to replicate these dietary and physical activity patterns in the 24 h before each subsequent experimental trial. Experimental trials took place following an overnight fast from 2100 h, with the exception of the ingestion of 500 mL of water approximately 90 min before the arrival at the laboratory, in an attempt to ensure a consistent and adequate hydration status.

Following arrival to the laboratory, participants were asked to completely empty their bladder into a container, of which 5 mL was retained for later analysis. Following a measurement of body mass, participants lay in a semi-supine position while an intravenous cannula was inserted into an antecubital vein. This remained in place for the duration of the experimental trial and was kept patent by the infusion of saline after each blood sample collection. Participants completed a 10 cm visual analogue scale (VAS), assessing their level of hunger, fullness, and prospective food consumption. A baseline 5 mL blood sample was collected before participants ingested 595 mL of the test solution over a maximum period of two minutes. Test solutions contained water only (W), 39.6 g glucose monohydrate (G), 36 g fructose (F), 36 g sucrose (S), or 19.8 g glucose monohydrate + 18 g fructose (C). Test solutions were prepared to a volume of 600 mL and a 5 mL sample was retained for osmolality analysis. Participants remained in a semi-supine position for 60 min following drink ingestion. Further assessment of subjective feelings of appetite using a VAS were taken at 10 min intervals throughout this period and blood samples were collected 10, 20, 30, and 60 min after ingestion. Time-points for blood analysis were selected based on previous studies that showed that the ingestion of 75 g of fructose elicits peak concentrations of glucose and GLP-1 at approximately 30 min, before progressively declining to near baseline levels by 60 min [3]. Following the last sample collection, the cannula was removed and a second urine sample was collected before participants were allowed to leave the laboratory.

2.3. Sample Analysis

Urine, drink, and serum samples were analysed for osmolality by freezing point depression (Gonotec Osmomat 030, Gonotec, Berlin, Germany). Analysis was performed in duplicate. Upon collection of blood samples, 50 μL of Pefabloc (Roche Diagnostics Limited, Burgess Hill, UK) was immediately added to the blood to prevent the degradation of acylated ghrelin. Blood samples were centrifuged at $1500 \times g$ for 15 min and the serum was aliquoted then stored at $-80\ °C$ until analysis was performed. Serum glucose, lactate, triglyceride, NEFA, and D-3 hydroxybutyrate concentrations were determined in duplicate using a clinical chemistry analyser (Randox Daytona, Crumlin, UK), while serum fructose concentration was determined using a colorimetric assay (EnzyChrom™ EFRU-100; BioAssay Systems, Hayward, CA, USA). The circulating concentration of acylated ghrelin, insulin, and glucose dependent insulinotropic polypeptide (GIP) were determined using multiplex analysis (Luminex 200, Luminex Corporation, Austin, TX, USA), with kits purchased from Merck-Millipore (Milliplex MAP, Merck Millipore Ltd., Feltham, UK). The circulating concentrations of total GLP-1 were determined in duplicate, using Enzyme Linked Immunoassay (Merck Millipore Ltd., Feltham, UK).

2.4. Statistical Analysis

The incremental area under the curve (iAUC) for gut hormone and hepatic metabolism data was calculated using the trapezoid method. Differences in pre-trial body mass, pre-trial urine osmolality, drink osmolality, and gut hormone concentration iAUC were examined using one-way repeated analysis of variance (ANOVA). Significant *F*-tests were followed by Bonferroni-adjusted pairwise comparisons. Two-way repeated ANOVA were used to examine differences in urine osmolality, serum osmolality, blood glucose and fructose concentrations, gut hormone concentrations, hepatic metabolism concentrations, and subjective appetite VAS scores. Significant *F*-tests were followed with the appropriate paired Student's *t*-tests or one-way repeated ANOVA and Bonferroni-adjusted pairwise comparisons. Sphericity for repeated measures was assessed, and where appropriate, Greenhouse-Geisser corrections were applied for epsilon <0.75 and the Huynh-Feldt correction was applied for less severe asphericity. All variables had full data sets with the exception of serum fructose for which eight samples (4.6% of total) were unable to be analysed and were therefore missing from the data analysis. Consequently, one data value (2.9% of total) was missing from the serum fructose iAUC data set. All data were analysed using SPSS Statistics for Windows (IBM, New York, NY, USA). Statistical significance was accepted at the 5% level and results were presented as means ± standard deviation (SD).

3. Results

3.1. Body Mass, Urine, and Drink Analysis

No change in body mass (Table 1) occurred during the study period ($p = 0.638$). Pre-trial urine volume and osmolality (Table 1) were not different between trials ($p = 0.863$ and $p = 0.504$, respectively). Post-trial urine volume was not different between trials ($p = 0.231$), and drinking resulted in reductions in urine osmolality in W, G, F, and S ($p < 0.05$), but not in C ($p = 0.221$).

The osmolality of ingested drinks were 13 ± 1, 370 ± 6, 368 ± 4, 204 ± 1, and 369 ± 4 mOsm/kg for W, G, F, S, and C, respectively. Drink osmolality for W was lower than all other solutions ($p < 0.001$) and drink osmolality for S was lower than G, F, and C ($p < 0.001$).

Table 1. Pre-trial body mass and urine characteristics pre- and post-trial.

	Water		Glucose		Fructose		Sucrose		Combined	
	Mean	SD	Mean	SD	Mean	SD	Mean	SD	Mean	SD
Body mass (kg)	81.52	12.03	81.84	11.77	81.80	12.31	81.93	12.06	81.54	12.42
Pre urine volume (mL)	174	114	199	178	143	136	164	120	179	197
Post urine volume (mL)	613	268	639	226	411	254	577	400	596	331
Pre urine osmolality (mOsmol/kg)	461	232	375	224	431	174	593	309	465	260
Post urine osmolality (mOsmol/kg)	161 [a]	101	137 [a]	59	233 [a]	148	185 [a]	157	269	299

[a] Significantly lower than pre urine osmolality ($p < 0.05$). Values are means and standard deviations (SD).

3.2. Serum Glucose, Fructose, and Lactate

Baseline serum glucose concentrations (Table 2) were not different between trials ($p = 0.288$). Effects of trial ($p < 0.001$), time ($p < 0.001$), and interaction ($p < 0.001$), were present for serum glucose concentration (Figure 1a). Concentrations were elevated from pre-ingestion values at 10, 20, and 30 min after the ingestion of G, S, and C ($p < 0.05$). No difference was observed from baseline after the ingestion of W and F. At 10 min, blood glucose concentrations for G, S, and C, were greater than W ($p < 0.05$) and the concentration for S was greater than for F ($p < 0.05$). At 20 min after ingestion, blood glucose concentrations were greater for G, S, and C, than for W and F ($p < 0.05$). Furthermore, at 30 min after ingestion, blood glucose concentrations were greater for G, S, C, and F, compared to W ($p < 0.05$), while the concentration for S was greater than F ($p < 0.05$). Incremental AUC values for serum glucose concentration were -7.48 ± 12.17, 96.73 ± 55.64, 7.81 ± 9.78, 73.36 ± 24.39, and 66.61 ± 38.33 mmol/L 1 h, for W, G, F, S, and C, respectively. Trials G, S, and C were greater than W ($p < 0.05$), and S was greater than F ($p = 0.005$).

Baseline serum fructose concentrations (Table 2) were not different between trials ($p = 0.912$). Effects of trial ($p < 0.001$), time ($p = 0.001$), and interaction ($p < 0.001$), were present for the serum fructose concentration (Figure 1b). Concentrations were lower at 10 min ($p = 0.032$) and 30 min ($p = 0.012$) compared to pre-ingestion values for W. Serum fructose concentrations were greater than pre-ingestion values at 20, 30, and 60 min for F, and at 30 and 60 min for S ($p < 0.05$). At 10 min after ingestion, serum fructose concentration was greater for S compared to G ($p = 0.036$). At 20 min after ingestion, the concentration was greater for F compared to W ($p = 0.043$) and G ($p = 0.038$). At 30 min post ingestion, concentrations for F and S were greater than W and G ($p < 0.05$). At 60 min after ingestion, concentrations were greater for F and S compared to G ($p < 0.05$) and F was greater than C ($p = 0.041$). Incremental AUC values for the serum fructose concentration were -1194.12 ± 587.20, -451.19 ± 513.01, $15{,}780.52 \pm 4156.57$, $10{,}480.64 \pm 4631.63$, and 8788.90 ± 4665.14 µmol/L 1 h, for W, G, F, S, and C, respectively. Trials F, S, and C were greater than both W and G ($p < 0.05$).

Baseline serum lactate concentrations (Table 2) were not different between trials ($p = 0.074$). Effects of trial ($p < 0.001$), time ($p < 0.001$), and interaction ($p < 0.001$), were present for serum lactate concentration (Figure 1c). Concentrations were elevated from pre-ingestion values at all time-points for S ($p < 0.05$), and for F at 20, 30, and 60 min ($p < 0.01$). Elevations from baseline concentrations were observed for C at 30 ($p = 0.043$) and 60 min ($p = 0.004$), and for G at 60 min only. At 20 min after ingestion, concentrations were greater for S, compared to W, F, and G ($p < 0.05$), and at 30 min, concentrations were greater for S and F, compared to W and G ($p < 0.05$). At 60 min, the concentration for W was lower than all other trials ($p < 0.05$), and the concentration for F was greater than G ($p < 0.05$). Incremental AUC values were greater for F, S, and C compared to W and G ($p < 0.05$), with values 53.38 ± 6.32, 60.49 ± 18.45, 54.42 ± 27.10, -2.18 ± 8.21, and 8.88 ± 8.22 mmol/L 1 h, respectively.

Table 2. Baseline concentrations for blood serum measures.

	Water		Glucose		Fructose		Sucrose		Combined	
	Mean	SD	Mean	SD	Mean	SD	Mean	SD	Mean	SD
Glucose (mmol/L)	5.15	0.39	5.11	0.28	5.27	0.21	5.25	0.18	5.12	0.26
Fructose (µM/L)	67.34	19.59	60.70	41.81	51.75	37.31	57.95	36.73	64.62	40.65
Lactate (mmol/L)	0.93	0.27	1.13	0.30	0.91	0.23	0.94	0.18	0.88	0.24
Insulin (pg/mL)	191.4	88.5	216.9	163.1	192.1	102.3	172.4	103.4	177.7	89.4
GIP (pg/mL)	8.81	3.33	12.67	7.71	9.31	5.26	12.12	8.82	13.15	7.20
GLP-1 (pg/mL)	58.4	6.3	61.7	4.2	64.1	12.5	62.9	11.4	69.2	14.2
Ghrelin (pg/mL)	232.1	79.6	200.9	80.2	189.0	68.8	220.7	84.2	189.9	65.1
Triglycerides (mmol/L)	1.20	0.47	1.19	0.59	1.29	0.62	1.13	0.56	1.13	0.52
D-3 Hydroxybutyrate (mmol/L)	0.12	0.06	0.11	0.09	0.11	0.05	0.10	0.03	0.10	0.02
NEFA (mmol/L)	0.74	0.35	0.60	0.22	0.64	0.32	0.50	0.12	0.62	0.56

Values are means and standard deviations (SD).

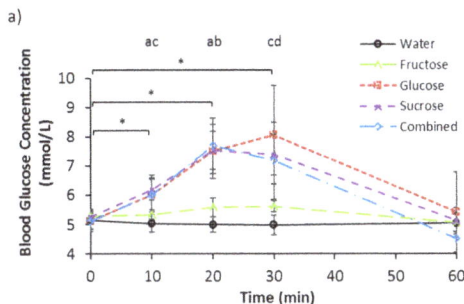

Figure 1. *Cont.*

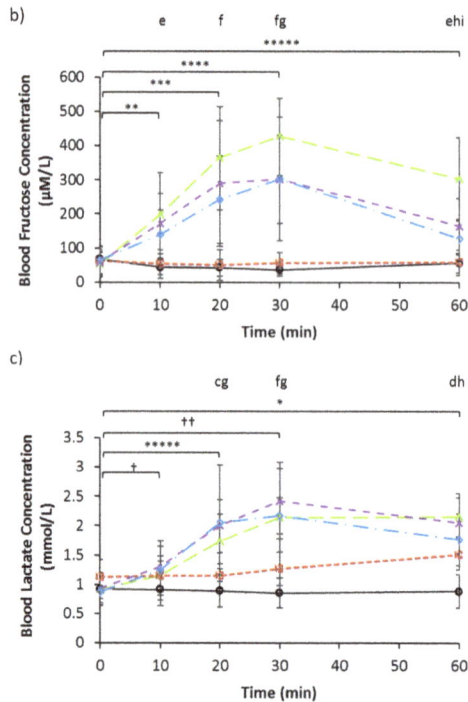

Figure 1. Serum (a) glucose (b) fructose and (c) lactate concentrations at baseline and following ingestion of 595 mL of water (W), 6% fructose (F), 6% glucose (G), 6% sucrose (S) and 6% combined glucose and fructose (C) solutions. [a] G, S, and C are greater than W; [b] G, S, and C are greater than F; [c] S is greater than F; [d] All carbohydrate trials are greater than W; [e] S is greater than G; [f] F is greater than W and G; [g] S is greater than W and G; [h] F is greater than G; [I] F is greater than C; * Increase from baseline for G, S, and C; ** Decrease from baseline for W; *** Increase from baseline for F; **** Decrease from baseline for W, and increase for F and S; ***** Increase from baseline for F and S; † Increase from baseline for S; †† Increase from baseline for S and C. All $p < 0.05$. Values are mean ± standard deviation.

3.3. Serum Insulin, GIP, GLP-1, and Ghrelin

Baseline serum insulin concentrations (Table 2) were not different between trials ($p = 0.587$). Effects of trial ($p = 0.032$), time ($p = 0.014$), and interaction ($p < 0.001$), were present for serum insulin concentration (Figure 2a). Insulin concentrations were elevated from pre-ingestion values for G and S at 10 min after ingestion ($p < 0.05$). For G, the concentration at 60 min was lower than at 20 and 30 min ($p < 0.05$). No other differences were observed over time or between trials at the different time-points. Incremental AUC values were -1856.2 ± 2166.8, $59,342.5 \pm 55,279.2$, 6510.6 ± 3449.0, $37,052.1 \pm 25,605.6$, and $39,270.8 \pm 33,159.7$ pg/mL 1 h, for W, G, F, S, and C, respectively. Incremental AUC was greater for F than W ($p = 0.028$).

Baseline serum GIP concentrations (Table 2) were not different between trials ($p = 0.246$). Effects of trial ($p < 0.001$), time ($p < 0.001$), and interaction ($p < 0.001$), were present for serum GIP concentration (Figure 2b). Concentrations were elevated ($p < 0.05$) from pre-ingestion values for G at all time points ($p < 0.05$). For S, the concentration tended to increase 10 min after ingestion ($p = 0.052$), and were elevated at 20 ($p = 0.049$) and 30 ($p = 0.036$) min after ingestion. This was followed by a decrease at 60 min compared to 20 ($p = 0.047$) and 30 min ($p = 0.036$). For C, concentrations were increased at 10 ($p = 0.020$) and 30 min ($p = 0.014$) compared to baseline. At 10 min after ingestion, concentrations for W and F were lower than G, S, and C ($p < 0.05$), while at 20 min, they were lower than G and S

($p < 0.05$). At 30 min after ingestion, concentrations for W and F were again lower than G, S, and C ($p < 0.05$), and the concentration for G was greater than S ($p = 0.035$). At 60 min after ingestion, the concentration for W was lower than G, S, and C ($p < 0.05$), while the concentration for G was greater than S ($p = 0.044$) and C ($p = 0.034$), and tended to be greater than F ($p = 0.052$). Incremental AUC values were -5.9 ± 111.9, 2224.8 ± 937.2, 50.8 ± 135.0, 1172.3 ± 701.8, and 1252.8 ± 720.7 pg/mL 1 h, for W, G, F, S, and C, respectively. Incremental AUC for G, S, and C, were greater than W ($p < 0.05$), and iAUC for G was greater than F ($p = 0.014$) and S ($p = 0.033$).

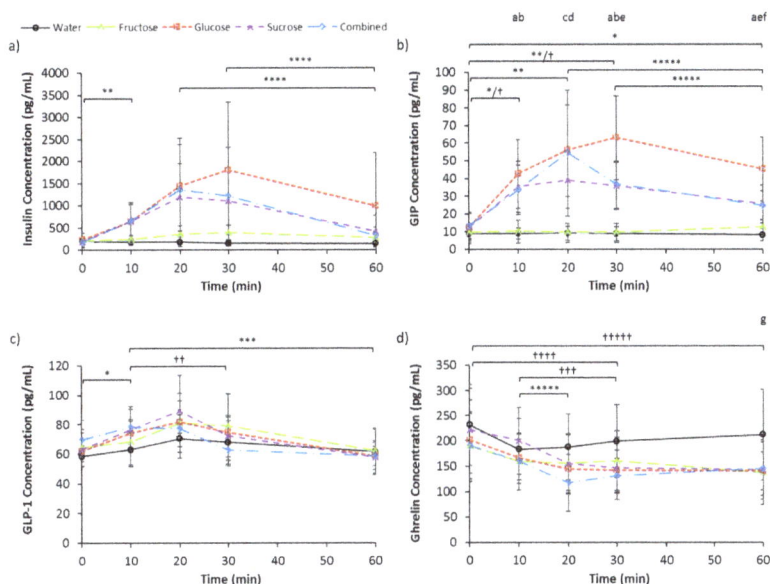

Figure 2. Serum (**a**) Insulin (**b**) glucose dependent insulinotropic polypeptide (GIP) (**c**) glucagon like peptide-1 (GLP-1) and (**d**) ghrelin concentrations at baseline and following ingestion of 595 mL of water (W), 6% fructose (F), 6% glucose (G), 6% sucrose (S) and 6% combined glucose and fructose (C) solutions. [a] W is less than G, S, and C; [b] Fructose is less than G, S, and C; [c] W is less than G and S; [d] F is less than G and S; [e] S is less than G; [f] C is less than G; [g] W is greater than F; * Increase from baseline for G; ** Increase from baseline for G and S; *** Decrease from time-point for G, S, and C; **** Decrease from time-point for G; ***** Decrease from time-point for S; [†] Increase from baseline for C; [††] Decrease from time-point for C; [†††] Decrease from time-point for C and S; [††††] Decrease from baseline for S and C; [†††††] Decrease from baseline for F and S. All $p < 0.05$. Values are mean $\pm$ standard deviation.

Baseline serum GLP-1 concentrations (Table 2) were not different between trials ($p = 0.092$). An effect of time ($p < 0.001$), an interaction effect tending to significance ($p = 0.078$), and no main effect of trial ($p = 0.354$), were present for serum GLP-1 concentration (Figure 2c). GLP-1 concentration was elevated from pre-ingestion values after 10 min ($p = 0.023$), and was lower at 60 min compared to 10 min ($p = 0.005$) for G. Concentrations were also lower at 60 min compared to 10 min for S ($p = 0.008$), and lower at 30 and 60 min compared to 10 min for C ($p < 0.05$). Incremental AUC values for W, G, F, S, and C, were 403.2 ± 655.7, 519.8 ± 345.8, 447.9 ± 390.7, 499.3 ± 574.2, and -131.6 ± 516.3 pg/mL 1 h, respectively. There were no differences in iAUC ($p = 0.152$).

Baseline serum ghrelin concentrations (Table 2) were not different between trials ($p = 0.066$). Effects of trial ($p = 0.016$), time ($p < 0.001$), and interaction ($p = 0.001$), were present for serum ghrelin concentration (Figure 2d). Ghrelin concentration tended to be reduced from pre-ingestion at 20 min for F ($p = 0.064$), and was reduced from pre-ingestion at 60 min ($p = 0.006$). For S and C, reductions from baseline were observed at 30 and 60 min, and 30 min, respectively ($p < 0.05$). Concentrations were also lower at 20 and 30 min, and at 30 min, compared to 10 min for S and C, respectively. No differences over time were present for W and G, although a decrease tending to significance at 60 min compared to 10 min was present for G ($p = 0.072$). At 60 min, W was higher than F ($p = 0.014$). Incremental AUC values were -1892.4 ± 1488, -3028.6 ± 2530.0, -2063.3 ± 1106.9, -3546.1 ± 2073.6, and -2898.5 ± 2007.8 pg/mL 1 h, for W, G, F, S, and C, respectively. No differences were seen in iAUC ($p = 0.209$).

3.4. Serum Triglycerides, D-3 Hydroxybutyrate, and NEFA

Baseline serum triglyceride concentrations (Table 2) were not different between trials ($p = 0.673$). An interaction effect ($p = 0.032$) was indicated for serum triglyceride concentration (Figure 3a). No main effects of trial ($p = 0.425$) or time ($p = 0.254$) were present. A difference at 10 min between trials tended to significance ($p = 0.099$). Differences over time tended to significance for G ($p = 0.053$), S ($p = 0.092$), and C ($p = 0.073$). A difference over time was indicated for W ($p = 0.039$), but no pairwise differences were located, and no change over time was seen for F ($p = 0.279$). Incremental AUC values were -1.81 ± 3.00, -0.65 ± 1.74, 0.54 ± 5.56, -1.97 ± 1.75, and -2.09 ± 3.56 mmol/L 1 h, for W, G, F, S, and C, respectively. No differences were present for iAUC ($p = 0.534$).

Baseline serum D-3 hydroxybutyrate concentrations (Table 2) were not different between trials ($p = 0.753$). No effect of trial ($p = 0.220$), an effect of time tending to significance ($p = 0.098$), and no interaction effect ($p = 0.891$) was present for serum D-3 hydroxybutyrate concentration (Figure 3b). Also, no difference was present for iAUC ($p = 0.828$), where the areas were -0.19 ± 3.05, 1.58 ± 4.30, -1.11 ± 2.89, -1.50 ± 1.72, and -0.99 ± 0.90 mmol/L 1 h, for W, G, F, S, and C, respectively.

Baseline serum NEFA concentrations (Table 2) were not different between trials ($p = 0.544$). No effect of trial ($p = 0.411$) or interaction effect ($p = 0.431$) was present for serum NEFA concentration (Figure 3c), but an effect of time was revealed ($p = 0.002$). Concentrations decreased over time for W, G, and C. For W, the concentrations at 20 and 30 min were lower than baseline ($p < 0.05$). For G, the concentrations at 20, 30, and 60 min were lower than baseline ($p < 0.01$) and 10 min ($p < 0.05$), and in addition, the concentration at 60 min was lower than at 30 min ($p = 0.040$). For C, the concentrations at 20, 30, and 60 min were lower than baseline ($p < 0.05$), the concentrations at 30 and 60 min were lower than at 10 min ($p < 0.05$), and additionally, the concentration at 60 min was lower than at 20 min ($p = 0.003$). No difference was present for iAUC ($p = 0.512$), where the areas were -7.70 ± 5.02, -10.68 ± 3.61, -14.26 ± 13.47, -9.22 ± 9.97, and -11.38 ± 3.96, for W, G, F, S, and C, respectively.

a)

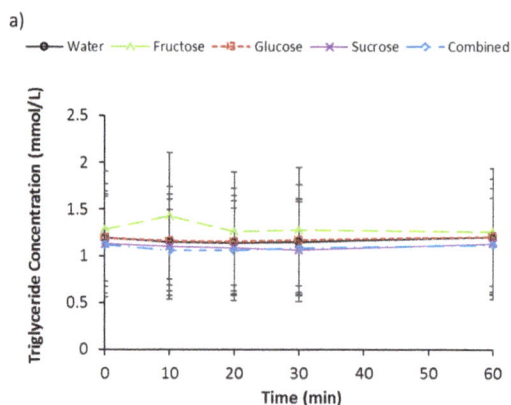

Figure 3. *Cont.*

b)

c)

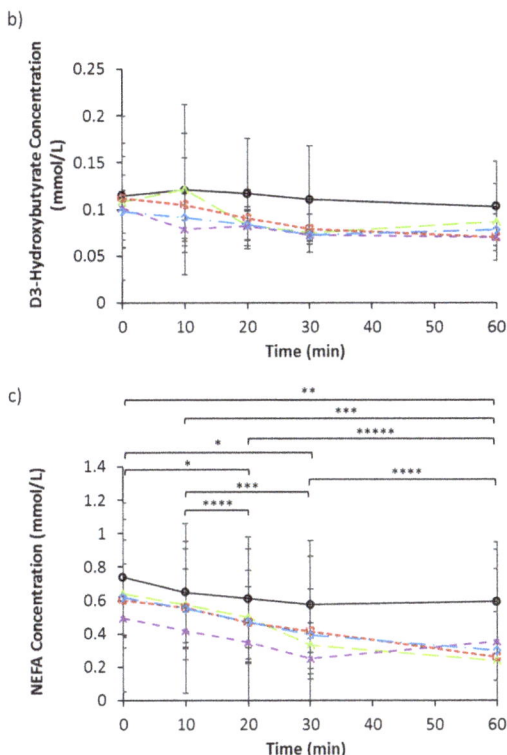

Figure 3. Serum (**a**) triglycerides (**b**) D-3 hydroxybutyrate and (**c**) non esterified fatty acids (NEFA) concentrations at baseline and following ingestion of 595 mL of water (W), 6% fructose (F), 6% glucose (G), 6% sucrose (S) and 6% combined glucose and fructose (C) solutions. * Decrease from baseline for W, G, and C; ** Decrease from baseline for G and C; *** Decrease from 10 min for G and C; **** Decrease from time-point for G; ***** Decrease from time-point for C. All $p < 0.05$. Values are mean ± standard deviation.

3.5. Subjective Measurements of Appetite

A transient pattern of decreased hunger and prospective food consumption ratings occurred at 10 min post drink ingestion followed by a gradual increase thereafter for all trials. Furthermore, consistent with the above, fullness ratings transiently increased at 10 min post ingestion then gradually decreased thereafter. No effect of trial ($p = 0.337$), an effect of time tending to significance ($p = 0.091$), and no interaction effect ($p = 0.492$), were present for hunger ratings (Figure 4a). For fullness ratings, no effects of trial ($p = 0.455$), time ($p = 0.106$), or interaction ($p = 0.288$), were present (Figure 4b). No main effect of trial ($p = 0.652$) or interaction effect ($p = 0.430$) was present for prospective food consumption, but a main effect of time ($p = 0.001$) was seen (Figure 4c). An effect of time was indicated for trial G with 20 min tending to be lower than 60 min ($p = 0.078$). An effect of time also tended to significance for C ($p = 0.051$).

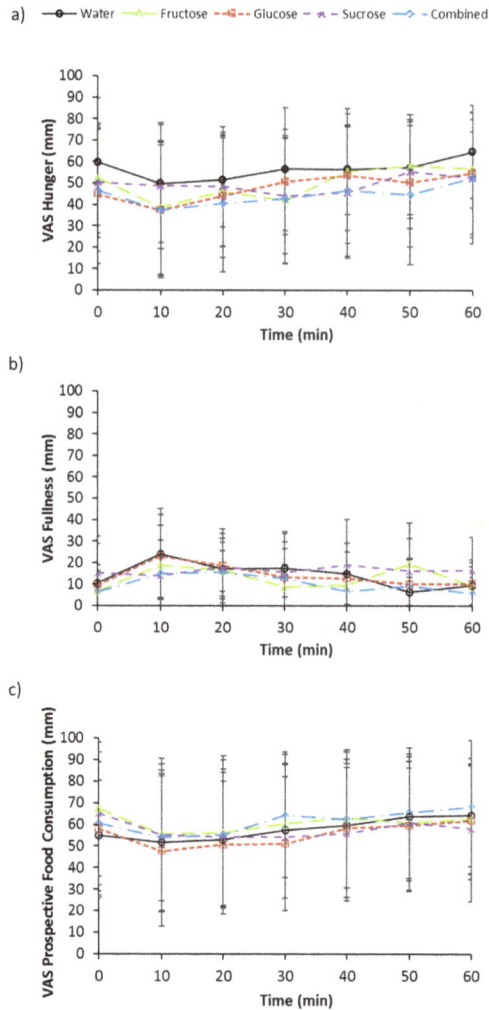

Figure 4. Visual analogue scale (VAS) scores for (**a**) hunger (**b**) fullness and (**c**) prospective food consumption at baseline and following ingestion of 595 mL of water (W), 6% fructose (F), 6% glucose (G), 6% sucrose (S) and 6% combined glucose and fructose (C) solutions. Values are mean ± standard deviation.

4. Discussion

The ingestion of glucose and the ingestion of fructose resulted in respective increases in blood glucose and blood fructose concentration in a dose-related fashion with peak concentrations being attained at 30 min by the glucose alone and fructose alone trials, correspondingly. The similar sucrose and combined solutions resulted in comparable blood glucose and blood fructose concentration responses. Whilst the ingestion of glucose alone resulted in no changes to blood fructose concentration, the ingestion of fructose alone saw a significant increase in blood glucose above water control values at 30 min. This can be explained by the evidence that a moderate amount of fructose undergoes conversion to glucose [19,20]. The ingestion of fructose alone resulted in a significantly lower blood glucose concentration than glucose alone ingestion at 20 min but no significantly lower overall (iAUC) blood glucose response. This result is therefore partially inconsistent with the findings of Kong et al. [3], although the large number of comparisons in this present study may have concealed any statistical difference. A significantly greater blood glucose response was seen with sucrose compared to fructose alone, however, suggesting an interaction of glucose co-ingestion that was not present with the mixed glucose-fructose ingestion. One possibility is the effect of lower osmolality in sucrose resulting in a faster gastric emptying rate and thus a greater increase in the blood glucose concentration. The blood glucose response to different sugars was mirrored by both insulin and GIP responses. However, the pattern of response for GLP-1 did not follow. It is thought that GLP-1 plays a more potent role in glucose-stimulated insulin release, but the results of this study potentially suggest a predominant role of the incretin GIP.

The ingestion of solutions containing fructose resulted in significant increases in blood lactate concentration at a faster rate than the ingestion of glucose alone. This increase in lactate concentration occurred even with the relatively small amount of fructose ingestion (18 g) within the S and C trials. Furthermore, the ingestion of sucrose, and combined glucose and fructose, resulted in similar iAUCs, compared to fructose ingestion alone, despite containing half of the amount of fructose. This may be due to a differential fate of fructose when co-ingested with glucose. The presence of glucose in the ingested solutions may have led to the preferential oxidation of glucose within the Krebs cycle, as well as the conversion to glycogen, thus limiting this pathway for fructose oxidation and resulting in greater lactate production. It is unlikely that this was due to reduced insulin action, which is reported to result in less pyruvate entering the mitochondria for oxidation and thus causing a corresponding increase of anaerobic metabolism to lactate [21], because insulin secretion following both S and C were pronounced in comparison to fructose. Another potential explanation is related to the observations that fructose absorption is augmented when ingested with glucose [22]. However, it is unlikely that the observed results were due to a greater or more efficient absorption of fructose when co-ingested with glucose, as serum fructose concentration increased significantly from baseline following fructose alone ingestion but not for the fructose-glucose solutions.

The ingestion of all four sugar solutions resulted in similar acylated ghrelin suppression, unlike the finding by Teff et al. [6] that fructose ingestion results in less suppression following fructose ingestion when compared to glucose ingestion. Furthermore, little difference between sugars was observed for GLP-1 response. This is in contrast to previous findings by Kong et al. [3] and Kuhre et al. [23] where participants were fed 75 g of sugar in both studies. Although it is noted that a potential limitation of the present study is that we measured total GLP-1, and not the specific active form GLP-1$^{7-36}$, the reported difference seen by Kuhre et al. [23] was also for total GLP-1, indicating the contrasting findings are likely due to the lower amount of sugar ingestion (36 g) in the present study. However, a marked difference between sugars was seen with GIP responses. The ingestion of fructose induced virtually no GIP response in contrast to the other sugar solutions, and was comparable to the effects of water. Although insulin concentrations significantly increased and then decreased following glucose and sucrose ingestion, whilst no significant changes over time was observed for fructose ingestion, there were no significant differences detected between sugars at different time-points or for the overall (iAUC) response. The insulin results are therefore inconsistent with those of previous studies that have shown significantly lower responses following fructose ingestion compared to glucose ingestion [3–5]. This may be due to the large number of comparisons in the present study masking any differences. Alternatively, this may have been due to the large standard deviations observed. The large inter-individual variability may be due to the differences in the body mass index of the participants, which ranged from normal to obese classifications. The range of participants utilised in this study is a limitation as insulin and metabolic responses may differ in participants with different levels of adiposity. However, as this study utilised a repeated measures design, each participant acted as their own control. In line with the absence of response differences in the gut-derived appetite hormones ghrelin and GLP-1, no subsequent difference or effect of sugar ingestion was observed for any of the appetite ratings.

Triglyceride concentrations were unchanged following ingestion of the sugar solutions, and no difference was found between trials, suggesting that the acute ingestion of simple sugars in typical amounts does not result in immediate increases in the rate of de novo lipogenesis. However, it may be that the 60 min postprandial measurement period in the present study was not long enough to detect any changes, as triglyceride concentrations have been shown to be significantly elevated 2–3 h after fructose ingestion [24]. The one-hour postprandial measurement period was selected based on the main responses of blood glucose, GLP-1, and insulin, occurring within 60 min after the ingestion of a much larger bolus of fructose (75 g) in studies with two-hour [3] and four-hour [4] measurement periods. In addition, whilst significant decreases in NEFA concentrations for W, G, and C trials were observed over time, no differences in NEFA or D-3-hydroxybutyrate concentration suppression was seen between sugar trials, indicating that the ingestion of the different sugars resulted in similar reductions in lipolysis and NEFA metabolism. This is consistent with the studies by Ngo Sock et al. [16], Teff et al. [5], and Teff et al. [6]. For the trials involving glucose ingestion, this is consistent with the elevation and action of insulin. However, this is unlikely to be the mechanism for reduced NEFA concentrations following fructose ingestion as insulin secretion was relatively unchanged. Instead, the mechanism relating to this may be explained by the increased lactate production seen with fructose ingestion. Lactate has been shown to inhibit lipolysis in adipocytes [25].

Whilst the participants were asked to record their food intake and physical activity in the 24 h prior to their first experimental trial, for the purpose of standardisation by repeating these in subsequent trials, no dietary information was collected on the habitual consumption of sugar-sweetened beverages. Long periods of high fructose intake at 25% of the energy requirements can alter glucose and insulin responses within ten weeks, and markers of lipid metabolism within two weeks [13,14]. However, during the relatively short period of study, it would have been unlikely that any participants had such a large change in their habitual diet in the present study. Furthermore, as it was a repeated measures design, each participant acted as their own control so this would not affect the conclusions made. A limitation of the current study is the generalisability of these novel results on the effect of ingestion of simple sugars in amounts reflective of typical consumption, as only healthy men were studied in the present study. Hormonal and metabolic responses to simple sugar ingestion in women may differ, and future research in this area should explore whether there are any sex differences, in addition to the responses of those who are obese or who have other metabolic disorders.

5. Conclusions

The acute ingestion of simple sugars in typical amounts induced marked differences in the circulating GIP response, and blood glucose and fructose responses, but not acylated ghrelin, total GLP-1, or insulin responses. No effects on appetite scores were seen as a result. The acute ingestion of a solution containing typical amounts of sugar does not result in significantly increased triglyceride synthesis over the postprandial period investigated. Furthermore, no differences between sugars in these smaller quantities were seen for lipolysis and NEFA metabolism suppression but fructose ingestion results in significantly increased lactate production that is augmented with glucose co-ingestion.

Acknowledgments: The authors would like to acknowledge Dave Maskew and Saeed Ahmad of Manchester Metropolitan University for their technical support in the laboratory. A.M.W.Y. was supported by a Manchester Metropolitan University Ph.D. studentship. This research received no specific grant from any funding agency in the public, commercial, or not-for-profit sectors.

Author Contributions: A.M.W.Y., G.H.E., J.M., R.J.M. and W.G. conceived and designed the experiments; A.M.W.Y. and G.H.E. performed the experiments; A.M.W.Y. analysed the data; A.M.W.Y. wrote the paper with contributions from G.H.E., J.M., R.J.M. and W.G. All authors have read and approved the final manuscript.

Conflicts of Interest: The authors declare no conflict of interest.

Nutrients **2017**, *9*, 135

References

1. Johnson, R.J.; Murray, R. Fructose, Exercise, and Health. *Curr. Sports Med. Rep.* **2010**, *9*, 253–258. [CrossRef] [PubMed]
2. Lindqvist, A.; Baelemans, A.; Erlanson-Albertsson, C. Effects of sucrose, glucose and fructose on peripheral and central appetite signals. *Regul. Pept.* **2008**, *150*, 26–32. [CrossRef] [PubMed]
3. Kong, M.F.; Chapman, I.; Goble, E.; Wishart, J.; Wittert, G.; Morris, H.; Horowitz, M. Effects of oral fructose and glucose on plasma GLP-1 and appetite in normal subjects. *Peptides* **1999**, *20*, 545–551. [CrossRef]
4. Bowen, J.; Noakes, M.; Clifton, P.M. Appetite hormones and energy intake in obese men after consumption of fructose, glucose and whey protein beverages. *Int. J. Obes.* **2007**, *31*, 1696–1703. [CrossRef] [PubMed]
5. Teff, K.L.; Grudziak, J.; Townsend, R.R.; Dunn, T.N.; Grant, R.W.; Adams, S.H.; Keim, N.L.; Cummings, B.P.; Stanhope, K.L.; Havel, P.J. Endocrine and Metabolic Effects of Consuming Fructose- and Glucose-Sweetened Beverages with Meals in Obese Men and Women: Influence of Insulin Resistance on Plasma Triglyceride Responses. *J. Clin. Endocrinol. Metab.* **2009**, *94*, 1562–1569. [CrossRef] [PubMed]
6. Teff, K.L.; Elliott, S.S.; Tschop, M.; Kieffer, T.J.; Rader, D.; Heiman, M.; Townsend, R.R.; Keim, N.L.; D'alessio, D.; Havel, P.J. Dietary fructose reduces circulating insulin and leptin, attenuates postprandial suppression of ghrelin, and increases triglycerides in women. *J. Clin. Endocrinol. Metab.* **2004**, *89*, 2963–2972. [CrossRef] [PubMed]
7. Marriott, B.P.; Cole, N.; Lee, E. National estimates of dietary fructose intake increased from 1977 to 2004 in the United States. *J. Nutr.* **2009**, *139*, S1228–S1235. [CrossRef] [PubMed]
8. Scientific Advisory Committee on Nutrition. Carbohydrates and Health Report. 2015. Available online: https://www.gov.uk/government/uploads/system/uploads/attachment_data/file/445503/SACN_Carbohydrates_and_Health.pdf (accessed on 1 July 2016).
9. Scientific Advisory Committee on Nutrition. Dietary Reference Values for Energy. 2011. Available online: https://www.gov.uk/government/uploads/system/uploads/attachment_data/file/339317/SACN_Dietary_Reference_Values_for_Energy.pdf (accessed on 1 July 2016).
10. Vos, M.B.; Lavine, J.E. Dietary fructose in nonalcoholic fatty liver disease. *Hepatology* **2013**, *57*, 2525–2531. [CrossRef] [PubMed]
11. Tappy, L.; Le, K.A. Does fructose consumption contribute to non-alcoholic fatty liver disease? *Clin. Res. Hepatol. Gastroenterol.* **2012**, *36*, 554–560. [CrossRef] [PubMed]
12. Yilmaz, Y. Review article: Fructose in non-alcoholic fatty liver disease. *Aliment. Pharmacol. Ther.* **2012**, *35*, 1135–1144. [CrossRef] [PubMed]
13. Stanhope, K.L.; Bremer, A.A.; Medici, V.; Nakajima, K.; Ito, Y.; Nakano, T.; Chen, G.; Fong, T.H.; Lee, V.; Menorca, R.I.; et al. Consumption of fructose and high fructose corn syrup increase postprandial triglycerides, LDL-cholesterol, and apolipoprotein-B in young men and women. *J. Clin. Endocrinol. Metab.* **2011**, *96*, E1596–E1605. [CrossRef] [PubMed]
14. Stanhope, K.L.; Schwarz, J.M.; Keim, N.L.; Griffen, S.C.; Bremer, A.A.; Graham, J.L.; Hatcher, B.; Cox, C.L.; Dyachenko, A.; Zhang, W.; et al. Consuming fructose-sweetened, not glucose-sweetened, beverages increases visceral adiposity and lipids and decreases insulin sensitivity in overweight/obese humans. *J. Clin. Investig.* **2009**, *119*, 1322–1334. [CrossRef] [PubMed]
15. Stanhope, K.L.; Griffen, S.C.; Bair, B.R.; Swarbrick, M.M.; Keim, N.L.; Havel, P.J. Twenty-four-hour endocrine and metabolic profiles following consumption of high-fructose corn syrup-, sucrose-, fructose-, and glucose-sweetened beverages with meals. *Am. J. Clin. Nutr.* **2008**, *87*, 1194–1203. [PubMed]
16. Ngo Sock, E.T.; Lê, K.A.; Ith, M.; Kreis, R.; Boesch, C.; Tappy, L. Effects of a short-term overfeeding with fructose or glucose in healthy young males. *Br. J. Nutr.* **2010**, *103*, 939–943. [CrossRef] [PubMed]
17. Bidwell, A.J.; Holmstrup, M.E.; Doyle, R.P.; Fairchild, T.J. Assessment of endothelial function and blood metabolite status following acute ingestion of a fructose-containing beverage. *Acta Physiol.* **2010**, *200*, 35–43. [CrossRef] [PubMed]
18. Parks, E.J.; Skokan, L.E.; Timlin, M.T.; Dingfelder, C.S. Dietary sugars stimulate fatty acid synthesis in adults. *J. Nutr.* **2008**, *138*, 1039–1046. [PubMed]
19. Sun, S.Z.; Empie, M.W. Fructose metabolism in humans—What isotopic tracer studies tell us. *Nutr. Metab.* **2012**, *9*, 89. [CrossRef] [PubMed]

20. Delarue, J.; Normand, S.; Pachiaudi, C.; Beylot, M.; Lamisse, F.; Riou, J.P. The contribution of naturally labeled C-13 fructose to glucose appearance in humans. *Diabetologia* **1993**, *36*, 338–345. [CrossRef] [PubMed]
21. Mueller, W.M.; Stanhope, K.L.; Gregoire, F.; Evans, J.L.; Havel, P.J. Effects of metformin and vanadium on leptin secretion from cultured rat adipocytes. *Obes. Res.* **2000**, *8*, 530–539. [CrossRef] [PubMed]
22. Truswell, A.S.; Seach, J.M.; Thorburn, A.W. Incomplete absorption of pure fructose in healthy-subjects and the facilitating effect of glucose. *Am. J. Clin. Nutr.* **1988**, *48*, 1424–1430. [PubMed]
23. Kuhre, R.E.; Gribble, F.M.; Hartmann, B.; Reimann, F.; Windeløv, J.A.; Rehfeld, J.F.; Holst, J.J. Fructose stimulates GLP-1 but not GIP secretion in mice, rats, and humans. *Am. J. Physiol. Gastrointest. Liver Physiol.* **2014**, *306*, G622–G630. [CrossRef] [PubMed]
24. Dushay, J.R.; Toschi, E.; Mitten, E.K.; Fisher, F.M.; Herman, M.A.; Maratos-Flier, E. Fructose ingestion acutely stimulates circulating FGF21 levels in humans. *Mol. Metab.* **2014**, *4*, 51–57. [CrossRef] [PubMed]
25. Liu, C.; Wu, J.; Zhu, J.; Kuei, C.; Yu, J.; Shelton, J.; Sutton, S.W.; Li, X.; Yun, S.J.; Mirzadegan, T.; et al. Lactate inhibits lipolysis in fat cells through activation of an orphan G-protein-coupled receptor, GPR81. *J. Biol. Chem.* **2009**, *284*, 2811–2828. [CrossRef] [PubMed]

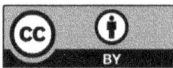

nutrients

MDPI

Article

The Effect of Short-Term Dietary Fructose Supplementation on Gastric Emptying Rate and Gastrointestinal Hormone Responses in Healthy Men

Adora M. W. Yau [1], John McLaughlin [2], Ronald J. Maughan [3], William Gilmore [1,4] and Gethin H. Evans [1,*]

[1] School of Healthcare Science, Manchester Metropolitan University, Manchester, Greater Manchester M1 5GD, UK; a.yau@mmu.ac.uk (A.M.W.Y.); b.gilmore@mmu.ac.uk or ws.gilmore@ulster.ac.uk (W.G.)
[2] Institute of Inflammation and Repair, Faculty of Medical and Human Sciences, University of Manchester, Manchester, Greater Manchester M13 9PT, UK; john.mclaughlin@manchester.ac.uk
[3] School of Sport, Exercise and Health Sciences, Loughborough University, Loughborough, Leicestershire LE11 3TU, UK; R.J.Maughan@lboro.ac.uk
[4] School of Biomedical Sciences, Ulster University, Cromore Road, Coleraine, Co Londonderry BT52 1SA, UK
[*] Correspondence: gethin.evans@mmu.ac.uk; Tel.: +44-161-247-1208

Received: 7 February 2017; Accepted: 7 March 2017; Published: 10 March 2017

Abstract: This study aimed to examine gastric emptying rate and gastrointestinal hormone responses to fructose and glucose ingestion following 3 days of dietary fructose supplementation. Using the ^{13}C-breath test method, gastric emptying rates of equicaloric fructose and glucose solutions were measured in 10 healthy men with prior fructose supplementation (fructose supplement, FS; glucose supplement, GS) and without prior fructose supplementation (fructose control, FC; glucose control, GC). In addition, circulating concentrations of acylated ghrelin (GHR), glucagon-like peptide-1 (GLP-1), glucose-dependent insulinotropic polypeptide (GIP), and insulin were determined, as well as leptin, lactate, and triglycerides. Increased dietary fructose ingestion resulted in accelerated gastric emptying rate of a fructose solution but not a glucose solution. No differences in GIP, GLP-1, or insulin incremental area under curve (iAUC) were found between control and supplement trials for either fructose or glucose ingestion. However, a trend for lower ghrelin iAUC was observed for FS compared to FC. In addition, a trend of lower GHR concentration was observed at 45 min for FS compared to FC and GHR concentration for GS was greater than GC at 10 min. The accelerated gastric emptying rate of fructose following short-term supplementation with fructose may be partially explained by subtle changes in delayed postprandial ghrelin suppression.

Keywords: fructose supplementation; glucose; fructose; sugar ingestion; gastric emptying; gastrointestinal adaptation; gastrointestinal hormones

---

1. Introduction

Gastric emptying is a rate-limiting step in the delivery and absorption of nutrients and fluids in the small intestine. Therefore, the rate at which nutrients empty from the stomach directly affects the period of gastric distension and nutrient sensing. Gastric distension causes both satiation and satiety [1] and a prolonged period of gastric distension due to delayed emptying may lead to a prolonged satiety period. A number of hormones secreted from the gastrointestinal tract involved in appetite regulation have also been to shown to influence gastric emptying rate. Ghrelin, the only orexigenic hormone, accelerates gastric emptying rate [2,3] whilst satiety hormones such as glucagon-like peptide-1 (GLP-1), peptide tyrosine tyrosine (PYY), and cholecystokinin (CCK) inhibit gastric emptying rate [4–8].

The gastrointestinal tract has been shown to be a highly adaptive organ. Gastric emptying in humans has been shown to be influenced by previous dietary intake. Increases in the gastric emptying rate of a high-fat test meal following three days of a high-fat diet [9] and increases in the gastric emptying rate of a glucose test solution following 3 days of high glucose intake [10,11] have been shown. More recently, three days of dietary fructose supplementation has been shown to result in a monosaccharide specific acceleration of a fructose solution but not a glucose solution [12]. One potential mechanism for this adaptation is an alteration in gastrointestinal hormone response.

A small number of studies that have investigated the effects of previous dietary intake on gut hormone responses in humans have shown changes in the secretion of gut-derived hormones. Most of this work to date has been conducted on the effects of a high-fat diet, however, and few have simultaneously measured gastric emptying rate. Following the observations by Cunningham et al. [13] where emptying rate of a fatty meal was accelerated as a result of a high-fat diet for two weeks, it was reported that a high-fat diet resulted in an increase in postprandial CCK concentration [14]. Fasting levels of CCK have also been shown to be altered in humans following three weeks of a high-fat diet compared to an isoenergetic low-fat diet [15]. The effect of a high-fat diet has also been shown by others to suppress postprandial ghrelin response to a greater extent [16], but result in unaltered fasting concentration and postprandial response for GLP-1 [17].

With regards to increased dietary intake of carbohydrates, increased glucose ingestion for 4–7 days resulted in accelerated gastric emptying of glucose and fructose solutions but differential gut hormones responses [11]. Greater glucose-dependent insulinotropic polypeptide (GIP) hormone responses were observed following the glucose-supplemented diet for both sugar solutions [11]. However, insulin response was greater following glucose ingestion but unchanged following fructose ingestion in the glucose-supplemented trials [11]. In addition, it followed that glycaemic response was lower for glucose ingestion but not for fructose ingestion following glucose supplementation [11]. The only study to our knowledge that has investigated the effects of increased fructose consumption on gut hormones showed that two weeks of a high-fructose diet in rats increased fasting ghrelin levels by 40% [18]. The effect of increased fructose consumption over a shorter period of time on moderations of postprandial gut hormone responses in relation to adaptations of gastric emptying rate in humans is unknown. Therefore, the aim of this study was to investigate the effect of a short-term increase in dietary fructose ingestion on gastric emptying rate and associated gastrointestinal hormone responses in healthy men.

2. Materials and Methods

2.1. Participants

Ten healthy men (mean ± standard deviation, age 26 ± 7 years, height 179.0 ± 6.3 cm, body mass 81.2 ± 11.1 kg, body mass index 25.3 ± 3.1 kg·m^{-2}, and estimated body fat 23.2% ± 8.1%) volunteered to take part in this investigation. All participants were non-smokers, had no history of chronic gastrointestinal disease, were not consuming medication with any known effect on gastrointestinal function and had no medical conditions as assessed by a medical screening questionnaire. The participants provided written informed consent prior to participation and ethical approval was provided via the Institutional Ethical Advisory Committee (Reference: SE111228).

2.2. Experimental Protocol

Experimental trials were conducted in a single-blind, randomised, crossover fashion commencing between 0800 and 0900 h following an overnight fast from 2100 h with the exception of drinking 500 mL of water approximately 90 min before arrival at the laboratory. Participants reported to the laboratory on four occasions to complete four experimental trials; fructose with supplementation (FS), fructose with water control (FC), glucose with supplementation (GS) and glucose with water control (GC) as previously conducted by Yau et al. [12]. Experimental trials were separated by a minimum period of 7 days. A 3-day dietary and physical activity maintenance period preceded each experimental trial. Participants were asked to record their diet and physical activity prior to their first trial then to replicate them in the remaining three trials. The purpose of this was to ensure standardisation and consistency of macronutrient intake and metabolic status in the days leading up to each trial. Furthermore, participants were asked to refrain from alcohol and caffeine consumption and the performance of strenuous physical activity in the 24 h preceding each experimental trial. In addition to their normal dietary intake, participants were asked to consume either four 500 mL bottles of water (control trials) or four 500 mL solutions, each containing 30 g fructose (supplement trials) per day over the 3-day dietary maintenance period. Participants were instructed to consume these drinks evenly throughout the day in between meals.

Upon arrival at the laboratory, participants were asked to completely empty their bladder into a container from which a 5 mL urine sample was retained for later analysis of osmolality. Body mass was subsequently recorded before an intravenous cannula was inserted into an antecubital vein. This remained in place for the duration of the experimental trial and was kept patent with infusion of saline after each blood sample collection. A baseline 5 mL blood sample was collected before participants ingested 595 mL of a fructose solution (36 g dissolved in water and prepared to a volume of 600 mL) or an equicaloric glucose monohydrate solution (39.6 g dissolved in water and prepared to a volume of 600 mL). A 5 mL sample of the test solutions was retained for osmolality analysis. Participants were given a maximum of two minutes to consume the test solution and instructed to consume it as quickly as they were able to. Participants remained in a semi-supine position for 60 min following drink ingestion where further blood samples were collected at 10, 20, 30, 45 and 60 min post ingestion. Ratings of appetite (hunger, fullness, prospective food consumption) were assessed at baseline and at 10-min intervals following drink ingestion for 60 min using a 100-mm visual analogue scale (VAS). Following the last sample collection the cannula was removed before participants left the laboratory.

2.3. Gastric Emptying Measurement

Gastric emptying was assessed using the ^{13}C-acetate breath method as described in Yau et al. [12]. Prior to ingestion of the fructose or glucose test drink containing 100 mg ^{13}C-sodium acetate (Cambridge Isotope Laboratories Inc., Andover, MA, USA), a basal end-expiratory breath sample was collected. Further end-expiratory breath samples were collected at 10-min intervals over a period of 60 min following drink ingestion. Breath samples were collected into a 100-mL foil bag on each occasion by exhalation through a mouthpiece. Bags were then sealed with a plastic stopper and stored for later analysis.

Breath samples were analysed by non-dispersive infra-red spectroscopy (IRIS, Wagner Analyzen-Technik, Bremen, Germany) for the ratio of $^{13}CO_2$:$^{12}CO_2$. The differences in the ratio of $^{13}CO_2$:$^{12}CO_2$ from baseline breath to post breath samples are expressed as delta over baseline (DOB). Half emptying time ($T_{1/2}$) and time of maximum emptying rate (T_{lag}) were calculated using the manufacturer's integrated software evaluation embedded with the equations of Ghoos et al. [19]. Each participant's own physiological CO_2 production assumed as 300 mmol CO_2 per m^2 body surface per hour was set as default and body surface area was calculated by the integrated software according to the formula of Haycock et al. [20].

2.4. Sample Analysis

Urine, drink and serum samples were analysed in duplicate for osmolality by freezing point depression (Gonotec Osmomat 030, Gonotec, Berlin, Germany). To prevent the degradation of acylated ghrelin, 50 μL of Pefabloc (Roche Diagnostics Limited, Burgess Hill, UK) was immediately added to blood samples. Blood samples were centrifuged at 1500× *g* for 15 min at 4 °C and the serum aliquoted and stored at −80 °C until analysis was performed. Serum glucose, lactate, and triglyceride concentrations were determined in duplicate using a clinical chemistry analyser

(Randox Daytona, Crumlin, UK). Serum fructose concentration was determined using a colorimetric assay (EnzyChrom™ EFRU-100; BioAssay Systems, Hayward, CA, USA). Circulating concentrations of acylated ghrelin, insulin, GIP, and leptin were determined using multiplex analysis (Luminex 200, Luminex Corporation, Austin, TX, USA) with kits purchased from Merck-Millipore (HMHMAG-34K, Milliplex MAP, Merck Millipore Ltd., Feltham, UK). Circulating concentrations of total GLP-1 were determined in duplicate using Enzyme Linked Immunoassay (EZGLP1T-36K, Merck Millipore Ltd., Feltham, UK).

2.5. Data and Statistical Analysis

The trapezoid method was utilised to calculate incremental area under curve (iAUC). Differences in pre-ingestion body mass, pre-ingestion urine osmolality, drink osmolality and iAUC for serum blood measures were examined using one-way repeated analysis of variance (ANOVA). Post-hoc analysis consisted of Bonferroni adjusted pairwise comparisons. Two-way repeated ANOVA were used to examine differences in gastric emptying DOB values, serum blood measures, and subjective appetite VAS scores. Sphericity for repeated measures was assessed, and where appropriate, Greenhouse–Geisser corrections were applied for epsilon <0.75, and the Huynh–Feldt correction adopted for less severe asphericity. Significant *F*-tests were followed by dependent Student's *t*-Tests or one-way repeated ANOVA and Bonferroni adjusted pairwise comparisons as appropriate. Gastric emptying $T_{1/2}$ and T_{lag} data were examined with dependent Student's *t*-Tests to test the hypothesis of interest (i.e., effect of supplementation on gastric emptying rate of fructose and of glucose). All data were analysed using SPSS Statistics for Windows version 21 (IBM, New York, NY, USA). Statistical significance was accepted at the 5% level and results presented as means and standard deviations.

3. Results

3.1. Body Mass, Hydration Status and Drink Osmolality

Body mass (Table 1) remained stable over the duration of the study ($p = 0.338$). Pre-ingestion urine osmolality (Table 1) was generally lower in each supplement trial compared to the control trials but was not statistically significant ($p = 0.067$). Drink osmolalities were 368 ± 3, 367 ± 4, 371 ± 3 and 370 ± 4 mOsmol/kg ($p = 0.010$) for FC, FS, GC and GS, respectively. Post hoc analysis indicated no significant differences between trials.

Table 1. Pre-trial body mass and urine osmolality as a marker of hydration status.

	FC		FS		GC		GS	
	Mean	SD	Mean	SD	Mean	SD	Mean	SD
Body mass (kg)	80.87	11.15	81.13	11.04	81.48	11.46	80.95	10.80
Urine osmolality (mOsmol/kg)	560	262	397	271	504	266	356	193

FC, fructose ingestion control trial; FS, fructose ingestion supplement trial; GC, glucose ingestion control trial; GS, glucose ingestion supplement trial; SD, standard deviation.

3.2. Gastric Emptying

Gastric emptying $T_{1/2}$ for fructose ingestion was accelerated after the period of dietary supplementation with fructose compared to the control (FC, 59 ± 13 min vs. FS, 51 ± 10 min; $p = 0.004$). The same was also observed for T_{lag}, with dietary fructose supplementation accelerating fructose ingestion T_{lag} (FC, 37 ± 3 min vs. FS, 32 ± 7 min; $p = 0.026$). In contrast, gastric emptying $T_{1/2}$ for glucose ingestion did not change with fructose supplementation (GC, 75 ± 18 min vs. GS, 68 ± 16 min; $p = 0.245$), and neither did T_{lag} (GC, 38 ± 7 min vs. GS, 40 ± 7 min; $p = 0.679$). Breath DOB values for fructose ingestion (Figure 1a) revealed no main effect of trial ($p = 0.912$), a significant main effect of time ($p < 0.001$) and no interaction effect ($p = 0.376$). The ratio of $^{13}CO_2$ to $^{12}CO_2$ was significantly increased at all post-ingestion time-points compared to baseline and 10 min ($p < 0.01$) for FC. The ratio of $^{13}CO_2$ to $^{12}CO_2$ was significantly increased at all post-ingestion time-points compared to baseline ($p < 0.01$) and from 20 to 40 min compared to 10 min ($p < 0.01$) for FS. Breath DOB for glucose ingestion (Figure 1b) showed no main effect of trial ($p = 0.537$), a significant main effect of time ($p < 0.001$) and no interaction effect ($p = 0.282$). The ratio of $^{13}CO_2$ to $^{12}CO_2$ was significantly increased at all post-ingestion time-points compared to baseline and at 10 min ($p < 0.01$) for GC and GS. Data for dose/h ($\%^{13}C$) are provided in Figure 1c,d.

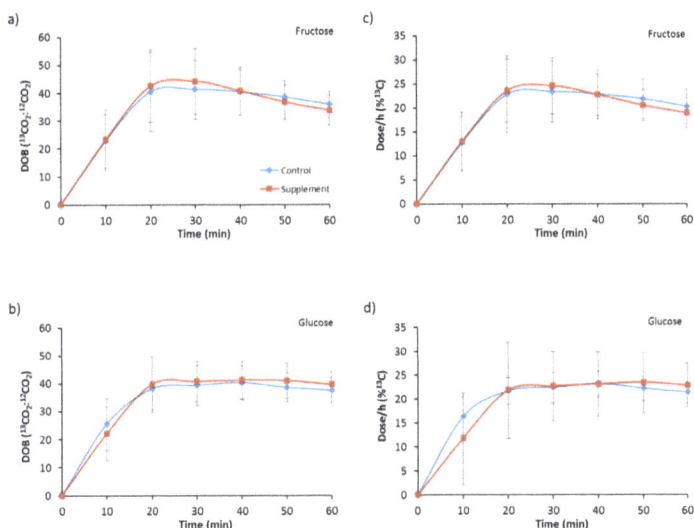

Figure 1. Gastric emptying delta over baseline (DOB) for 60 min following ingestion of (**a**) a 6% fructose solution and (**b**) a 6% glucose solution, and dose/h ($\%^{13}C$) following ingestion of (**c**) a 6% fructose solution and (**d**) a 6% glucose solution. Treatments were control without fructose supplementation and with three days of supplementation with 120 g fructose per day. Values are mean ± standard deviation.

3.3. Gut Hormones

3.3.1. Ghrelin

Baseline ghrelin concentrations (Table 2) were not different between any of the four trials ($p = 0.131$). However, there was a pattern for higher baseline levels following supplementation compared to each respective control trial. For fructose ingestion, this tended to significance ($p = 0.089$). Analysis of fructose ingestion (Figure 2a) revealed no main effect of supplementation ($p = 0.264$) but an effect of time ($p < 0.001$) and a trend of an interaction ($p = 0.065$). Post-hoc analysis revealed that ghrelin concentration significantly decreased between 10 min and 60 min in FC whilst the decrease from baseline levels in FS occurred from 20 min after ingestion. A trend of lower ghrelin concentration was also indicated for FS compared to FC at 45 min after ingestion ($p = 0.063$). There was a trend in a lower iAUC for FS compared to FC (FC, -1506.94 ± 1704.50 pg/mL vs. FS, -2514.09 ± 1151.33 pg/mL; $p = 0.053$). Analysis for glucose ingestion (Figure 3a) revealed a trend of a supplementation effect ($p = 0.080$), an effect of time ($p < 0.001$) and no interaction effect ($p = 0.276$). Post-hoc analysis showed ghrelin concentration significantly decreased from baseline levels at 20 min to 60 min after ingestion in both GC and GS. Furthermore, ghrelin concentration was significantly higher in GS compared to GC at 10 min after ingestion ($p = 0.019$). There was no difference in iAUC between GC and GS (GC, -2535.20 ± 1530.65 pg/mL vs. GS, -2826.96 ± 1499.31 pg/mL; $p = 0.478$).

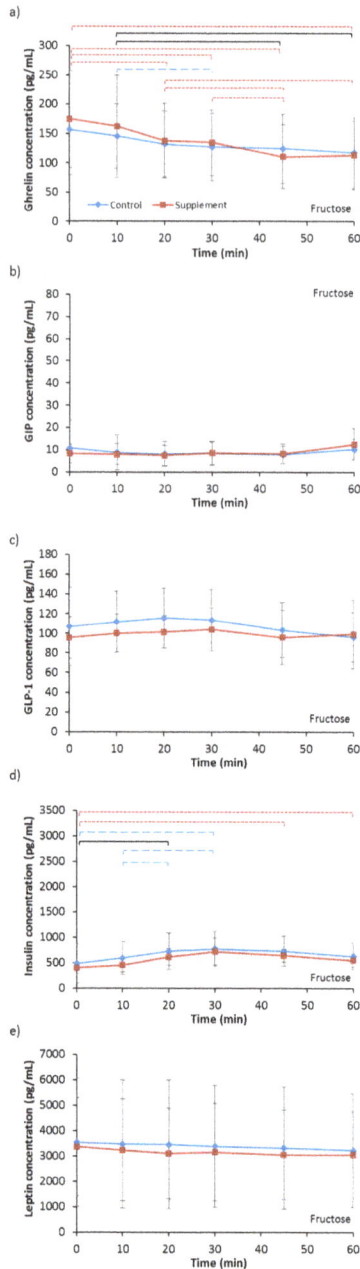

Figure 2. Serum concentrations of (**a**) ghrelin; (**b**) glucose-dependent insulinotropic polypeptide (GIP); (**c**) glucagon-like peptide-1 (GLP-1); (**d**) insulin and (**e**) leptin for 60 min following ingestion of a 6% fructose solution. Treatments were control without fructose supplementation and with three days of supplementation with 120 g fructose per day. Brackets denote significant difference between time-points, blue long dashed for control trial only, red small dashed for supplement trial only and black solid for both trials ($p < 0.05$). Values are mean ± standard deviation.

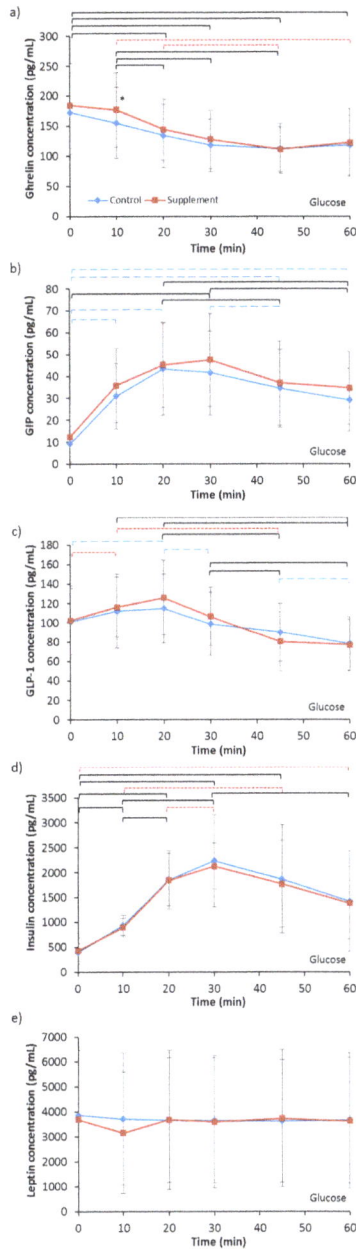

Figure 3. Serum concentrations of (**a**) ghrelin; (**b**) GIP; (**c**) GLP-1; (**d**) insulin and (**e**) leptin for 60 min following ingestion of a 6% glucose solution. Treatments were control without fructose supplementation and with three days of supplementation with 120 g fructose per day. * Significantly greater for supplement compared to control ($p < 0.05$). Brackets denote significant difference between time-points, blue long dashed for control trial only, red small dashed for supplement trial only and black solid for both trials ($p < 0.05$). Values are mean ± standard deviation.

Table 2. Baseline concentrations for blood serum measures.

	FC		FS		GC		GS	
	Mean	SD	Mean	SD	Mean	SD	Mean	SD
Ghrelin (pg/mL)	156.65	77.25	174.64	82.47	172.06	68.19	184.05	71.00
GIP (pg/mL)	10.78	12.44	8.26	4.13	9.31	8.18	12.47	15.20
GLP-1 (pg/mL)	106.78	40.07	95.49	21.29	101.12	34.41	102.55	35.53
Insulin (pg/mL)	438.05	383.64	396.53	93.16	396.20	180.37	425.87	260.60
Leptin (pg/mL)	3542.36	2525.04	3371.53	1934.44	3857.64	2711.35	3687.42	2767.98
Glucose (mmol/L)	5.21	0.46	5.28	0.30	5.21	0.40	5.11	0.25
Fructose (µM)	137.0	48.8	115.8	39.6	129.8	36.6	139.4	38.4
Lactate (mmol/L)	1.12	0.41	1.11	0.30	1.08	0.39	1.00	0.30
Triglycerides (mmol/L)	1.03	0.53	1.12	0.44	0.92	0.40	1.25	0.45

FC, fructose ingestion control trial; FS, fructose ingestion supplement trial; GC, glucose ingestion control trial; GS, glucose ingestion supplement trial; SD, standard deviation.

3.3.2. GIP

Baseline GIP concentrations (Table 2) were not different between any of the four trials ($p = 0.545$). Analysis for fructose ingestion (Figure 2b) showed no effect of supplementation ($p = 0.760$), time ($p = 0.121$) or interaction ($p = 0.368$). There was no difference in iAUC between FC and FS (FC, -124.98 ± 435.74 pg/mL vs. FS, 22.04 ± 169.69 pg/mL; $p = 0.346$). Analysis for glucose ingestion (Figure 3b) revealed a trend of a supplementation effect ($p = 0.076$), a main effect of time ($p < 0.001$) but no interaction effect ($p = 0.707$). GIP concentration for GC significantly increased from baseline values by 10 min then decreased from 20 min but remained significantly higher than baseline at 60 min. GIP concentration for GS, on the other hand, significantly increased from baseline at 30 min and remained elevated from baseline at 60 min but not significantly. There was no difference in iAUC between GS and GC (GC, 1485.26 ± 644.97 pg/mL vs. GS, 1518.83 ± 1275.25 pg/mL; $p = 0.911$).

3.3.3. GLP-1

Baseline GLP-1 concentrations (Table 2) were not different between any of the four trials ($p = 0.719$). Analysis for fructose ingestion (Figure 2c) showed no main effect of supplementation ($p = 0.339$), an effect of time tending to significance ($p = 0.081$) and no interaction effect ($p = 0.328$). No difference in iAUC was seen between FC and FS (FC, -80.46 ± 142.16 pg/mL vs. FS, 27.70 ± 142.48 pg/mL; $p = 0.178$). Analysis for glucose ingestion (Figure 3c) showed no main effect of supplementation ($p = 0.747$), an effect of time ($p < 0.001$) and an interaction effect tending to significance ($p = 0.064$). Post hoc analysis revealed GLP-1 concentration increased significantly from baseline at 20 min then decreased significantly at every time-point in GC. For GS, concentrations significantly increased from baseline at 10 min, then increased further non-significantly at 20 min before significantly decreasing. No difference in iAUC was observed (GC, -152.36 ± 667.66 pg/mL vs. 100.16 ± 908.36 pg/mL; $p = 0.492$).

3.3.4. Insulin

Baseline insulin concentrations (Table 2) were not different between any of the four trials ($p = 0.750$). Analysis for fructose ingestion (Figure 2d) showed no main effect of supplementation ($p = 0.341$), an effect of time ($p < 0.001$) and no interaction effect ($p = 0.778$). Post hoc analysis showed a significant increase in insulin from baseline levels for both FC and FS. No difference in iAUC was observed between FC and FS (FC, 1079.96 ± 2019.57 pg/mL vs. FS, 1109.93 ± 793.25 pg/mL; $p = 0.958$). Analysis for glucose ingestion (Figure 3d) showed no main effect of supplementation ($p = 0.975$), an effect of time ($p < 0.001$) and no interaction effect ($p = 0.844$). Post hoc analysis showed insulin concentrations increased significantly from baseline values at 30 min then significantly decreased thereafter for both GC and GS. No difference in iAUC was present (GC, $72,133.17 \pm 32,863.68$ pg/mL vs. GS, $68,512.93 \pm 15,821.44$ pg/mL; $p = 0.626$).

3.3.5. Leptin

Baseline leptin concentrations (Table 2) were not different between any of the four trials ($p = 0.484$). Analysis for fructose ingestion (Figure 2e) showed no effect of supplementation ($p = 0.302$), time ($p = 0.100$) or interaction ($p = 0.466$). No difference in iAUC between FC and FS was present (FC, -2389.11 ± 3623.58 pg/mL vs. FS, -2387.77 ± 3522.92 pg/mL; $p = 0.999$). Analysis for glucose ingestion (Figure 3e) also showed no effect of supplementation ($p = 0.934$), time ($p = 0.378$) or interaction ($p = 0.294$. No difference in iAUC was present between GC and GS (GC, $-10,592.99 \pm 13,423.93$ pg/mL vs. GS, $-3557.61 \pm 10,977.20$ pg/mL; $p = 0.147$).

3.4. Blood Glucose and Fructose

Baseline serum glucose concentrations (Table 2) were not different between any of the four trials ($p = 0.591$). Analysis for fructose ingestion (Figure 4a) revealed no effect of supplementation ($p = 0.880$), an effect of time ($p = 0.024$) and no interaction effect ($p = 0.928$). Post-hoc analysis showed serum glucose concentration significantly increased at 20 min from baseline concentrations then decreased significantly at 60 min for FC. A similar response pattern over time for FS was not significantly different ($p = 0.174$). No difference in iAUC was observed between FC and FS (FC, 9.75 ± 5.39 mmol/L vs. FS, 5.53 ± 19.02 mmol/L; $p = 0.438$). Analysis for glucose ingestion (Figure 4b) showed no effect of supplementation ($p = 0.428$), an effect of time ($p < 0.001$) and no interaction effect ($p = 0.658$). Post hoc analysis revealed serum glucose concentrations significantly increased from baseline, peaking at 30 min, and then decreased significantly to near baseline levels at 60 min for both GC and GS. No difference in iAUC existed (GC, 95.07 ± 56.21 mmol/L vs. GS, 88.17 ± 54.12 mmol/L; $p = 0.711$).

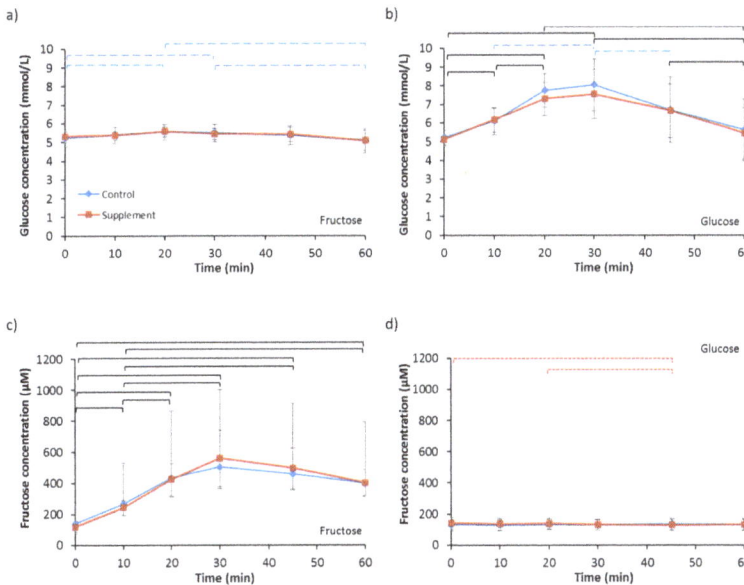

Figure 4. Serum concentrations of glucose for 60 min following ingestion of (**a**) a 6% fructose solution and (**b**) a 6% glucose solution and serum concentrations of fructose following ingestion of (**c**) a 6% fructose solution and (**d**) a 6% glucose solution. Treatments were control without fructose supplementation and with three days of supplementation with 120 g fructose per day. Brackets denote significant difference between time-points, blue long dashed for control trial only, red small dashed for supplement trial only and black solid for both trials ($p < 0.05$). Values are mean $\pm$ standard deviation.

Baseline serum fructose concentrations (Table 2) were not different between any of the four trials ($p = 0.163$). Analysis for fructose ingestion (Figure 4c) showed no main effect of supplementation ($p = 0.948$), an effect of time ($p < 0.001$) and an interaction effect ($p = 0.011$). Post hoc analysis revealed serum fructose concentrations increased rapidly from baseline concentrations within the first 10 min for both FC and FS. There was a strong tendency for iAUC to be higher in FS compared to FC (FC, $15,505.00 \pm 4377.39$ µM vs. FS, $17,583.45 \pm 4597.19$ µM; $p = 0.050$). Analysis for glucose ingestion (Figure 4d) showed no main effect of supplementation ($p = 0.547$), no effect of time ($p = 0.172$) but an interaction effect ($p = 0.036$). Post-hoc analysis revealed serum fructose concentrations did not change over time in GC ($p = 0.645$), but in GS, concentrations were significantly lower at 45 min compared to baseline ($p = 0.041$) and 20 min ($p = 0.017$). No difference in iAUC was observed (GC, 41.73 ± 889.46 µM vs. GS, -409.76 ± 457.67 µM; $p = 0.226$).

3.5. Lactate and Triglycerides

Baseline serum lactate concentrations (Table 2) were not different between any of the four trials ($p = 0.686$). Analysis for fructose ingestion (Figure 5a) revealed no effect of supplementation ($p = 0.511$), an effect of time ($p < 0.001$) and no interaction effect ($p = 0.457$). Lactate concentrations increased significantly from baseline values from 10 min for both FC and FS. No difference in iAUC was observed (FC, 51.63 ± 22.84 mmol/L vs. FS, 47.86 ± 15.17 mmol/L; $p = 0.482$). Analysis for glucose ingestion (Figure 5b) showed no effect of supplementation ($p = 0.198$), an effect of time ($p < 0.001$) and no interaction effect ($p = 0.621$). Lactate concentrations increased significantly from 45 min onwards compared to baseline for both GC and GS. No difference in iAUC was observed (GC, 8.14 ± 7.84 mmol/L vs. 6.30 ± 10.65 mmol/L; $p = 0.331$).

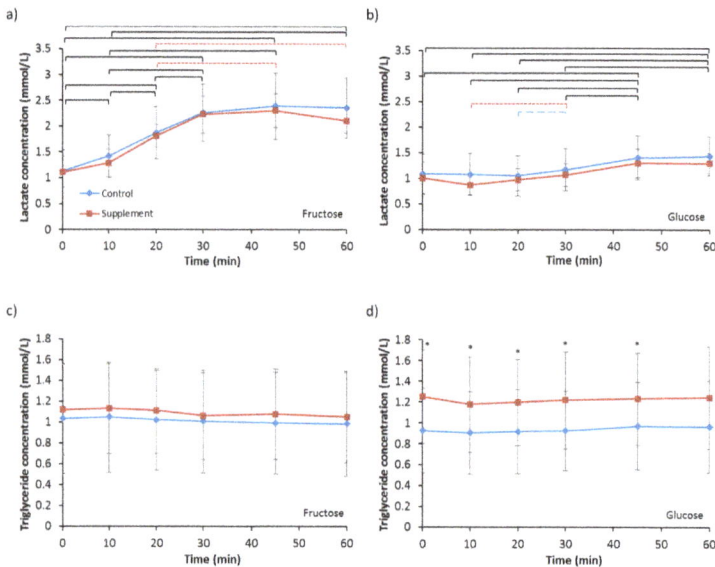

Figure 5. Serum concentrations of lactate following ingestion of (**a**) a 6% fructose solution and (**b**) a 6% glucose solution and serum concentrations of triglyceride following ingestion of (**c**) a 6% fructose solution and (**d**) a 6% glucose solution. Treatments were control without fructose supplementation and with three days of supplementation with 120 g fructose per day. Brackets denote significant difference between time-points, blue long dashed for control trial only, red small dashed for supplement trial only and black solid for both trials ($p < 0.05$). * Significantly greater for supplement compared to control ($p < 0.05$). Values are mean ± standard deviation.

Baseline triglyceride concentrations (Table 2) were not different between any of the four trials ($p = 0.082$). Analysis for fructose ingestion (Figure 5c) revealed no effect of supplementation ($p = 0.944$), a trend for an effect of time ($p = 0.069$) and no interaction effect ($p = 0.726$). No difference in iAUC was seen (FC, -1.31 ± 5.01 mmol/L vs. FS, -1.30 ± 5.21 mmol/L; $p = 0.998$). Analysis for glucose ingestion (Figure 5d) showed a main effect of supplementation ($p = 0.021$), but no significant effect of time ($p = 0.287$) or interaction ($p = 0.596$). Triglyceride concentration was significantly greater for GS compared to GC at all time points ($p < 0.05$) except at 60 min where it was strongly tending to significance ($p = 0.051$). Incremental AUC was not different between GC and GS (GC, 0.69 ± 2.45 mmol/L vs. GS, -1.49 ± 5.55 mmol/L; $p = 0.243$).

3.6. Appetite Ratings

Hunger ratings for fructose ingestion (Figure 6a) showed a trend of a supplementation effect ($p = 0.090$), and no main effect of time ($p = 0.106$) or interaction ($p = 0.477$). Ingestion of a glucose solution (Figure 6b) also showed no main effect of supplementation ($p = 0.231$), time ($p = 0.410$) or interaction ($p = 0.237$).

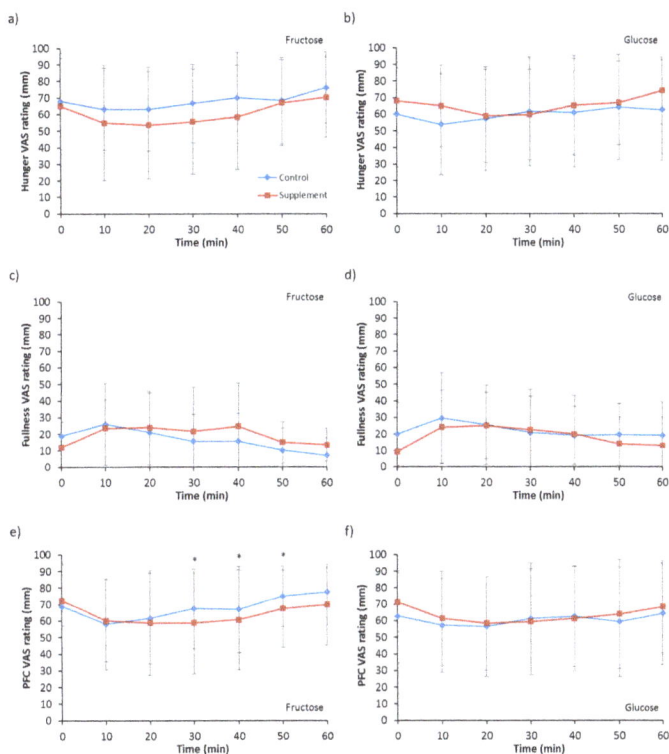

Figure 6. Visual analogue scale (VAS) appetite ratings of hunger following ingestion of (**a**) a 6% fructose solution and (**b**) a 6% glucose solution, ratings of fullness following ingestion of (**c**) a 6% fructose solution and (**d**) a 6% glucose solution, and ratings of prospective food consumption (PFC) following ingestion of (**e**) a 6% fructose solution and (**f**) a 6% glucose solution. Treatments were control without fructose supplementation and with three days of supplementation of 120 g fructose per day. * Significantly greater for control trial compared to supplement ($p < 0.05$). Values are mean ± standard deviation.

Analysis on feeling of fullness for fructose ingestion (Figure 6c) showed no effect of supplementation ($p = 0.231$), time ($p = 0.144$) or interaction ($p = 0.236$). For glucose ingestion (Figure 6d), a trend of a main effect of supplementation was observed for fullness ($p = 0.083$) but no main effect of time ($p = 0.235$) or interaction ($p = 0.523$).

No main effect of time ($p = 0.101$) or interaction ($p = 0.205$) was seen for prospective food consumption with fructose ingestion (Figure 6e) but a main effect of supplementation was present ($p = 0.027$). Post hoc analysis revealed ratings were temporarily lower for FS compared to FC from 30 to 50 min. For glucose ingestion (Figure 6f), no effect of supplementation ($p = 0.550$), time ($p = 0.370$) or interaction ($p = 0.661$) was observed.

4. Discussion

The gastric emptying results of this study are in agreement to previous findings showing a monosaccharide-specific adaptation in gastric emptying rate following short-term dietary supplementation of fructose [12]. Gastric emptying rate of a solution containing 36 g of fructose was accelerated whilst emptying rate of an equicaloric glucose solution was unchanged. These results may be partially explained by subtle changes in gut hormone responses seen in this present study. Whilst a larger sugar load, such as the typically used load of 75 g, would have resulted in more pronounced effects on secretory endocrine and enteroendocrine hormone responses, these modest loads were utilized in the present study to reflect more commonly ingested amounts of sugar ingestion.

Supplementation of the diet with fructose for three days resulted in a short delay in the postprandial suppression of ghrelin following the ingestion of a fructose solution and a greater ghrelin concentration at 10 min with the ingestion of a glucose solution. Although not significantly different, fasting ghrelin levels were also slightly elevated by 7%–11% after the supplementation period. This is in agreement, proportionally, with the results of Lindqvist et al. [18] who reported a 40% increase in fasting ghrelin concentrations following two weeks of a high-fructose diet in rats. Since ghrelin is known to accelerate gastric emptying rate [2,3], these fasting and postprandial observations would suggest a slight initial acceleration of emptying rate for both fructose and glucose solution ingestion. Therefore, this does not explain the specific acceleration of fructose emptying rate only. However, the differences in the other hormone responses to counter the changes in ghrelin response may offer some explanation.

One potential explanation is that there was no difference in GIP response for fructose ingestion whilst there was a trend for significantly greater GIP response for glucose ingestion following supplementation. This difference in supplementation effect may have been because GIP secretion is comparatively limited in response to fructose ingestion as seen in the present study and as reported by Kuhre et al. [21] who used a much greater amount of fructose at 75 g. These results contrast those of Horowitz et al. [11] who showed GIP response increased for both glucose and fructose ingestion following dietary glucose supplementation. However, whether these GIP results in the present study indicate a potential mechanism for the specific acceleration of fructose but not glucose emptying is questionable as the influence of GIP on gastric emptying rate is unclear with mixed results. Administration of pharmacological doses of GIP in healthy men have been shown to have no effect on gastric emptying rate [22] as well as moderately accelerating emptying [4]. It may be, therefore, the differences observed in GLP-1 response between fructose ingestion and glucose ingestion that hold the key to the specific gastrointestinal adaptation results. The ingestion of a fructose solution resulted in no significant changes over time in circulating GLP-1 concentration, and although not significantly different, lower concentrations were seen for the supplement trial with a difference tending to significance at 20 min. In addition to greater responses as a result of glucose ingestion compared to fructose ingestion, faster elevations in GLP-1 concentration was observed in the supplement trial compared to the control trial. However, the overall response to glucose ingestion seen in the present study was lower than other studies such as Kuhre et al. [21]. This is likely due to the smaller quantity of sugar ingested in this study compared to 75 g utilised by others. As GLP-1 is known to strongly inhibit gastric emptying and has been termed as an "ileal brake" [4,5,23], this would suggest a greater ileal brake effect to counter the ghrelin increases for glucose ingestion but not for fructose ingestion, resulting in faster fructose emptying rate. Alternatively, other gut hormones not measured in this study may play a more important role. A further potential limitation of the hormones included in the present study is that total GLP-1 and not the active form GLP-1$^{7-36amide}$ was measured.

Changes in CCK and ghrelin concentrations following high protein or high fat diets have previously been shown to be associated with complementary changes in mRNA levels [24,25]. It is unknown whether any changes in circulating concentrations of gut hormones in this present study were simply changes in hormone release and intestinal feedback or whether the three days of increased dietary fructose load led to up- or down-regulation of genes and associated changes in mRNA levels leading to increased hormone production. This should be investigated further. In terms of the potential mechanism of altered hormone release and intestinal feedback, the increased consumption of fructose may have led to changes in the sensitivity or stimulation to the presence of fructose. This may have been through increased expression of gut sweet taste receptors T1R2/T1R3 which have been detected in the intestinal tract and enteroendocrine cells [26,27] and may potentially be involved in the secretion of gut hormones [28]. It is noted, however, that ingested solutions were not considered to be equisweet and, consequently, activation of sweet taste receptors in the tongue and intestine may have been different between solutions. Equicaloric doses of fructose and glucose were favoured in this study in order to avoid any potential effects of energy density on gastric emptying rate as well as potential effects of different caloric intakes on the secretion of gut-derived hormone response. Alternatively, enhanced absorption of fructose as a result of glucose transporter 5 (GLUT5) up-regulation and consequently greater transporter activity may be involved in the mediation of gut hormone release.

Three days of fructose supplementation did not result in a change in leptin concentration in this study. This is most likely because there was no change in body mass and thus assumed no change in body fat/adiposity occurred over this short study period where only an extra 1440 kcal was consumed over the three days. This result is in contrast to the results of Le et al. [29] who reported a significant increase in leptin levels within one week of a high-fructose diet. The longer supplementation period with an approximate mean extra 2898 kcal consumption may have accounted for this difference. However, the authors of that study also reported no change in body weight and body fat percentage.

The rate of gastric emptying is expected to have an important impact on the magnitude of both glycaemic and insulinaemic responses. Despite the faster emptying rate, however, serum glucose response to fructose ingestion was not different after supplementation. This suggests that the capacity to metabolise fructose into glucose is not altered and is further supported with the observation that there were no differences in lactate concentration, suggesting that lactate production was also unaltered. Alternatively, greater uptake of glucose by cells may have occurred, though this may be unlikely as no differences were seen for insulin secretion for either fructose or glucose ingestion despite slight variations in incretin hormone responses. The faster gastric emptying of fructose did result in a slightly higher, albeit insignificant, peak serum fructose concentration at 30 min, however. The implications of this, if any, are unknown at this stage.

Triglyceride concentration was significantly elevated at baseline and remained elevated at all postprandial time-points for glucose ingestion following fructose supplementation. However, no difference was found between the fructose ingestion trials. Taking the glucose ingestion results alone extends the observations that increased fructose intake for seven days can cause significant increases in fasting triglyceride levels [30]. These levels were still far from dyslipidaemia values, however. It is uncertain as to why no differences were also evident at baseline between the fructose control and fructose supplement trials. The results of this short-term feeding study, therefore, do not suggest a link between excessive fructose intake and metabolic dysfunction. It is possible that some of the observations seen by others in more chronic feeding studies, such as elevated fasting concentrations of low density lipoprotein , glucose and insulin [31,32], and decreased insulin sensitivity [32] could be related to changes in gastric emptying rate and gut hormone responses measured in this present study. However, as the present study involved only three days of dietary supplementation, it is difficult to extrapolate the results of the present study to those aforementioned and longer-term studies are required.

The accelerated emptying of fructose resulted in a trend of greater hunger suppression. It is unlikely that this was due to the hormones studied in the present study as greater ghrelin concentrations are inconsistent with the observed hunger effects. A greater length of exposure of the intestine to fructose may have resulted in greater release of other hormones not measured in the present study that are known to decrease appetite, such as PYY and CCK. In line with the lesser feelings of hunger, lower prospective food consumption was also observed with fructose ingestion following supplementation. The satiety effects of fructose ingestion were therefore greater following increased dietary intake of fructose. The absence of differences in appetite measures with glucose ingestion suggests gastric emptying is an important modulatory process linked to appetite. Whether these changes in subjective feelings of appetite translate to changes in food intake need to be investigated further.

5. Conclusions

In conclusion, the results of this study show that three days of dietary supplementation with 120 g fructose per day results in an accelerated gastric emptying rate of a fructose solution but not a glucose solution. This monosaccharide specific adaptation may be partly explained by moderations of ghrelin secretion, though larger participant numbers may be required to elucidate clearer differences in gut-derived hormone responses following supplementation. The adaptability of the gut and the mechanisms responsible for this should be further investigated with both short- and longer-term studies, along with the subsequent effects on food intake.

Acknowledgments: The authors would like to acknowledge Dave Maskew of Manchester Metropolitan University for his technical support in the laboratory; and the staff at Salford Royal Hospital's Gastrointestinal Physiology department for their co-operation with breath sample analysis. A.M.W.Y. was supported by a Manchester Metropolitan University Ph.D. studentship. This research received no specific grant from any funding agency in the public, commercial or not-for-profit sectors.

Author Contributions: A.M.W.Y., G.H.E., J.M., R.J.M. and W.G. conceived and designed the experiments; A.M.W.Y. and G.H.E. performed the experiments; A.M.W.Y. analysed the data; and A.M.W.Y. wrote the paper with contributions from G.H.E., J.M., R.J.M. and W.G. All authors have read and approved the final manuscript.

Conflicts of Interest: The authors declare no conflict of interest.

References

1. Geliebter, A.; Westreich, S.; Gage, D. Gastric distension and gastric capacity in relation to food intake in humans. *Physiol. Behav.* **1988**, *44*, 665–668. [CrossRef]
2. Falken, Y.; Webb, D.-L.; Abraham-Nordling, M.; Kressner, U.; Hellstrom, P.M.; Naslund, E. Intravenous ghrelin accelerates postoperative gastric emptying and time to first bowel movement in humans. *Neurogastroent. Motil.* **2013**, *25*, 474–480. [CrossRef] [PubMed]
3. Levin, F.; Edholm, T.; Schmidt, P.T.; Gryback, P.; Jacobsson, H.; Degerblad, M.; Hoybye, C.; Holst, J.J.; Rehfeld, J.F.; Hellstrom, P.M.; et al. Ghrelin stimulates gastric emptying and hunger in normal-weight humans. *J. Clin. Endocrin. Metab.* **2006**, *91*, 3296–3302. [CrossRef] [PubMed]
4. Edholm, T.; Degerblad, M.; Gryback, P.; Hilsted, L.; Holst, J.J.; Jacobsson, H.; Efendic, S.; Schmidt, P.T.; Hellstrom, P.M. Differential incretin effects of GIP and GLP-1 on gastric emptying, appetite, and insulin-glucose homeostasis. *Neurogastroent. Motil.* **2010**, *22*, 1191–1201. [CrossRef] [PubMed]
5. Wettergren, A.; Schjoldager, B.; Mortensen, P.E.; Myhre, J.; Christiansen, J.; Holst, J.J. Truncated glp-1 (proglucagon 78-107-amide) inhibits gastric and pancreatic functions in man. *Digest. Dis. Sci.* **1993**, *38*, 665–673. [CrossRef] [PubMed]
6. Witte, A.-B.; Gryback, P.; Holst, J.J.; Hilsted, L.; Hellstrom, P.M.; Jacobsson, H.; Schmidt, P.T. Differential effect of PYY1-36 and PYY3-36 on gastric emptying in man. *Regul. Peptides* **2009**, *158*, 57–62. [CrossRef] [PubMed]

7. Schwizer, W.; Borovicka, J.; Kunz, P.; Fraser, R.; Kreiss, C.; D'Amato, M.; Crelier, G.; Boesiger, P.; Fried, M. Role of cholecystokinin in the regulation of liquid gastric emptying and gastric motility in humans: Studies with the CCK antagonist loxiglumide. *Gut* **1997**, *41*, 500–504. [CrossRef] [PubMed]

8. Liddle, R.A.; Morita, E.T.; Conrad, C.K.; Williams, J.A. Regulation of gastric emptying in humans by cholescystokinin. *J. Clin. Investig.* **1986**, *77*, 992–996. [CrossRef] [PubMed]

9. Clegg, M.E.; McKenna, P.; McClean, C.; Dabison, G.W.; Trinick, T.; Duly, E.; Shafat, A. Gastrointestinal transit, post-prandial lipaemia and satiety following 3 days high-fat diet in men. *Eur. J. Clin. Nutr.* **2011**, *65*, 240–246. [CrossRef] [PubMed]

10. Cunningham, K.M.; Horowitz, M.; Read, N.W. The effect of short-term dietary supplementation with glucose on gastric-emptying in humans. *Br. J. Nutr.* **1991**, *65*, 15–19. [CrossRef] [PubMed]

11. Horowitz, M.; Cunningham, K.M.; Wishart, J.M.; Jones, K.L.; Read, N.W. The effect of short-term dietary supplementation with glucose on gastric emptying of glucose and fructose and oral glucose tolerance in normal subjects. *Diabetologia* **1996**, *39*, 481–486. [CrossRef] [PubMed]

12. Yau, A.M.W.; McLaughlin, J.; Maughan, R.J.; Gilmore, W.; Evans, G.H. Short-term dietary supplementation with fructose accelerates gastric emptying of a fructose but not a glucose solution. *Nutrition* **2014**, *30*, 1344–1348. [CrossRef] [PubMed]

13. Cunningham, K.M.; Daly, J.; Horowitz, M.; Read, N.W. Gastrointestinal adaptation to diets of differing fat composition in human volunteers. *Gut* **1991**, *32*, 483–486. [CrossRef] [PubMed]

14. French, S.J.; Murray, B.; Rumsey, R.D.E.; Fadzlin, R.; Read, N.W. Adaptation to high-fat diets—Effects on eating behavior and plasma cholecystokinin. *Br. J. Nutr.* **1995**, *73*, 179–189. [CrossRef] [PubMed]

15. Little, T.J.; Feltrin, K.L.; Horowitz, M.; Meyer, J.H.; Wishart, J.; Chapman, I.M.; Feinle-Bisset, C. A high-fat diet raises fasting plasma CCK but does not affect upper gut motility, PYY, and ghrelin, or energy intake during CCK-8 infusion in lean men. *Am. J. Physiol. Regul. Integr. Comp. Physiol.* **2007**, *294*, R45–R51. [CrossRef] [PubMed]

16. Robertson, M.D.; Henderson, R.A.; Vist, G.E.; Rumsey, R.D. Plasma ghrelin response following a period of acute overfeeding in normal weight men. *Int. J. Obes.* **2004**, *28*, 727–733. [CrossRef] [PubMed]

17. Boyd, K.A.; O'Donovan, D.G.; Doran, S.; Wishart, J.; Chapman, I.M.; Horowitz, M.; Feinle, C. High-fat diet effects on gut motility, hormone, and appetite responses to duodenal lipid in healthy men. *Am. J. Physiol. Gastrointest. Liver* **2003**, *284*, G188–G196. [CrossRef] [PubMed]

18. Lindqvist, A.; Baelemans, A.; Erlanson-Albertsson, C. Effects of sucrose, glucose and fructose on peripheral and central appetite signals. *Regul. Pept.* **2008**, *150*, 26–32. [CrossRef] [PubMed]

19. Ghoos, Y.F.; Maes, B.D.; Geypens, B.J.; Mys, C.; Hiele, M.I.; Rutgeerts, P.J.; Vantrappen, G. Measurement of gastric-emptying rate of solids by means of a carbon-labeled octanoic-acid breath test. *Gastroenterology* **1993**, *104*, 1640–1647. [CrossRef]

20. Haycock, G.B.; Schwartz, G.J.; Wisotsky, D.H. Geometric method for measuring body surface area: A height-weight formula validated in infants, children, and adults. *J. Pediatr.* **1978**, *93*, 62–66. [CrossRef]

21. Kuhre, R.E.; Gribble, F.M.; Hartmann, B.; Reimann, F.; Windeløv, J.A.; Rehfeld, J.F.; Holst, J.J. Fructose stimulates GLP-1 but not GIP secretion in mice, rats, and humans. *Am. J. Physiol. Gastrointest. Liver Physiol.* **2014**, *306*, G622–G630. [CrossRef] [PubMed]

22. Meier, J.J.; Goetze, O.; Anstipp, J.; Hagemann, D.; Holst, J.J.; Schmidt, W.E.; Gallwitz, B.; Nauck, M.A. Gastric inhibitory polypeptide does not inhibit gastric emptying in humans. *Am. J. Physiol. Endocrinol. Metab.* **2004**, *286*, E621–E625. [CrossRef] [PubMed]

23. Wishart, J.M.; Horowitz, M.; Morris, H.A.; Jones, K.L.; Nauck, M.A. Relation between gastric emptying of glucose and plasma concentrations of glucagon-like peptide-1. *Peptides* **1998**, *19*, 1049–1053. [CrossRef]

24. Lee, H.M.; Wang, G.Y.; Englander, E.W.; Kojima, M.; Greeley, G.H. Ghrelin, a new gastrointestinal endocrine peptide that stimulates insulin secretion: Enteric distribution, ontogeny, influence of endocrine, and dietary manipulations. *Endocrinology* **2002**, *143*, 185–190. [CrossRef] [PubMed]

25. Liddle, R.A.; Carter, J.D.; McDonald, A.R. Dietary regulation of rat intestinal cholecystokinin gene expression. *J. Clin. Investig.* **1988**, *81*, 2015–2019. [CrossRef] [PubMed]

26. Bezencon, C.; le Coutre, J.; Damak, S. Taste-signaling proteins are coexpressed in solitary intestinal epithelial cells. *Chem. Senses* **2007**, *32*, 41–49. [CrossRef] [PubMed]

27. Dyer, J.; Salmon, K.S.H.; Zibrik, L.; Shirazi-Beechey, S.P. Expression of sweet taste receptors of the T1R family in the intestinal tract and enteroendocrine cells. *Biochem. Soc. Trans.* **2005**, *33*, 302–305. [CrossRef] [PubMed]

28. Gerspach, A.C.; Steinert, R.E.; Schonenberger, L.; Graber-Maier, A.; Beglinger, C. The role of the gut sweet taste receptor in regulating GLP-1, PYY, and CCK release in humans. *Am. J. Physiol. Endocrinol. Metab.* **2011**, *301*, E317–E325. [CrossRef] [PubMed]

29. Le, K.A.; Faeh, D.; Stettler, R.; Ith, M.; Kreis, R.; Vermathen, P.; Boesch, C.; Ravussin, E.; Tappy, L. A 4-wk high-fructose diet alters lipid metabolism without affecting insulin sensitivity or ectopic lipids in healthy humans. *Am. J. Clin. Nutr.* **2006**, *84*, 1374–1379. [PubMed]

30. Ngo Sock, E.T.; Le, K.-A.; Ith, M.; Kreis, R.; Boesch, C.; Tappy, L. Effects of a short-term overfeeding with fructose or glucose in healthy young males. *Brit. J. Nutr.* **2010**, *103*, 939–943. [CrossRef] [PubMed]

31. Stanhope, K.L.; Bremer, A.A.; Medici, V.; Nakajima, K.; Ito, Y.; Nakano, T.; Chen, G.; Fong, T.H.; Lee, V.; Menorca, R.I.; et al. Consumption of fructose and high fructose corn syrup increase postprandial triglycerides, LDL-cholesterol, and apolipoprotein-B in young men and women. *J. Clin. Endocrinol. Metab.* **2011**, *96*, E1596–E1605. [CrossRef] [PubMed]

32. Stanhope, K.L.; Schwarz, J.M.; Keim, N.L.; Griffen, S.C.; Bremer, A.A.; Graham, J.L.; Hatcher, B.; Cox, C.L.; Dyachenko, A.; Zhang, W.; et al. Consuming fructose-sweetened, not glucose-sweetened, beverages increases visceral adiposity and lipids and decreases insulin sensitivity in overweight/obese humans. *J. Clin. Investig.* **2009**, *119*, 1322–1334. [CrossRef] [PubMed]

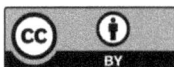

nutrients

MDPI

Article

Metabolic Impact of Light Phase-Restricted Fructose Consumption Is Linked to Changes in Hypothalamic AMPK Phosphorylation and Melatonin Production in Rats

Juliana de Almeida Faria [1], Thiago Matos F. de Araújo [2], Daniela S. Razolli [2],
Letícia Martins Ignácio-Souza [3], Dailson Nogueira Souza [1], Silvana Bordin [4]
and Gabriel Forato Anhê [1,*]

[1] Department of Pharmacology, Faculty of Medical Sciences, State University of Campinas,
   #105 Alexander Fleming St., Campinas SP 13092-140, Brazil; ju.almeidafaria@gmail.com (J.d.A.F.);
   dailson.ns@gmail.com (D.N.S.)
[2] Laboratory of Cell Signaling, Faculty of Medical Sciences, State University of Campinas,
   Carl von Linnaeus St., Campinas SP 13083-864, Brazil; thiagomatosaraujo@gmail.com (T.M.F.d.A.);
   danirazolli@yahoo.com.br (D.S.R.)
[3] Faculty of Applied Sciences, State University of Campinas, #1300 Pedro Zaccaria St., Limeira SP 13484-350,
   Brazil; leticia.isouza@gmail.com
[4] Department of Physiology and Biophysics, Institute of Biomedical Sciences, University of Sao Paulo,
   Sao Paulo SP 05508-900, Brazil; silvana.bordin@gmail.com
* Correspondence: anhegf@fcm.unicamp.br; Tel.: +55-19-3521-9527; Fax: +55-19-3289-2968

Received: 15 February 2017; Accepted: 16 March 2017; Published: 27 March 2017

Abstract: Recent studies show that the metabolic effects of fructose may vary depending on the phase of its consumption along with the light/dark cycle. Here, we investigated the metabolic outcomes of fructose consumption by rats during either the light (LPF) or the dark (DPF) phases of the light/dark cycle. This experimental approach was combined with other interventions, including restriction of chow availability to the dark phase, melatonin administration or intracerebroventricular inhibition of adenosine monophosphate-activated protein kinase (AMPK) with Compound C. LPF, but not DPF rats, exhibited increased hypothalamic AMPK phosphorylation, glucose intolerance, reduced urinary 6-sulfatoxymelatonin (6-S-Mel) (a metabolite of melatonin) and increased corticosterone levels. LPF, but not DPF rats, also exhibited increased chow ingestion during the light phase. The mentioned changes were blunted by Compound C. LPF rats subjected to dark phase-restricted feeding still exhibited increased hypothalamic AMPK phosphorylation but failed to develop the endocrine and metabolic changes. Moreover, melatonin administration to LPF rats reduced corticosterone and prevented glucose intolerance. Altogether, the present data suggests that consumption of fructose during the light phase results in out-of-phase feeding due to increased hypothalamic AMPK phosphorylation. This shift in spontaneous chow ingestion is responsible for the reduction of 6-S-Mel and glucose intolerance.

Keywords: fructose; out-of-phase feeding; AMPK; corticosterone; melatonin

1. Introduction

Impaired glucose tolerance (defined for humans as 2 h values in the oral glucose tolerance test ranging between 140 mg/dL and 199 mg/dL) [1] and insulin resistance (resistance to insulin-stimulated glucose uptake) [2] can be induced in rodents and humans by excessive fructose consumption. For instance, Sprague–Dawley rats fed a fructose-enriched diet develop impaired glucose tolerance and whole body insulin resistance [3]. In mice, fructose-enriched diets were found to cause impaired glucose tolerance with concomitant hepatic triglyceride accumulation and insulin resistance [4]. Interventional experiments with humans have also demonstrated that overweight subjects display impaired glucose tolerance after a 10-week interval of consumption of fructose sweetened beverages [5]. Among the myriad of endocrine changes that putatively underlie these metabolic effects, the consumption of a fructose-enriched diet was shown to reduce nocturnal melatonin production in rats [6].

The relationship between melatonin and the control of energy metabolism has been supported by several studies using distinct experimental approaches. Surgical ablation of the pineal gland was reported to result in impaired glucose tolerance and insulin resistance with increased nocturnal levels of glycemia and gluconeogenesis [7–9]. Accordingly, the aging-related reduction of melatonin levels was shown to mediate the enhanced adiposity in middle-aged rats [10]. In turn, exogenous melatonin administration is able to improve the metabolic control in rodents rendered glucose intolerant either by high-fat diets or fructose administration [11–13].

Recent studies have revealed that metabolic outcomes caused by fructose and high-fat diet intake is influenced by their out-of-phase consumption. Mice allowed to consume a high-fat diet exclusively during the dark-phase fail to develop abrupt body weight gain and impaired glucose tolerance relative to those subjected to ad libitum or light phase-restricted consumption [14,15]. In addition, fructose consumption by mice exclusively during the light phase, but not during the dark phase, resulted in increased body weight, adiposity and insulin levels [16]. However, the precise mechanism by which fructose induces these changes are not known. We have previously demonstrated that short-term fructose injections in the central nervous system during the light phase leads to an increase in the endogenous glucose production (EGP) by hypothalamic AMP-activated protein kinase (AMPK) activation [17]. It was also shown that hypothalamic AMPK activation by fructose is also important to acutely stimulate food intake [18].

Depending on its intensity and frequency, out-of-phase food intake by humans can be classified as the night eating syndrome (NES) [19]. The prevalence of NES is relatively low in the general population but ranges between 8.9% and 27% in obese subgroups [20]. Cohort studies have shown that NES positively correlates with the diagnosis of metabolic syndrome, increased triglycerides and waist circumference [21]. Among several adaptations, the circadian endocrine profile of NES patients is characterized by reduced melatonin levels during the night and increased morning cortisol concentrations [22].

Given the mentioned observations, the present study was conducted to investigate whether the metabolic impact resulting from fructose consumption during different phases of the light/dark cycle is dependent on changes in hypothalamic AMPK activation and in the circadian pattern of food intake in rats. We also collected results suggesting that disruption of melatonin production is a key event in the mechanism linking the light phase-restricted fructose consumption and its metabolic outcomes.

2. Materials and Methods

2.1. Animals and Treatments

The experimental procedures were approved by the State University of Campinas Committee for Ethics in Animal Experimentation (protocol No. 3506-1) and were conducted in accordance with the guidelines of the Brazilian College for Animal Experimentation.

Three-week-old male Sprague–Dawley rats were obtained from the Animal Breeding Center at the University of Campinas (CEMIB, Campinas, Sao Paulo, Brazil) and were housed at 22 ± 2 °C under a 12:12 h light:dark cycle (lights on at 7:00 a.m.) with free access to food and water for 5 weeks. At 8 weeks of age, rats were assigned to the experimental groups for an additional 8 weeks of treatment with fructose and/or melatonin. Measurements of chow consumption and body mass were made twice and once a week during the period of treatment, respectively. When specified in the results section, one of the three experimental strategies was combined with the fructose treatment: (i) chow availability was restricted to the dark phase (Chow-R rats) during the 8 weeks of treatment; (ii) compound C was administered during the last week of treatment through a cannula placed in the lateral ventricle or (iii) melatonin dissolved in the drinking water was administrated during the dark phase during the 8 weeks of treatment.

Fructose was dissolved in regular water to produce a 70% stock solution (w/v). The fructose stock solution was further diluted to 10% (w/v) with regular water immediately before treatment. Fructose was made available exclusively during the light or the dark phases (LPF and DPF rats, respectively). Bottles containing just water were offered to the rats only when fructose was absent.

Melatonin (Cat. A9525; Sigma-Aldrich, St. Louis, MO, USA) was initially diluted in 100% ethanol to generate a 100 mg/mL stock solution that was kept protected from the light in -20 °C for no longer than 7 days. The melatonin stock solution was further diluted (1:50) with distilled water every 3 days of treatment to generate a 2 mg/mL solution. Variable volumes of this solution were added to the drinking water bottle to yield a 0.5 mg/kg ingestion of melatonin. Bottles with melatonin were placed on the cages 30 min before "lights off" and removed 30 min after "lights on". The individual calculations of the required volumes of melatonin solution were based on the body weight (weekly assessed) and nocturnal water intake (daily assessed) and were adjusted daily.

2.2. Surgical Procedure and Intracerebroventricular Treatment

Six weeks after the beginning of treatment using fructose solution, rats were anesthetized with diazepam and ketamine (2 and 50 mg/kg, respectively) and placed in a stereotaxic apparatus to insert a stainless-steel cannula into the lateral ventricle. Stereotaxic coordinates were 0.8 mm (anteroposterior), 1.5 mm (lateral), and 4.0 mm (depth) [23]. The localization of the cannula was tested by evaluating the dipsogenic response to an intracerebroventricular (icv) angiotensin II injection (5 ng/μL saline; Sigma, St. Louis, MO, USA) 1 week after the surgical procedure (7th week of fructose treatment). Only animals that presented a positive response in these tests were used for further experimentation.

The pharmacological inhibitor of AMPK, Compound C (Cat. 171260; EMD4 Biosciences, Gibbstown, NJ, USA) was diluted in 5% dimethylsulfoxide (DMSO) to a final concentration of 200 mM and was injected daily through the cannula for five days during the last week of treatment with fructose. Injections (2 μL) were performed 1 h after lights on Zeitgeber Time 1 (ZT 1) and equal volumes of vehicle were injected in the controls. Experiments with these rats were carried out two hours before lights off (ZT 10) on the day of the last icv injection. Fasting prior to the analyses and sample collection started immediately after the last injection (between ZT 1 and ZT 2).

2.3. Intraperitoneal Pyruvate Tolerance Test (pTT)

Rats were fasted for 10 h, and a sodium pyruvate solution (250 mg/mL) was injected intraperitoneal (i.p.) at a dosage of 2 g/kg. Pyruvate injections were made two hours before lights off. Glucose concentration was determined in blood extracted from the tail before (0 min) and 15, 30, 60, 90, and 120 min after pyruvate injection. The area under the curve (AUC) of glycemia vs. time was calculated using each individual baseline (basal glycemia) to estimate glucose clearance after pyruvate injection.

2.4. Intraperitoneal Glucose Tolerance Test (GTT)

Rats were fasted for 10 h prior to i.p. glucose injection (2 g/kg of a 25% solution of D-glucose) two hours before lights off. The blood samples were collected from the tail at 0, 10, 15, 30, 60 and 120 min to determine the blood glucose concentration. The area under the curve (AUC) of glycemia vs. time was calculated from each individual baseline (basal glycemia) to estimate glucose tolerance.

2.5. Intraperitoneal Insulin Tolerance Test (ITT)

Rats were fasted for 10 h prior to i.p. insulin injection (2 IU/kg) two hours before "lights off". Blood glucose was measured before and 5, 10, 15, 20, 25 and 30 min after insulin injection to determine the sensitivity of insulin-responsive tissues. Blood glucose values were converted to a logarithmic scale, and the slope of the curve was calculated. This value multiplied by 100 was assumed to be the glucose decay constant (KITT).

2.6. Protein Extraction and Immunoblotting

Anesthetized rats were decapitated, and the hypothalamus was removed and processed for Western blotting as previously described [17]. The hypothalamic tissue removed for Western blot analysis contained approximately 4.0 mm^3 and had the optic chiasm as the rostral limit (bregma −0.25 mm), the infundibular stem as the caudal limit (bregma −4.20 mm) and were 4.0 mm wide and 3.0 mm deep [24]. The extractions occurred two hours before lights off (ZT 10). The primary antibodies used were as follows: anti-pAMPK alpha (T172) from Cell Signaling Technology (Cat. 2531S, Danvers, MA, USA) and anti-GAPDH from Cell Signaling (Cat. 2118S, Danvers, MA, USA). Secondary antibodies conjugated with horseradish peroxidase (Bio-Rad Laboratories, Hercules, CA, USA) were used, followed by chemiluminescent detection of the bands on X-ray-sensitive films. Optical densitometry was performed using the Scion Image analysis software (version, Scion Corp., Frederick, MD, USA).

2.7. Immunofluorescent Staining

Initial perfusion of the anesthetized rats with saline was followed by perfusion with 4% paraformaldehyde. After perfusion, the animals were decapitated and they had the encephalon excised. Each fixed encephalon was cut into a fragment limited by the bregma −0.25 mm (rostral) and bregma −4.20 mm (caudal). The sections (5.0 micrometer thick) used for staining were between bregma −2.50 and −2.80. The atrium of the central, third and lateral ventricles as well as the hippocampus served as indicators for the sections within this antero-posterior interval [24]. Sections were incubated with primary antibody against pAMPK (Thr 172) (Cat. 2535, Cell Signaling Technology, Danvers, MA, USA) overnight at −4 °C and with secondary antibody conjugated to Alexafluor 546 for 2 h (Cat. A10040, Thermo Fisher Scientific, Waltham, MA, USA). The 4′,6-diamidino-2-phenylindole (DAPI) stain (Cat. H-1200, Vector Laboratories, Burlingame, CA, USA) was used for nuclear staining and images were captured with a Leica Confocal microscope TCS SP5 II (Leica Microsystems, Mannheim, Germany). Hypothalamic areas were defined according to the Paxinos and Watson rat brain atlas [24]. Images were acquired in high (400×) magnification.

2.8. Hormone Measurements

Trunk blood was collected two hours before lights off and plasma was extracted with heparin and stored at −80 °C for corticosterone determination with a commercially available ELISA kit (Cat. #402810; Neogen, Lexington, KY, USA). For urine collection, rats were placed in a metabolic cage during the dark phase. Urine was allowed to accumulate overnight in a glass tube placed under the cages. Urine samples were used for 6-sulfatoxi-melatonin (6-S-Mel) determination using a commercially available ELISA kit (Cat. #RE54031; IBL International, Hamburg, Germany).

2.9. RNA Extraction and Real Time pCR

Fragments of liver were homogenized in Trizol (50 mg/mL) and the total RNA was extracted and quantified using a Nanodrop 8000 device (Thermo Scientific, Wilmington, DE, USA). The cDNA was synthesized using 2 µg of the total RNA and the High-Capacity cDNA Reverse Transcription Kit (Cat. 4368813). PCR was performed for cytochrome P450 1A2 (*cyp1a2*) and cytosolic sulfotransferase 1A1 (*sult1a1*) genes using the respective Taqman primers assays rn00561082_m1 and rn01510633_m1 and the Taqman Gene Expression Master Mix (Cat. 4369016) in a Step One Plus sequence detection system (Applied Biosystems, Carlsbad, CA, USA). All reagents for reverse transcription and PCR were obtained from Applied Biosystems. Values of mRNA expression were normalized to *gapdh* (rn99999916) gene expression using the ΔΔCT method.

2.10. Statistical Analysis

The results are presented as the mean ± standard error of the mean Comparisons were performed using one-way Analysis of Variance followed by Tukey–Kramer post hoc testing or Student's *t*-test (version, GraphPad Prism Software, Inc., San Diego, CA, USA). Values of $p < 0.05$ indicate a significant difference.

3. Results

3.1. Metabolic and Endocrine Changes in Rats Exposed to Fructose Consumption during the Light or the Dark Phases

Body weights of control CTL, LPF and DPF rats were similar at baseline, prior to the beginning of treatments. Body weight gain after the eight weeks of treatment did not differ among the experimental groups so that the final body weight was similar among rats assigned to the CTL, LPF and DPF groups (Figure 1A). Food intake was also assessed at the eighth week of treatment. The rats exhibited an expected nocturnal eating pattern so that, for every group, food intake during the dark phase was higher than that during the light phase ($p < 0.001$). Consumption of chow during the light phase, however, was increased in LPF rats (58% higher than CTL values; $p < 0.001$), but reduced in DPF rats (44% lower than CTL values; $p < 0.01$). Chow consumption during the dark phase was similarly reduced in LPF and DPF rats (23 and 31% lower than CTL, respectively; $p < 0.01$) (Figure 1B).

Increased glucose levels were found in LFP rats, but not in DFP rats, as evidenced by increased AUC values obtained from the GTTs (120% higher than CTL; $p < 0.05$) (Figure 1C). Conversely, the AUC values obtained from the curve glycemia vs. time after a pyruvate load were increased in both LPF and DPF rats (respectively, 114% and 42% higher than CTL; $p < 0.05$). The values of DPF were, however, 44% lower than those of LFP ($p < 0.001$) (Figure 1E). Apart from these changes in glucose levels during the GTT, our data revealed that neither LPF nor DPF rats exhibited insulin resistance as shown by similar K_{ITT} values (Figure 1G). Endocrine changes in LPF rats were hallmarked by increased levels of corticosterone (91% higher than CTL; $p < 0.05$) and reduced urinary levels of 6-S-Mel (63% lower than CTL; $p < 0.05$) (Figure 1D,F, respectively). Importantly, the expressions of the two main enzymes responsible for hepatic melatonin metabolism, *cyp1a2* and *sult1a1*, were similarly expressed in the liver of CTL, LPF and DPF at the end of treatment (Figure 1H). Thus, decreased urinary levels of 6-S-Mel are likely to result from reduced melatonin production rather than changes in hepatic melatonin metabolism.

Liquid ingestion (either water or 10% fructose) was also assessed. LPF rats ingested less water during the dark phase (19.5 ± 0.8 mL) as compared to CTL (26.2 ± 1.2 mL) ($p < 0.05$; $n = 5$). LPF rats, however, increased liquid ingestion during the light phase. LPF rats consumed a mean volume of 26.02 ± 4.1 mL of 10% fructose while CTL consumed a mean volume of 4.2 ± 0.4 mL of water during the light phase ($p < 0.05$; $n = 5$).

DPF increased liquid ingestion during the dark phase as compared to CTL (39.6 ± 1.2 mL of 10% fructose vs. 26.2 ± 1.2 mL of water; $p < 0.05$; $n = 5$). Water ingestion during the light phase, however, was similar between CTL and DPF.

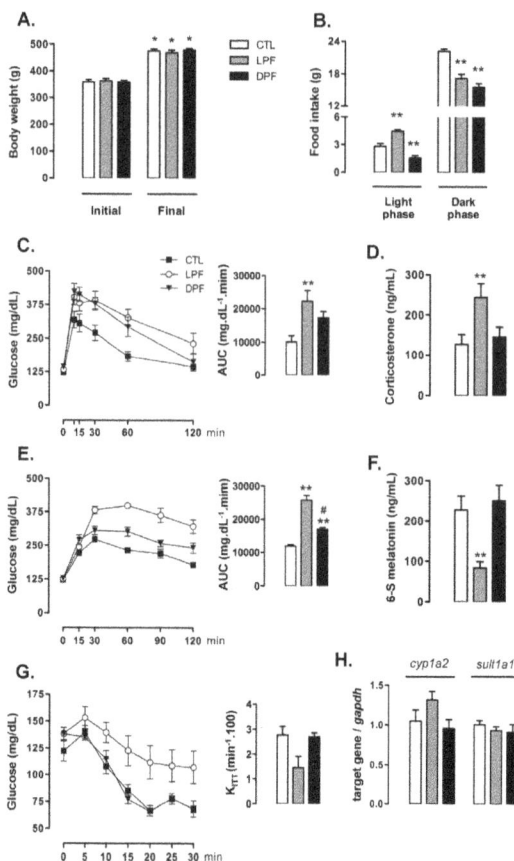

Figure 1. Metabolic and endocrine changes in rats exposed to fructose consumption during the light or the dark phases. Rats assigned to the groups control (CTL), Light Phase Fructose (LPF) and Dark Phase Fructose (DPF) had their (**A**) body weights assessed before and after (8 weeks) treatments. (**B**) Food intake during the light and the dark phases were also assessed at the end of the treatments. After these measurements, the rats were subjected to (**C**) glucose tolerance tests, (**E**) pyruvate tolerance tests and (**G**) insulin tolerance tests. Tests were performed two hours before "lights off" and the area under the curve (AUC) was calculated. Euthanasia was performed two hours before "lights off" when fragments of liver and plasma were collected. (**D**) Plasma samples were used for the determination of corticosterone levels. (**F**) Urine was collected overnight before euthanasia for determination of 6-S-Mel concentration. Fragments of liver were used for relative determination of (**H**) *cyp1a2* and *sult1a1* mRNAs by real time PCR. The results are presented as the means $\pm$ standard error of the mean. * $p < 0.05$ vs. The same group before treatment; ** $p < 0.05$ vs. CTL at the same phase of the light/dark cycle; # $p < 0.05$ vs. LPF at the same phase of the light/dark cycle.

3.2. Hypothalamic AMpK Phosphorylation in Rats Exposed to Fructose Consumption during the Light or the Dark Phases

Western blot analyses of whole hypothalamus revealed that the levels of AMPK phosphorylation were increased in LPF but not in DPF rats (102% higher than CTL; $p < 0.05$) (Figure 2A). In contrast, the content of AMPK was not modulated in the hypothalamus of LPF rats but was increased in the hypothalamus of DPF (30% higher than CTL; $p < 0.05$) (Figure 2B).

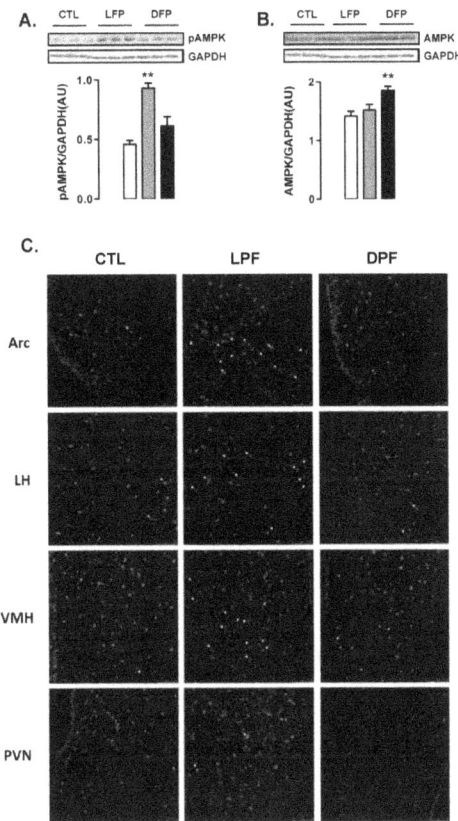

Figure 2. AMPK phosphorylation and content in hypothalamus of rats exposed to fructose consumption during the light or the dark phases. Rats assigned to the groups control (CTL), Light Phase Fructose (LPF) and Dark Phase Fructose (DPF) had their hypothalamus removed at the end of the eighth week of treatment. A first set of samples was used for (**A**) Western blot detection of phosphorylated Adenosine Monophosphate-activated protein kinase (AMPK) and (**B**) total AMPK. Target proteins were normalized to Glyceraldehyde 3-phosphate dehydrogenase (GAPDH). A second set of samples was processed for immunofluorescent staining. Sections were stained using an anti-pAMPK antibody followed by secondary antibody conjugated to Alexafluor 546 (red). Nuclear structures are visualized by 4′,6-diamidino-2-phenylindole (DAPI) probing (Blue). (**C**) Large magnification (400×) images are shown from the arcuate nucleus (ARC), lateral hypothalamus (LH), ventro medial hypothalamus (VMH) and paraventricular nucleus (PVN). The results are presented as the means ± standard error of the mean. ** $p < 0.05$ vs. CTL.

Immunofluorescent staining was performed to identify the hypothalamic areas that could account for the results seen in the Western blot experiments. We found that the number of cells with phosphorylated AMPK was evidently increased in the regions of the arcuate nucleus (ARC) and the ventro medial hypothalamus (VMH) from LPF rats. No evident of increase in the number of cells with phosphorylated AMPK was found in the regions of the lateral hypothalamus (LH) and the paraventricular nucleus (PVN). In agreement with the Western blot data, we found a similar number of cells with phosphorylated AMPK in the ARC, VMH, LH and PVN regions of the CTL and DPF rats (Figure 2C).

3.3. Increased Hypothalamic AMPK Phosphorylation in LPF Phase Advances Food Intake Resulting in Metabolic and Endocrine Changes

Hypothalamic AMPK activation was already reported to stimulate food intake and reduce melatonin production [25,26]. Thus, we decided to assess the relevance of the increased hypothalamic AMPK phosphorylation for LPF rats in a set of experiments in which they received icv injections with Compound C, a pharmacological AMPK inhibitor. The rats were assigned to four different groups in these experiments, as follows: CTL (rats that did not receive fructose and were treated with vehicle icv), LPF (rats that received fructose during the light phase and were treated with vehicle icv), Compound C (CC) (rats that did not receive fructose and were treated with Compound C icv) and LPF/CC (rats that received fructose during the light phase and were treated with Compound C icv). Icv treatments lasted for five days during the eighth week of treatment with fructose.

Icv treatments did not interfere with the final body weight so that similar values were obtained among the groups at the end of the eighth week of treatment. For the four groups, the final body weight reached values higher than in the beginning of treatments ($p < 0.05$) (Figure 3A). Before the beginning of icv treatments, food intake during the light phase was increased in animals assigned to both LPF and LPF/CC groups (139% and 119% higher than CTL, respectively; $p < 0.05$). Thus, surgical implantation of the cannula in the lateral ventricle alone did not affect the response to light phase fructose described in the previous experiments. After icv treatments, the LPF animals treated with vehicle, but not those treated with Compound C, maintained increased values of food intake during the light phase (200% higher than CTL after treatment with vehicle; $p < 0.05$) (Figure 3B).

Food intake during the dark phase was similarly not affected by cannula implantation per se so that, before icv treatments, the amount of chow ingested by LPF and LPF/CC groups during the dark phase was lower than that ingested by rats assigned to the CTL group (25% and 28% lower than CTL before icv treatment; $p < 0.05$). After icv treatments, food intake during the dark phase remained reduced in both LPF and LPF/CC groups (32% and 34% lower than CTL after icv treatment with vehicle; $p < 0.05$) (Figure 3C).

Glucose tolerance test performed after icv treatments showed that these injections with vehicle did not interfere with the metabolic effect of fructose consumption during the light phase. In these experiments, as in those described above, LPF animals treated with vehicle presented increased glucose levels as evidenced by the AUC values (114% higher than in CTL after icv treatment with vehicle; $p < 0.05$). When compared with CTL rats, the CC and the LPF/CC rats exhibited similar changes in glucose levels during the GTT (evidenced by similar values of AUC) (Figure 3D).

Corticosterone levels were increased in LPF rats treated with vehicle via icv (150% higher than in CTL treated with vehicle; $p < 0.05$). Corticosterone levels of LPF/CC and CC rats remained similar to those of CTL rats after icv treatments (Figure 3E). The urinary 6-S-Mel concentration in LPF rats, but not in LPF/CC and CC rats, was reduced after icv treatments (65% lower than CTL after icv treatment with vehicle; $p < 0.05$) (Figure 3F). The phosphorylation levels of hypothalamic AMPK were increased in LPF rats after treatment with vehicle (460% higher than in CTL treated with vehicle; $p < 0.05$). Treatment with Compound C icv blunted this response so that hypothalamic AMPK phosphorylation in LPF/CC rats was similar to that of CTL rats (Figure 3G).

Pharmacological inhibition of hypothalamic AMPK in LPF rats was able to blunt both the reduction in urinary 6-S-Mel levels and the changes hallmarked by increased corticosterone and increased glucose levels during the GTT. However, pharmacological AMPK inhibition in LPF also inhibited the shift in spontaneous chow ingestion to the light phase.

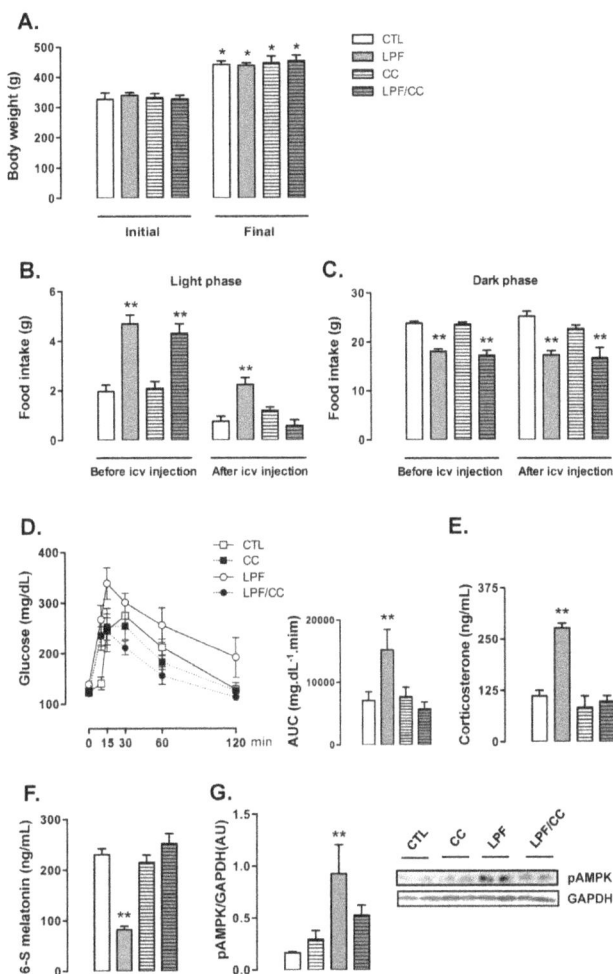

Figure 3. Pharmacological inhibition of adenosine monophosphate-activated protein kinase (AMPK) in the central nervous system of LPF rats. Rats were assigned to the groups control (CTL), Light Phase Fructose (LPF), Compound C (CC) and Light Phase Fructose with Compound C (LPF/CC). Cannula implantation and icv treatments (five days) occurred during the sixth and eighth weeks of fructose treatment, respectively. (**A**) Body weights were assessed before and after (8 weeks) fructose treatment. Food intake was assessed before and after icv injections during the last week of fructose treatment. Data were acquired separately during the (**B**) light and the (**C**) dark phases. After these measurements (**D**), the rats were subjected to glucose tolerance tests. Tests were performed two hours before "lights off" and area under the curve (AUC) was calculated. Euthanasia was performed two hours before lights off, and the hypothalamus and plasma were collected. (**E**) Plasma samples were used for corticosterone determinations. (**F**) Urine was collected overnight before euthanasia for determination of 6-S-Mel concentration. (**G**) Hypothalamus samples were used for Western blot detection of phosphorylated AMPK and normalization by Glyceraldehyde 3-phosphate dehydrogenase (GAPDH). The results are presented as the means ± standard error of the mean. * $p < 0.05$ vs. same group before fructose treatment; ** $p < 0.05$ vs. CTL at the same moment of icv treatment.

3.4. Increased Food Intake during the Light Phase Seen in LPF Contributes to Metabolic and Endocrine Changes

To investigate if the increase in food intake during the light phase was involved in the metabolic and endocrine changes observed in LPF animals, we designed an experimental protocol in which the animals were assigned to four different groups: CTL (rats that consumed chow ad libitum and did not receive fructose), LPF (rats that consumed chow ad libitum and received fructose during the light phase), Chow-R (rats that consumed chow exclusively during the dark phase and did not receive fructose) and LPF/Chow-R (rats that consumed chow exclusively during the dark phase and received fructose during the light phase).

The body weight of animals assigned to the four groups were similar at the beginning of the treatments. The four groups of animals exhibited a similar increase in body weight so that absolute body weights at the end of the treatments were also similar among the groups (Figure 4A). The increase in food intake during the light phase exhibited by LPF rats was replicated in this set of experiments (40% higher than food intake of CTL during the light phase; $p < 0.05$). The food intake during the dark phase was increased in Chow-R compared with CTL rats (26% higher; $p < 0.05$). Apart from that, consumption of fructose during the light phase resulted in reduced food intake during the dark phase irrespective of food restriction to this phase. Thus, food intake during the dark phase was reduced in LPF/Chow-R (14% lower than in Chow-R; $p < 0.05$) and in LPF (12% lower than in CTL; $p < 0.05$) (Figure 4B).

LPF animals exhibited consistent increased glucose levels during the GTT as evidenced by the AUC values (98% higher than CTL; $p < 0.05$). The glucose levels during the GTT were not modulated in Chow-R compared with CTL animals. Interestingly, increased glucose levels during the GTT were not replicated in LPF/Chow-R rats (Figure 4C). With regard to the endocrine profile, Chow-R exhibited corticosterone and urinary 6-S-Mel concentrations similar to those of CTL rats. The increase in circulating corticosterone levels (77%; $p < 0.05$) and the reduction in the urinary concentration of 6-S-Mel (74%; $p < 0.05$) observed in LPF rats when compared with CTL rats were not detected in LPF/Chow-R (respectively, Figure 4D,E). The hypothalamic AMPK phosphorylation levels observed in CTL and in LPF rats were not affected by restricting food availability to the dark phase. Thus, the amounts of phosphorylated AMPK were increased in LPF compared with CTL rats (72%; $p < 0.05$) and in LPF/Chow-R compared with Chow-R rats (41%; $p < 0.05$) (Figure 4F).

3.5. Reduced Melatonin Production in LPF Rats Leads to Increased Corticosterone Levels and Glucose Intolerance

To determine the metabolic relevance for reduced 6-S-Mel levels in LPF rats, we designed the next experimental protocol in which the animals were assigned to the following four different groups: CTL (rats that did not receive either fructose or melatonin), LPF (rats that received fructose during the light phase), Mel (rats that received melatonin exclusively during the dark phase) and LPF/Mel (rats that received fructose during the light phase and melatonin exclusively during the dark phase).

When compared to their initial body weights, the rats belonging to the four experimental groups exhibited increased body weight at the end of the treatment ($p < 0.05$). Treatment with melatonin did not affect the changes in body weights throughout the experimental period so that final body weights of the rats belonging to the CTL, LPF, Mel and LPF/Mel groups were similar (Figure 5A). The changes in the food intake profile observed in LPF animals, hallmarked by increased values during the light phase and reduced values during the dark phase, were not altered by melatonin treatment. Additionally, melatonin treatment per se did not affect food intake. Thus, food intake by both LPF and LPF/Mel rats was increased during the light phase (approximately 50% higher than CTL; $p < 0.05$) and reduced during the dark phase (approximately 17% lower than CTL; $p < 0.05$) (Figure 5B).

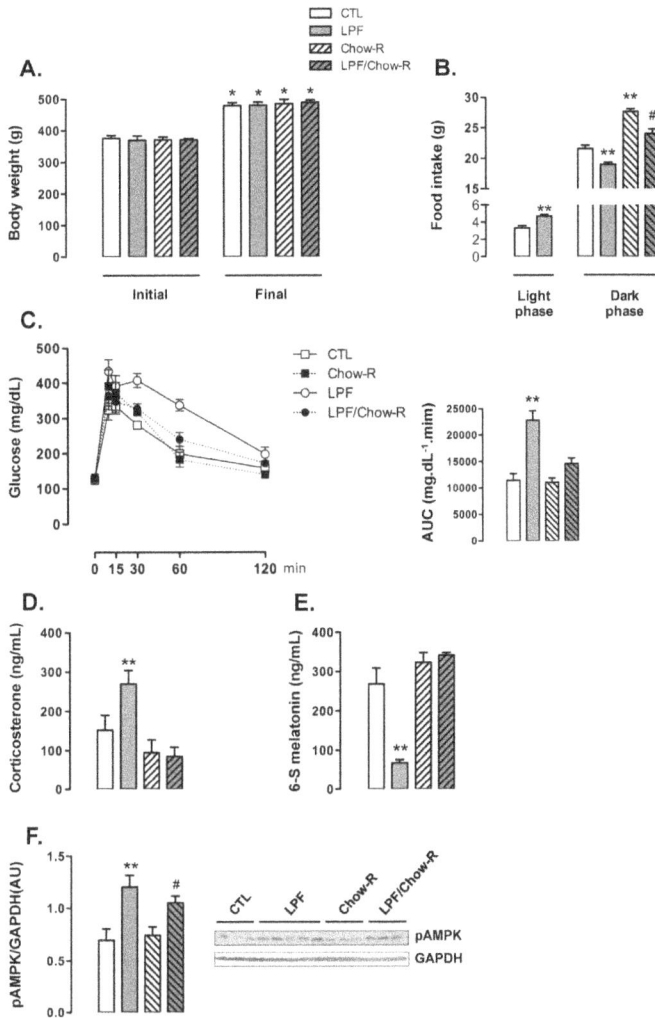

Figure 4. Dark-restricted feeding in rats exposed to fructose during the light phase. Rats were assigned to the groups Control (CTL), Light Phase Fructose (LPF), Chow restriction to the dark phase (Chow-R) and Light Phase Fructose with Chow restriction to the dark phase (LPF/Chow-R). (**A**) Body weights were assessed before and after (eight week) treatments; (**B**) Food intake during the light and the dark phases were also assessed at the end of the treatments; After these measurements (**C**), the rats were subjected to glucose tolerance tests. Tests were performed two hours before "lights off" and area under the curve (AUC) was calculated. Euthanasia was performed two hours before "lights off" and the hypothalamus and plasma were collected; (**D**) Plasma samples were used for the determination of corticosterone levels; (**E**) Urine was collected overnight before euthanasia for determination of the 6-S-Mel concentration; (**F**) Hypothalamus samples were used for Western blot detection of phosphorylated adenosine monophosphate-activated protein kinase and normalization by Glyceraldehyde 3-phosphate dehydrogenase (GAPDH). The results are presented as the means ± standard error of the mean. * $p < 0.05$ vs. same group before treatment; ** $p < 0.05$ vs. CTL at the same phase of the light/dark cycle; # $p < 0.05$ vs. Chow-R at the same phase of the light/dark cycle.

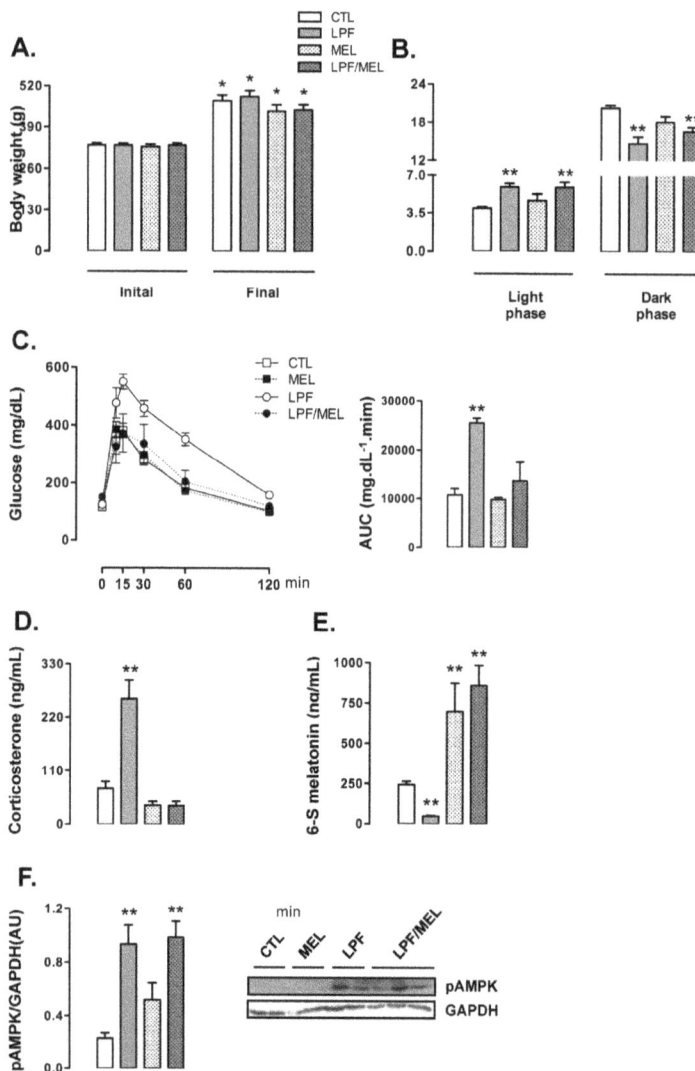

Figure 5. Nocturnal melatonin administration in rats exposed to fructose during the light phase. Rats were assigned to the groups control (CTL), Light Phase Fructose (LPF), melatonin (Mel) and Light Phase Fructose with melatonin (LPF/Mel). (**A**) Body weights were assessed before and after (eight week) treatments; (**B**) Food intake during the light and the dark phases were also assessed at the end of the treatments; After these measurements (**C**), the rats were subjected to glucose tolerance tests. Tests were performed two hours before "lights off" and area under the curve (AUC) was calculated. Euthanasia was performed two hours before "lights off" and the hypothalamus and plasma were collected; (**D**) Plasma samples were used for the determination of corticosterone levels; (**E**) Urine was collected overnight before euthanasia for determination of 6-S-Mel concentration; (**F**) Hypothalamus samples were used for Western blot detection of phosphorylated adenosine monophosphate-activated protein kinase and normalization by Glyceraldehyde 3-phosphate dehydrogenase (GAPDH). The results are presented as the means ± standard error of the mean. * $p < 0.05$ vs. same group before treatment; ** $p < 0.05$ vs. CTL at the same phase of the light/dark cycle.

Treatment with melatonin was able to blunt the increase in glucose levels induced by fructose consumption during the light phase. The AUC values obtained from the GTT were increased in LPF (138% higher than CTL; $p < 0.05$) but not in LPF/Mel rats. In turn, treatment with melatonin in fructose-naive rats did not alter glucose levels during the GTT (AUC values similar to CTL) (Figure 5C). As an example of what was observed for glucose levels along with the GTT, corticosterone levels were increased in LPF (249% higher than CTL; $p < 0.05$) but not in LPF/Mel animals. Melatonin treatment alone did not alter corticosterone concentrations (Figure 5D).

In this set of experiments, we also found that LPF rats had reduced urinary 6-S-Mel concentrations (80% lower than CTL; $p < 0.05$). Fructose consumption during the light phase, however, failed to reduce urinary 6-S-Mel concentrations in rats consuming melatonin (urinary 6-S-Mel concentration are similar between Mel and LPF/Mel groups). The urinary 6-S-Mel concentration was found to be similarly increased in both Mel and LPF/Mel groups (187% and 254% higher than CTL, respectively; $p < 0.05$) (Figure 5E).

Melatonin treatment alone did not interfere with hypothalamic AMPK phosphorylation so that these levels in rats belonging to the Mel group were similar to those of the CTL group. Melatonin treatment was also unable to modulate the increase in hypothalamic AMPK phosphorylation induced by the consumption of fructose during the light phase (LPF and LPF/Mel were, respectively, 302% and 325% higher than CTL; $p < 0.05$) (Figure 5F).

4. Discussion

The data presented herein show that rats receiving fructose during the light phase developed increased hypothalamic AMPK phosphorylation, reduced urinary 6-S-Mel, increased chow ingestion during the light phase and impaired glucose tolerance. Importantly, these combined changes were not observed in rats receiving fructose exclusively during the dark phase. Our data supports the conclusion that this shift in food intake is of pivotal relevance for metabolic outcomes because fructose ingestion during the light phase with simultaneous chow restriction to the dark phase fails to impair glucose tolerance. This finding is in accordance with recent publications showing that rats that increase their food intake during the light phase (either by forced activity protocols during the light phase or by simple restriction of food availability during dark phase) become glucose intolerant [27]. Out-of-phase feeding seems also to be relevant for human metabolism as subgroups of diabetic patients who display night eating behavior also have impaired glycemic control based on increased glycated hemoglobin levels [28].

The present data also allow us to conclude that hypothalamic AMPK activation (which takes place mainly in the ARC and VMH) is a key event induced by fructose ingestion during the light phase that increases out-of-phase feeding. This sequential cause/effect relationship is supported by our data which show: 1-pharmacological AMPK inhibition in the central nervous system using Compound C abrogates the shift in food intake and impaired glucose tolerance induced by fructose consumption during the light phase; and 2-fructose consumption during the light phase is still able to induce hypothalamic AMPK phosphorylation in rats for which food availability has been restricted to the dark phase. Accordingly, previous studies have already shown that a consistent increase in food intake occurs when hypothalamic AMPK is activated in the ARC and VMH [25,29] and that fructose metabolism in the hypothalamus results in a rapid reduction in ATP with parallel increase in the AMP/ATP ratio that activates AMPK and stimulates food intake [18,30]. To date, in vitro experiments have also shown that that fructose can directly activate AMPK in hypothalamic GT1-7 cells [31].

Previous publications have also shown that hypothalamic AMPK activation with pharmacological approaches triggers a counter-regulatory response hallmarked by increased EGP. The mechanisms for this response are not completely understood. However, it was demonstrated that hypothalamic AMPK activation in nuclei such as VMH and ARC is able to spread peripheral signals that lead to the secretion of glucocorticoids, glucagon and catecholamines [32–34]. These hormones are classically known to act in the liver by increasing gluconeogenesis and glycogenolysis, therefore stimulating EGP.

In this context, we have previously demonstrated that intra-cerebro ventricular injections with fructose during the light phase lead to an acute activation of hypothalamic AMPK in the central nervous system and consequently increases corticosterone levels that raise whole-body gluconeogenesis [17].

Increased corticosterone levels as an acute response to an oral fructose load have been formerly demonstrated by other groups [35,36]. The present data add further information to this field by revealing that chronic fructose consumption exclusively during the resting light phase can also increase corticosterone. As an example of glucose levels during the GTT, the increase of corticosterone levels was equally prevented by restricting chow availability to the dark phase and by pharmacological AMPK inhibition in the central nervous system. Thus, our data show that the ability of chronic fructose consumption during the light phase to increase corticosterone levels after eight weeks of treatment relies on the chronically light phase-shifted chow ingestion induced by hypothalamic AMPK activation.

Having established that hypothalamic AMPK activation and increased food intake during the light phase are important for the enhance in corticosterone levels observed in LPF rats, we next explored how changes in the central nervous system result in peripheral endocrine modulations. It was previously demonstrated that exposing Sprague–Dawley rats to a 60% fructose-enriched diet ad libitum resulted in a reduction of the levels of urinary 6-S-Mel [6]. 6-S-Mel is the most abundant melatonin metabolite. Its formation requires the conversion of melatonin into the intermediary 6-hydroxymelatonin that suffers subsequent sulfation. These two reactions (hydroxylation and sulfation) occur predominantly in the liver and, in rats, they are respectively catalyzed by cytochrome P450 1A2 (*cyp1a2*) and cytosolic sulfotransferase 1A1 (*sult1a1*) [37–39]. In this context, the determination of 6-S-Mel excretion in the urine is a well-recognized method to estimate melatonin production [40,41].

As LPF developed increased liquid and food intake during the light phase, we can presume that these rats may present a partial shift of global activity to the light phase. It is unlike, however, that increased activity during the light phase per se may account for the reduced melatonin metabolite concentration seen in LPF. This proposition is corroborated by studies showing that forced physical activity (swimming) during the light phase fails to modulate nocturnal melatonin production in rats [42]. We and others have also previously shown that light phase-restricted feeding with standard chow fail to reduce melatonin metabolite in the urine or melatonin circulating levels during the dark phase [43,44]. On the other hand, the daytime consumption of carbohydrates by rodents seems to be particularly relevant to yield reductions in nocturnal melatonin production. It was previously demonstrated that reduced amplitude of nocturnal melatonin levels was only achieved by offering a combination of a carbohydrate-enriched diet and standard chow during the light-resting phase [44]. Accordingly, the present data reveals that the consumption of fructose during the light phase fails to reduce 6-S-Mel production in rats subjected to restriction of chow availability to the dark phase. Our data from the experiments with Compound C further corroborates this hypothesis because the pharmacological inhibition of AMPK in the central nervous system abrogated both the shift in food intake to the light phase observed in LPF rats and the reduction in urinary 6-S-Mel. Importantly, LPF rats did not show any modulation of the hepatic expression of *cyp1a2* and *sult1a1*. Thus, it is unlikely that reduced urinary 6-S-Mel seen in LPF rats resulted from lower hepatic metabolism of melatonin.

The reduction in the concentration of melatonin metabolite seen in the urine of LPF rats cannot be attributed to an increase in water intake during the dark phase that could potentially increase urine volume and dilute melatonin metabolite. This can be concluded because LPF rats actually displayed reduced water intake during the dark phase, the period during which the urine samples were collected.

To date, the negative modulation of melatonin secretion secondary to hypothalamic AMPK activation has already been shown in other species. Menassol et al. demonstrated that acute icv injection with AICAR (a pharmacological AMPK activator) in ewes can actually reduce the amplitude of the nocturnal melatonin surge. This modulation occurred irrespective of changes in the rhythm of melatonin production [26]. As our data suggest, the ability of hypothalamic AMPK activation induced by fructose ingestion during the light phase to reduce melatonin production relies on changes in the rhythm of feeding behavior of the rat. Whether this applies to different species remains to be determined.

The causal relationship between the reduced urinary 6-S-Mel, impaired glucose tolerance and increased corticosterone were further examined in our experiments in which LPF rats were treated with melatonin. We have collected evidence to support the proposition that reduced urinary 6-S-Mel in rats consuming fructose during the light phase is likely to result from reduced melatonin production that is pivotal for the increase in corticosterone levels and impaired glucose tolerance as these adaptations were not observed in LPF rats receiving melatonin. Accordingly, melatonin has already been demonstrated to blunt insulin resistance induced by ad libitum consumption of a 60% fructose enriched diet in Wistar rats [12]. On the other hand, our data revealed that supplementation with melatonin had no effect on food intake. This is in accordance with other studies showing that, although melatonin is able to modulate the expression of orexigenic and anorexigenic neurotransmitters, this hormone has very discreet direct effect on food intake [13,45]. Altogether, our results indicate that increased food intake during the light phase seen in LPF animals is likely to be a cause, rather than a consequence, of reduced urinary 6-S-Mel.

The increased corticosterone levels observed in experimental conditions characterized by reduced melatonin production can be explained by the suppressive action that the pineal hormone exert on the Hypothalamus-Pituitary-Adrenal (HPA) axis. It has already been shown that melatonin acts through MT1 receptors to suppress adrenocorticotropic hormone-induced cortisol production in cultured adrenal glands isolated from primates [46]. This action of melatonin was reported to be dependent on the reduction of intracellular cAMP levels [46]. A similar response was found in adrenal glands from rats cultured with melatonin [47]. It is important to note that the suppressive action of melatonin over the HPA axis might not be restricted to direct action on the adrenal glands because rats treated with melatonin were also shown to have reduced corticotropin-releasing hormone and adrenocorticotropic hormone levels after a stress stimulus [48].

5. Conclusions

In summary, the present study demonstrates that fructose consumption during the light phase, but not during the dark phase, results in glucose intolerance and increased corticosterone levels. The effects of daytime consumption of fructose are secondary to hypothalamic AMPK activation that leads to upregulation of food intake during the light phase. We also show that the reduction of urinary 6-sulfatoxymelatonin (6-S-Mel) (probably indicative of reduced melatonin production) due to hypothalamic AMPK activation is a key event that mediates the increase in corticosterone and impaired glucose tolerance induced by the consumption of fructose during the light phase.

Acknowledgments: The authors would like to thank Miguel Borges da Silva, Antonio Vilson dos Santos and Agnaldo Fernando de Azevedo for their technical assistance (State University of Campinas). This study was supported by the Research Foundation of the State of Sao Paulo (FAPESP process number 2012/11409-4) and the National Council of Research (CNPq).

Author Contributions: Juliana de Almeida Faria designed and performed the experiments, acquired the data, contributed to data analysis/interpretation, and prepared and approved the manuscript. Thiago Matos F. de Araújo performed the experiments and approved the manuscript. Daniela S. Razolli performed the experiments and approved the manuscript. Letícia Martins I. de Souza performed the experiments and approved the manuscript. Dailson Nogueria Souza performed the experiments and approved the manuscript. Silvana Bordin prepared and approved the manuscript. Gabriel Forato Anhê designed the experiments, contributed to the data analysis/interpretation, and prepared and approved the manuscript.

Conflicts of Interest: The authors declare no conflict of interest, financial or otherwise, associated with this article. The authors are responsible for the writing and content of the article.

References

1. American Diabetes Association. Diagnosis and classification of diabetes mellitus. *Diabetes Care* **2010**, *33*, S62–S69.

2. Reaven, G.M. Banting lecture 1988. Role of insulin resistance in human disease. *Diabetes* **1988**, *37*, 1595–1607. [CrossRef] [PubMed]
3. Oron-herman, M.; Kamari, Y.; Grossman, E.; Yeger, G.; Peleg, E.; Shabtay, Z.; Shamiss, A.; Sharabi, Y. Metabolic syndrome: Comparison of the two commonly used animal models. *Am. J. Hypertens.* **2008**, *21*, 1018–1022. [CrossRef] [PubMed]
4. Chan, S.M.; Sun, R.Q.; Zeng, X.Y.; Choong, Z.H.; Wang, H.; Watt, M.J.; Ye, J.M. Activation of PPARα ameliorates hepatic insulin resistance and steatosis in high fructose-fed mice despite increased endoplasmic reticulum stress. *Diabetes* **2013**, *62*, 2095–2105. [CrossRef] [PubMed]
5. Stanhope, K.L.; Schwarz, J.M.; Keim, N.L.; Griffen, S.C.; Bremer, A.A.; Graham, J.L.; Hatcher, B.; Cox, C.L.; Dyachenko, A.; Zhang, W.; et al. Consuming fructose-sweetened, not glucose-sweetened, beverages increases visceral adiposity and lipids and decreases insulin sensitivity in overweight/obese humans. *J. Clin. Investig.* **2009**, *119*, 1322–1334. [CrossRef] [PubMed]
6. Leibowitz, A.; Peleg, E.; Sharabi, Y.; Shabtai, Z.; Shamiss, A.; Grossman, E. The role of melatonin in the pathogenesis of hypertension in rats with metabolic syndrome. *Am. J. Hypertens.* **2008**, *21*, 348–351. [CrossRef] [PubMed]
7. La Fleur, S.E.; Kalsbeek, A.; Wortel, J.; Van Der Vliet, J.; Buijs, R.M. Role for the pineal and melatonin in glucose homeostasis: Pinealectomy increases night-time glucose concentrations. *J. Neuroendocrinol.* **2001**, *13*, 1025–1032. [CrossRef] [PubMed]
8. Lima, F.B.; Machado, U.F.; Bartol, I.; Seraphim, P.M.; Sumida, D.H.; Moraes, S.M.; Hell, N.S.; Okamoto, M.M.; Saad, M.J.; Carvalho, C.R. Pinealectomy causes glucose intolerance and decreases adipose cell responsiveness to insulin in rats. *Am. J. Physiol.* **1998**, *275*, E934–E941. [PubMed]
9. Nogueira, T.C.; Lellis-Santos, C.; Jesus, D.S.; Taneda, M.; Rodrigues, S.C.; Amaral, F.G.; Lopes, A.M.; Cipolla-Neto, J.; Bordin, S.; Anhê, G.F. Absence of melatonin induces night-time hepatic insulin resistance and increased gluconeogenesis due to stimulation of nocturnal unfolded protein response. *Endocrinology* **2011**, *152*, 1253–1263. [CrossRef] [PubMed]
10. Wolden-Hanson, T.; Mitton, D.R.; McCants, R.L.; Yellon, S.M.; Wilkinson, C.W.; Matsumoto, A.M.; Rasmussen, D.D. Daily melatonin administration to middle-aged male rats suppresses body weight, intraabdominal adiposity, and plasma leptin and insulin independent of food intake and total body fat. *Endocrinology* **2000**, *141*, 487–497. [CrossRef] [PubMed]
11. Shieh, J.M.; Wu, H.T.; Cheng, K.C.; Cheng, J.T. Melatonin ameliorates high fat diet-induced diabetes and stimulates glycogen synthesis via a PKCzeta-Akt-GSK3beta pathway in hepatic cells. *J. Pineal Res.* **2009**, *47*, 339–344. [CrossRef] [PubMed]
12. Kitagawa, A.; Ohta, Y.; Ohash, K. Melatonin improves metabolic syndrome induced by high fructose intake in rats. *J. Pineal Res.* **2012**, *52*, 403–413. [CrossRef] [PubMed]
13. Cano, B.P.; Pagano, E.S.; Jiménez-Ortega, V.; Fernández-Mateos, P.; Esquifino, A.I.; Cardinali, D.P. Melatonin normalizes clinical and biochemical parameters of mild inflammation in diet-induced metabolic syndrome in rats. *J. Pineal Res.* **2014**, *57*, 280–290. [CrossRef] [PubMed]
14. Arble, D.M.; Bass, J.; Laposky, A.D.; Vitaterna, M.H.; Turek, F.W. Circadian timing of food intake contributes to weight gain. *Obesity* **2009**, *17*, 2100–2102. [CrossRef] [PubMed]
15. Hatori, M.; Vollmers, C.; Zarrinpar, A.; DiTacchio, L.; Bushong, E.A.; Gill, S.; Leblanc, M.; Chaix, A.; Joens, M.; Fitzpatrick, J.A.; et al. Time-restricted feeding without reducing caloric intake prevents metabolic diseases in mice fed a high-fat diet. *Cell Metab.* **2012**, *15*, 848–860. [CrossRef] [PubMed]
16. Morris, M.; Araujo, I.C.; Pohlman, R.L.; Marques, M.C.; Rodwan, N.S.; Farah, V.M. Timing of fructose intake: An important regulator of adiposity. *Clin. Exp. Pharmacol. Physiol.* **2012**, *39*, 57–62. [CrossRef] [PubMed]
17. Kinote, A.; Faria, J.A.; Roman, E.A.; Solon, C.; Razolli, D.S.; Ignacio-Souza, L.M.; Sollon, C.S.; Nascimento, L.F.; de Araújo, T.M.; Barbosa, A.P.; et al. Fructose-induced hypothalamic AMPK activation stimulates hepatic PEPCK and gluconeogenesis due to increased corticosterone levels. *Endocrinology* **2012**, *153*, 3633–3645. [CrossRef] [PubMed]
18. Cha, S.H.; Wolfgang, M.; Tokutake, Y.; Chohnan, S.; Lane, M.D. Differential effects of central fructose and glucose on hypothalamic malonyl-CoA and food intake. *Proc. Natl. Acad. Sci. USA* **2008**, *105*, 16871–16875. [CrossRef] [PubMed]
19. Stunkard, A.J.; Grace, W.J.; Wolff, H.G. The night-eating syndrome: A pattern of food intake among certain obese patients. *Am. J. Med.* **1955**, *19*, 78–86. [CrossRef]

20. Rand, C.S.; Macgregor, A.M.; Stunkard, A.J. The night eating syndrome in the general population and among postoperative obesity surgery patients. *Int. J. Eat. Disord.* **1997**, *22*, 65–69. [CrossRef]

21. Gallant, A.; Drapeau, V.; Allison, K.C.; Tremblay, A.; Lambert, M.; O'Loughlin, J.; Lundgren, J.D. Night eating behavior and metabolic heath in mothers and fathers enrolled in the QUALITY cohort study. *Eat. Behav.* **2014**, *15*, 186–191. [CrossRef] [PubMed]

22. Birketvedt, G.S.; Florholmen, J.; Sundsfjord, J.; Osterud, B.; Dinges, D.; Bilker, W.; Stunkard, A. Behavioral and neuroendocrine characteristics of the night-eating syndrome. *JAMA* **1999**, *282*, 657–663. [CrossRef] [PubMed]

23. Lin, Q.M.; Zhao, S.; Zhou, L.L.; Fang, X.S.; Fu, Y.; Huang, Z.T. Mesenchymal stem cells transplantation suppresses inflammatory responses in global cerebral ischemia: Contribution of TNF-α-induced protein 6. *Acta Pharmacol. Sin.* **2013**, *34*, 784–792. [CrossRef] [PubMed]

24. Paxinos, G.; Watson, C. *The Rat Brain in Stereotaxic Coordinates*; Academic Press: San Diego, CA, USA, 1997.

25. Kim, E.K.; Miller, I.; Aja, S.; Landree, L.E.; Pinn, M.; McFadden, J.; Kuhajda, F.P.; Moran, T.H.; Ronnett, G.V. C75, a fatty acid synthase inhibitor, reduces food intake via hypothalamic AMP-activated protein kinase. *J. Biol. Chem.* **2004**, *279*, 19970–19976. [CrossRef] [PubMed]

26. Menassol, J.B.; Tautou, C.; Collet, A.; Chesneau, D.; Lomet, D.; Dupont, J.; Malpaux, B.; Scaramuzzi, R.J. The effect of an intracerebroventricular injection of metformin or AICAR on the plasma concentrations of melatonin in the ewe: Potential involvement of AMPK? *BMC Neurosci.* **2011**, *12*, 76. [CrossRef] [PubMed]

27. Salgado-Delgado, R.C.; Saderi, N.; Basualdo M del, C.; Guerrero-Vargas, N.N.; Escobar, C.; Buijs, R.M. Shift work or food intake during the rest phase promotes metabolic disruption and desynchrony of liver genes in male rats. *PLoS ONE* **2013**, *8*, e60052. [CrossRef] [PubMed]

28. Hood, M.M.; Reutrakul, S.; Crowley, S.J. Night eating in patients with type 2 diabetes. Associations with glycemic control, eating patterns, sleep, and mood. *Appetite* **2014**, *79*, 91–96. [CrossRef] [PubMed]

29. Namkoong, C.; Kim, M.S.; Jang, P.G.; Han, S.M.; Park, H.S.; Koh, E.H.; Lee, W.J.; Kim, J.Y.; Park, I.S.; Park, J.Y.; et al. Enhanced hypothalamic AMP-activated protein kinase activity contributes to hyperphagia in diabetic rats. *Diabetes* **2005**, *54*, 63–68. [CrossRef] [PubMed]

30. Lane, M.D.; Cha, S.H. Effect of glucose and fructose on food intake via malonyl-CoA signaling in the brain. *Biochem. Biophys. Res. Commun.* **2009**, *382*, 1–5. [CrossRef] [PubMed]

31. Burmeister, M.A.; Ayala, J.; Drucker, D.J.; Ayala, J.E. Central glucagon-like peptide 1 receptor-induced anorexia requires glucose metabolism-mediated suppression of AMPK and is impaired by central fructose. *Am. J. Physiol. Endocrinol. Metab.* **2013**, *304*, E677–E685. [CrossRef] [PubMed]

32. Mccrimmon, R.J.; Shaw, M.; Fan, X.; Cheng, H.; Ding, Y.; Vella, M.C.; Zhou, L.; McNay, E.C.; Sherwin, R.S. Key role for AMP-activated protein kinase in the ventromedial hypothalamus in regulating counterregulatory hormone responses to acute hypoglycemia. *Diabetes* **2008**, *57*, 444–450. [CrossRef] [PubMed]

33. Han, S.M.; Namkoong, C.; Jang, P.G.; Park, I.S.; Hong, S.W.; Katakami, H.; Chun, S.; Kim, S.W.; Park, J.Y.; Lee, K.U.; et al. Hypothalamic AMP-activated protein kinase mediates counter-regulatory responses to hypoglycaemia in rats. *Diabetologia* **2005**, *48*, 2170–2178. [CrossRef] [PubMed]

34. Alquier, T.; Kawashima, J.; Tsuji, Y.; Kahn, B.B. Role of hypothalamic adenosine 5'-monophosphate-activated protein kinase in the impaired counterregulatory response induced by repetitive neuroglucopenia. *Endocrinology* **2007**, *148*, 1367–1375. [CrossRef] [PubMed]

35. Brindley, D.N.; Cooling, J.; Glenny, H.P.; Burditt, S.L.; McKechnie, I.S. Effects of chronic modification of dietary fat and carbohydrate on the insulin, corticosterone and metabolic responses of rats fed acutely with glucose, fructose or ethanol. *Biochem. J.* **1981**, *200*, 275–283. [CrossRef] [PubMed]

36. Brindley, D.N.; Saxto, J.; Shahidullah, H.; Armstrong, M. Possible relationships between changes in body weight set-point and stress metabolism after treating rats chronically with D-fenfluramine. Effects of feeding rats acutely with fructose on the metabolism of corticosterone, glucose, fatty acids, glycerol and triacylglycerol. *Biochem. Pharmacol.* **1985**, *34*, 1265–1271. [PubMed]

37. Skene, D.J.; Papagiannidou, E.; Hashemi, E.; Snelling, J.; Lewis, D.F.; Fernandez, M.; Ioannides, C. Contribution of CYP1A2 in the hepatic metabolism of melatonin: Studies with isolated microsomal preparations and liver slices. *J. Pineal Res.* **2001**, *31*, 333–342. [CrossRef] [PubMed]

38. Semak, I.; Korik, E.; Antonova, M.; Wortsman, J.; Slominski, A. Metabolism of melatonin by cytochrome P450s in rat liver mitochondria and microsomes. *J. Pineal Res.* **2008**, *45*, 515–523. [CrossRef] [PubMed]

39. Honma, W.; Kamiyama, Y.; Yoshinari, K.; Sasano, H.; Shimada, M.; Nagata, K.; Yamazoe, Y. Enzymatic characterization and interspecies difference of phenol sulfotransferases, ST1A forms. *Drug Metab. Dispos.* **2001**, *29*, 274–281. [PubMed]

40. Pääkkönen, T.; Mäkinen, T.M.; Leppäluoto, J.; Vakkuri, O.; Rintamäki, H.; Palinkas, L.A.; Hassi, J. Urinary melatonin: A noninvasive method to follow human pineal function as studied in three experimental conditions. *J. Pineal Res.* **2006**, *40*, 110–115. [CrossRef] [PubMed]

41. Stieglitz, A.; Spiegelhalter, F.; Klante, G.; Heldmaier, G. Urinary 6-sulphatoxymelatonin excretion reflects pineal melatonin secretion in the Djungarian hamster (Phodopus sungorus). *J. Pineal Res.* **1995**, *18*, 69–76. [CrossRef] [PubMed]

42. Golombek, D.A.; Burin, L.; Cardinali, D.P. Time-dependency for the effect of different stressors on rat pineal melatonin content. *Acta Physiol. Pharmacol. Ther. Latinoam.* **1992**, *42*, 35–42. [PubMed]

43. De Almeida Faria, J.; de Araújo, T.M.; Mancuso, R.I.; Meulman, J.; da Silva Ferreira, D.; Batista, T.M.; Vettorazzi, J.F.; da Silva, P.M.; Rodrigues, S.C.; Kinote, A.; et al. Day-restricted feeding during pregnancy and lactation programs glucose intolerance and impaired insulin secretion in male rat offspring. *Acta Physiol.* **2016**, *217*, 240–253. [CrossRef] [PubMed]

44. Selmaoui, B.; Oguine, A.; Thibault, L. Food access schedule and diet composition alter rhythmicity of serum melatonin and pineal NAT activity. *Physiol. Behav.* **2001**, *74*, 449–455. [CrossRef]

45. Ríos-Lugo, M.J.; Jiménez-Ortega, V.; Cano-Barquilla, P.; Mateos, P.F.; Spinedi, E.J.; Cardinali, D.P.; Esquifino, A.I. Melatonin counteracts changes in hypothalamic gene expression of signals regulating feeding behavior in high-fat fed rats. *Horm. Mol. Biol. Clin. Investig.* **2015**, *21*, 175–183. [CrossRef] [PubMed]

46. Torres-Farfan, C.; Richter, H.G.; Rojas-García, P.; Vergara, M.; Forcelledo, M.L.; Valladares, L.E.; Torrealba, F.; Valenzuela, G.J.; Serón-Ferré, M. mt1 Melatonin receptor in the primate adrenal gland: Inhibition of adrenocorticotropin-stimulated cortisol production by melatonin. *J. Clin. Endocrinol. Metab.* **2003**, *88*, 450–458. [CrossRef] [PubMed]

47. Richter, H.G.; Torres-Farfan, C.; Garcia-Sesnich, J.; Abarzua-Catalan, L.; Henriquez, M.G.; Alvarez-Felmer, M.; Gaete, F.; Rehren, G.E.; Seron-Ferre, M. Rhythmic expression of functional MT1 melatonin receptors in the rat adrenal gland. *Endocrinology* **2008**, *149*, 995–1003. [CrossRef] [PubMed]

48. Konakchieva, R.; Mitev, Y.; Almeida, O.F.; Patchev, V.K. Chronic melatonin treatment and the hypothalamo-pituitary-adrenal axis in the rat: Attenuation of the secretory response to stress and effects on hypothalamic neuropeptide content and release. *Biol. Cell* **1997**, *89*, 587–596. [CrossRef] [PubMed]

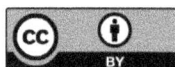

nutrients

MDPI

Article

Sweet Taste Receptor Activation in the Gut Is of Limited Importance for Glucose-Stimulated GLP-1 and GIP Secretion

Monika Y. Saltiel [1], Rune E. Kuhre [1], Charlotte B. Christiansen [1], Rasmus Eliasen [2], Kilian W. Conde-Frieboes [2], Mette M. Rosenkilde [1] and Jens J. Holst [1,*]

1   NNF Center for Basic Metabolic Research and Department of Biomedical Sciences, Panum Institute,
    Faculty of Health and Medical Sciences, University of Copenhagen, Blegdamsvej, DK-2200, Copenhagen N,
    Denmark; monika.yosifova@sund.ku.dk (M.Y.S.); kuhre@sund.ku.dk (R.E.K.);
    cbchristiansen@sund.ku.dk (C.B.C.); rosenkilde@sund.ku.dk (M.M.R.)
2   Protein & Peptide Chemistry, Novo Nordisk A/S, Novo Nordisk Park, DK-2760 Måløv, Denmark;
    rael@Nanotech.dtu.dk (R.E.); kcf@novonordisk.com (K.W.C.-F.)
*   Correspondence: jjholst@sund.ku.dk; Tel.: +45-2875-7518

Received: 28 February 2017; Accepted: 18 April 2017; Published: 22 April 2017

Abstract: Glucose stimulates the secretion of the incretin hormones: glucagon-like peptide-1 (GLP-1) and glucose-dependent insulinotropic peptide (GIP). It is debated whether the sweet taste receptor (STR) triggers this secretion. We investigated the role of STR activation for glucose-stimulated incretin secretion from an isolated perfused rat small intestine and whether selective STR activation by artificial sweeteners stimulates secretion. Intra-luminal administration of the STR agonists, acesulfame K (3.85% *w/v*), but not sucralose (1.25% *w/v*) and stevioside (2.5% *w/v*), stimulated GLP-1 secretion (acesulfame K: 31 ± 3 pmol/L vs. 21 ± 2 pmol/L, $p < 0.05$, $n = 6$). In contrast, intra-arterial administration of sucralose (10 mM) and stevioside (10 mM), but not acesulfame K, stimulated GLP-1 secretion (sucralose: 51 ± 6 pmol/L vs. 34 ± 4 pmol/L, $p < 0.05$; stevioside: 54 ± 6 pmol/L vs. 32 ± 2 pmol/L, $p < 0.05$, $n = 6$), while 0.1 mM and 1 mM sucralose did not affect the secretion. Luminal glucose (20% *w/v*) doubled GLP-1 and GIP secretion, but basolateral STR inhibition by gurmarin (2.5 µg/mL) or the inhibition of the transient receptor potential cation channel 5 (TRPM5) by triphenylphosphine oxide (TPPO) (100 µM) did not attenuate the responses. In conclusion, STR activation does not drive GIP/GLP-1 secretion itself, nor does it have a role for glucose-stimulated GLP-1 or GIP secretion.

Keywords: sweet taste receptor; GLP-1; GIP; glucose; sucralose

1. Introduction

A high consumption of sugar may lead to a higher prevalence of unhealthy metabolic conditions, like diabetes type 2, obesity, and metabolic syndrome. Therefore, it is of great importance to understand how sugars are metabolized in the body and which feedback mechanisms regulate this process, and thus how it could be controlled or manipulated. As an alternative to sugars, artificial sweeteners have attracted considerable interest in the battle with obesity and diabetes, as they do not elevate blood glucose levels and are not a source of additional calories. Nevertheless, epidemiological studies show that their consumption may still be associated with weight gain and diabetes type 2 due to adaptive mechanisms [1,2], although randomized controlled trials, investigating the effects of sweeteners on body weight, show that they may reduce weight compared to groups consuming water [3,4].

In response to meal ingestion, several hormones that regulate blood sugar levels and appetite are secreted. The incretin peptide hormones, glucose-dependent insulinotropic hormone (GIP) and glucagon-like peptide 1 (GLP-1), secreted from the intestinal K- and L-cells, respectively, play an important role in this process, as they both stimulate insulin secretion, and GLP-1 suppresses appetite and slows gastric emptying [5].

Glucose is an efficacious stimulus for the secretion of both GLP-1 and GIP, stimulating secretory responses that are comparable to the response after the intake of an isocaloric mixed meal [6]. While it is well established that glucose stimulates the secretion of GIP and GLP-1, several different molecular sensors may be involved. A main driver for secretion appears to be glucose transportation through sodium-glucose dependent transporter 1 (SGLT1) [7–12], triggering hormone secretion by the depolarization of the K/L-cell plasma membrane and the opening of voltage sensitive calcium channels [7]. Electroneutral GLUT2-mediated uptake may potentiate glucose-stimulated GLP-1 secretion [7], potentially by the closure of the K_{ATP} channel upon intracellular glucose metabolism to ATP [7,13]. Another molecular sensor that has been suggested to be implicated in the secretory response is the sweet-taste receptor (STR). It is activated by glucose and other sweet-taste molecules, and is found not only in the taste buds, but also in the enteroendocrine K- and L-cells along the gastrointestinal tract, with the highest expression rates found in the proximal intestine [14–17].

The STR is a heterodimer, formed by the subunits T1R2 and T1R3, coupled to the G-proteins α-gustducin and/or transducin [18]. Around one fifth of the cells expressing α-gustducin co-express GLP-1 and GIP [16,19,20]. Depending on the ligand, receptor activation activates adenylate cyclase and the formation of cAMP (Gαs-coupling), or mobilizes calcium from intracellular stores (Gq-coupling) by the activation of phospholipase C (PLC) and inositol triphosphate (IP3) [21]. The increase in intracellular Ca2+ opens the nonselective transient receptor potential monovalent cation channel 5 (TRPM5), which plays a critical role in sweet, bitter, and umami taste signal transduction, leading to Na+ influx, depolarization of the cell, and eventual hormone or neurotransmitter secretion [22]. Natural sweeteners (sucrose, glucose, fructose) activate STR in the range of 100 mM, while less than 10 mM of the artificial sweeteners is sufficient for activation [18]. Studies on incretin secreting cell lines (derived from human and mouse gut carcinomas) have shown that STR activation by artificial sweeteners elicits GLP-1 secretion [16,17], and in humans, the inhibition of the gut sweet taste receptor by lactisole attenuated the glucose-stimulated GLP-1 secretion [19]. However, these findings remain inconclusive, as other studies found no effect of artificial sweeteners on GLP-1 secretion in humans [11,23–27] and rats (in vivo and using isolated perfused intestine preparations) [7,28]. The only studies in humans that found an increase in GLP-1 secretion after artificial sweetener consumption investigated combinations of artificial sweeteners in diet drinks or studied whether sweeteners potentiated glucose-stimulated GLP-1 secretion rather than driving secretion per se [29,30]. An important question, which none of the studies explored by means other than immunohistochemistry, is whether the sweet receptors are located apically or at the basolateral side of the L-cells, which might play a role in the lack of a response in vivo as artificial sweeteners, like sucralose, are incompletely absorbed.

The purpose of this study was to investigate the importance of sweet taste receptor activation for glucose-stimulated hormone secretion, with a primary focus on GLP-1 secretion and a secondary focus on GIP secretion. For this investigation, we used the isolated perfused rat small intestine, which is a physiological model, maintaining the enteroendocrine cells in their normal environment, polarized form with preserved vascular circulation and contact to normal neighbor cells, paracrine cells, and neurons, while the input and output from the organ was strictly controlled. Due to the preservation of natural polarity, this model also has the advantage that it can be used to investigate whether the stimulus has an effect on the apical or basolateral membrane of the cell.

2. Materials and Methods

2.1. Perfusion of the Proximal Small Intestine

Studies were performed with permission from the Danish Animal Experiments Inspectorate (2013-15-2934-00833) and the local ethics committee (EMED, P-15-408) in accordance with the guidelines of the Danish legislation governing animal experimentation (1987) and the National Institutes of Health. The experimental method and protocol have been described elsewhere in detail [7]. In brief, male Wistar rats (weight: mean + SEM = 283 ± 28.8 g) were obtained from Janvier labs (Le Genest-Saint-Isle, France), and were housed two per cage on a 12:12 h light/dark cycle, with ad libitum access to standard chow and water. On the experimental day, animals (non-fasted) were anesthetized with a subcutane Hypnorm/Midazolam injection and placed on a 37 °C heating plate. The abdominal cavity was opened; the entire large intestine and the distal half of the small intestine was carefully removed, leaving 44 ± 5.2 cm of the upper small intestine in situ (approximately half of the entire small intestine). A plastic tube was inserted into the proximal part of the lumen and the intestinal content was carefully removed by flushing with isotonic saline (room temperature). Next, the lumen was perfused with saline at a steady flow of 0.5 mL/min. A catheter was placed in the superior mesenteric artery and the intestine was vascularly perfused with gassed perfusion buffer (95% O_2−5% CO_2) warmed to 37 °C at a rate of 7.5 mL/min. Perfusion effluent was collected each minute from a catheter inserted in the vena portae and samples were instantly transferred to ice and stored at −20°C until analysis. The perfusion buffer consisted of a Krebs-Ringer bicarbonate buffer supplemented with 0.1% BSA (albumin fraction V; Merck, cat. no. 1.12018.0500, Ballerup, Denmark), 3.5 mmol/L glucose, 5% dextran T-70 (to balance oncotic pressure; Pharmacosmos, Holbaek, Denmark), 5 mmol/L pyruvate, 10 μmol/L 3-Isobutyl-1-methylxanthine (IBMX) (Sigma-Aldrich, cat. no. 5879), fumarate, glutamate, and 2 mL/L of Vamin (cat. no. 11338; Fresenius Kabi, Uppsala, Sweden). The pH was adjusted with hydrochloric acid to 7.4–7.5. After the successful perfusion of the proximal small intestine, rats were sacrificed by cardiac perforation and the preparation was left to stabilize hormone secretion for approximately 30 min before the samples were collected.

2.2. Perfusion Protocol and Test Substances

Each experimental protocol started with ten minutes of baseline collection (pre-stimulatory period), followed by a stimulation for ten minutes, either luminally or vascularly. The intestine was stimulated luminally with 20% (*w/v*) glucose (1.1 mol/L) (Sigma-Aldrich, cat. no. G8270), 1.25% (*w/v*) sucralose (31.4 mmol/L) (Sigma-Aldrich, cat. no. 69293), 3.85% (*w/v*) acesulfame K (191.3 mmol/L) (Sigma-Aldrich, cat. no. 04054), or 2.5% (*w/v*) stevioside (31.1 mmol/L) (Sigma-Aldrich cat. no. CDS020802). The concentrations of the sweeteners employed correspond to 50 times the sweetness of 20% (*w/v*) glucose, given that sucralose, acesulfame K, and stevioside are 800, 260, and 400 times sweeter, respectively [31,32], and are all far beyond their respective EC50 values (0.3 mM for sucralose, 1 mM for acesulfame K, and 0.1 mM for stevioside [33]). Therefore, all of the solutions maximally activated the receptor. Luminal test stimulants were dissolved in isotonic saline without the addition of detergents and were applied at an initial rate of 2.5 mL/min for the first three minutes, followed by a rate of 0.5 mL/min during the rest of the stimulation. After the stimulation, isotonic saline was infused in the same pattern to replace test stimulant solution and reestablish baseline conditions. Vascular test stimulants (acefulfame K, sucralose, and stevioside) were dissolved in perfusion buffer to a final concentration of 10 mM (for sucralose also concentration 1 mM and 0.1 mM). To allow hormone secretion to return to the baseline after test stimulant application, stimulant applications were separated by 15 min. In separate experiments, the murine sweet taste receptor inhibitor gurmarin [34] (2.5 μg/mL) (provided by Rasmus Eliasen, synthetized at Novo Nordisk A/S as previously described [35]), was infused on the vascular side mixed with sucralose (10 mM) or simultaneously with glucose 20% (*w/v*) on the luminal side. Before the stimulation, the sweet taste receptor was primed with gurmarin for 15 min to ensure full inhibition at the time of test substance application. Using the same protocol, the TRPM5 channel was inhibited by the vascular administration (100 μM) of triphenylphosphine oxide (TPPO) (IC_{50} = 30 μM) (Sigma-Aldrich, cat. No T84603) [36]. To dissolve TPPO, it was mixed in 1% dimethyl sulfoxid solution and perfusion buffer. At the end of each experiment, the intestine was stimulated vascularly with bombesin (10 nM) (a potent GLP-1 secretagogue), to ensure that the preparation was viable until the end of the experiments. The perfusion pressure and effluent output were measured continuously, in order to evaluate the gut integrity and health during the experiment. Since all experiments were conducted with constant perfusion flow rates, all effluent hormone or metabolite concentrations correspond to the total secretion or absorption rates.

2.3. Hormone Secretion Analysis

GLP-1 concentrations in the venous effluents were analyzed using an in-house radioimmunoassay (RIA), employing a rabbit antiserum directed against the C-terminus of GLP-1 (code no. 89390), thus reacting with all amidated forms of GLP-1 (1-36NH2, 7-36NH2 and 9-36NH2).

GIP concentrations were quantified with an ELISA assay for the rat total GIP (Millipore, Merck, cat. no. EZRMGIP-55K), following the provided instructions.

2.4. Statistical Analysis

Changes in the hormone secretion were assessed by comparing the mean concentrations during the stimulation period with the baseline mean concentrations calculated as a mean of five consecutive one-minute observations before the stimulation and five one-minute observations before the start of the following stimulation. The stimulation period was defined as the start of the stimulant application until the end of the application. Statistical significance was assessed by one-way ANOVA, followed by Bonferroni post hoc analysis or a paired *t*-test, in the case that only two groups were compared. In the experiments where responses to stimuli with or without the presence of an inhibitor were compared, differences were assessed by a two-way paired *t*-test. Statistical analysis was performed using GraphPad Prism 7 (La Jolla, CA, USA). Data are expressed as averaged means $\pm$ SEM. $p < 0.05$ was considered significant.

3. Results

3.1. Glucose-Induced Incretin Secretion

3.1.1. Glucose Stimulates GLP-1 and GIP Secretion from the Perfused Rat Small Intestine

Luminally administered glucose 20% (*w/v*) was rapidly absorbed, increasing venous effluent glucose concentrations by two to three times compared to the baseline (*glucose 1st*: 11.5 $\pm$ 0.9 mmol/L vs. *baseline 1st*: 5 $\pm$ 0.4 mmol/L, $p < 0.001$; *glucose 2nd*: 14.2 $\pm$ 0.9 mmol/L vs. *baseline 2nd*: 5.2 $\pm$ 0.5 mmol/L, $p < 0.001$, $n = 6$, Figure 1a,b). At the same time, we observed a doubling in the GLP-1 (*glucose 1st*: 50.7 $\pm$ 2.9 pmol/L vs. *baseline 1st*: 22.6 $\pm$ 3 pmol/L, $p < 0.0001$; *glucose 2nd*: 49.3 $\pm$ 4.4 pmol/L vs. *baseline 2nd*: 30.8 $\pm$ 3.5 pmol/L, $p < 0.01$, $n = 6$, Figure 1c,d) and GIP secretion rate (*glucose 1st*: 12.2 $\pm$ 1.2 pmol/L vs. *baseline 1st*: 6.7 $\pm$ 0.6 pmol/L, $p < 0.05$; *glucose 2nd*: 12.6 $\pm$ 0.2 pmol/L vs. *baseline 2nd*: 8.4 $\pm$ 0.7 pmol/L, $p < 0.01$, $n = 6$, Figure 1c,e), and in both cases, the second secretory response was not significantly different from the first (GLP-1 $p = 0.55$; GIP $p = 0.73$). GLP-1 and GIP showed a similar dynamic of secretion. In all experiments, a robust GLP-1 response to bombesin, administered at the end of the experiments (61–65 min), was observed, indicating that the experimental model was working until the end of the protocols (Figure 1c).

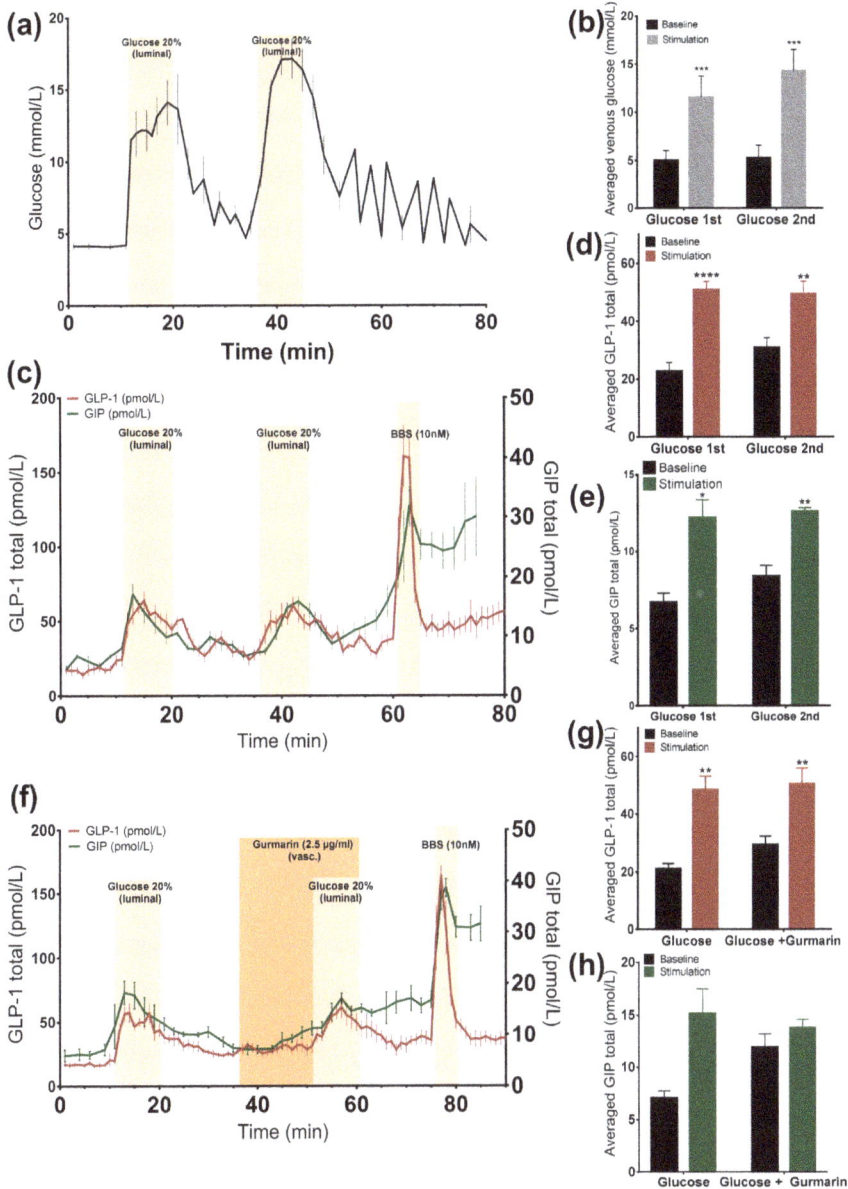

Figure 1. Glucose is a potent GLP-1 and GIP secretagogue and it is rapidly absorbed in the upper small intestine. Data is shown as averaged mean values ± SEM. (**a**) Glucose output in venous effluents in response to administration of luminal glucose. (**b**) Comparison between the venous glucose output upon glucose (stimulation) or saline (baseline). (**c**) GLP-1 (red line) and GIP (green line) secretion in response to luminal glucose. (**d,e**) Comparison between total GLP-1 or GIP output caused by glucose or saline. (**f**) GLP-1 (red line) and GIP (green line) secretion by luminal glucose administration and inhibition of the sweet taste receptor. (**g,h**) Comparison between the mean values of GLP-1 or GIP output upon glucose infusion ± gurmarin and saline. * $p < 0.05$, ** $p < 0.01$, *** $p < 0.001$. BBS bombesin; GLP-1 glucagon-like peptide 1; GIP glucose-dependent insulinotropic peptide.

3.1.2. Inhibition of the Murine Sweet Taste Receptor Does Not Change Glucose-Induced GLP-1 and GIP Secretion

In another series of experiments, the murine sweet taste receptor antagonist gurmarin was administered 15 min before and concomitantly with glucose (20% w/v). The inhibition of the sweet taste receptor did not attenuate glucose-induced GLP-1 secretion compared to glucose administration alone (Figure 1f), as the responses did not differ significantly ($p = 0.73$). Glucose increased GLP-1 secretion close by nearly two times, independently of whether it was added alone or concomitantly with gurmarin (*glucose*: 48.5 ± 4.6 pmol/L vs. *baseline 1*: 21.1 ± 1.9 pmol/L, $p < 0.01$; *glucose + gurmarin*: 50.3 ± 5.5 pmol/L vs. *baseline 2*: 29.4 ± 3 pmol/L, $p < 0.01$, $n = 6$, Figure 1f,g). The glucose-stimulated GIP response was also not significantly altered due to the presence of gurmarin ($p = 0.58$) (*glucose*: 15.1 ± 2.4 pmol/L vs. *baseline 1*: 7.1 ± 0.7 pmol/L, $p = 0.13$; *glucose + gurmarin*: 13.8 ± 0.8 pmol/L vs. *baseline 2*: 11.9 ± 1.3 pmol/L, $p = 0.24$, $n = 4$, Figure 1f,h).

3.2. Arificial Sweeteners and Incretin Secretion

3.2.1. Luminal Administration of Acesulfame K, but Not Sucralose or Stevioside, Stimulates GLP-1, but Not GIP Secretion

Intra-luminal administration of acesulfame K at a concentration that is thought to activate the sweet taste receptor resulted in a small, but significant, 1.5-fold increase in the GLP-1 concentrations (*acesulfame K*: 31.1 ± 2.5 pmol/L vs. *baseline*: 21.1 ± 2 pmol/L, $p < 0.05$, $n = 6$, Figure 2a,b), whereas it did not affect GIP secretion (*acesulfame K*: 4.6 ± 0.9 pmol/L vs. *baseline*: 5.1 ± 1 pmol/L, $p = 0.53$, $n = 5$, Figure 2a,c). Luminal infusion of sucralose and stevioside in matched concentrations with respect to sweetness, on the other hand, did not elevate the secretion of GLP-1 (Figure 2a,b,f,g).

3.2.2. Vascular Administration of Sucralose and Stevioside, but Not Acesulafme K, Stimulates GLP-1 and GIP Secretion

Intra-arterial administration of sucralose and stevioside significantly stimulated GLP-1 secretion (*sucralose*: 51.3 ± 5.9 pmol/L vs. *baseline*: 33.9 ± 3.9 pmol/L, $p < 0.05$, $n = 6$; *stevioside*: 54 ± 6.4 pmol/L vs. *baseline*: 31.5 ± 2.3 pmol/L, $p < 0.05$, $n = 6$, Figure 2d–g). However, vascular acesulfame K did not change the secretion rate (Figure 2d,e). The results were unchanged by the administration of acesulfame K before sucralose, suggesting that it is not the unavailability of the receptor that is responsible for the lack of the response to acesulfame K (data not shown). Sucralose slightly elevated GIP concentrations, although not significantly (*sucralose*: 9.3 ± 2 pmol/L vs. *baseline*: 7.2 ± 1.2 pmol/L, $p = 0.09$, $n = 5$, Figure 3c,e).

3.2.3. Sucralose Only Stimulates GLP-1 Secretion at High Doses

In order to evaluate whether sucralose also stimulates GLP-1 secretion from the vascular side at doses lower than 10 mM, we stimulated the gut with 10 mM, 1 mM, or 0.1 mM sucralose in a separate line of experiments. Only 10 mM sucralose stimulated secretion (Figure 3a,b).

Stimulating the intestine with 10 mM of sucralose resulted in two secretory responses that did not differ ($p = 0.25$) (*sucralose 1*: 45 ± 2.8 pmol/L vs. *baseline 1*: 23.5 ± 1.7 pmol/L, $p < 0.0001$; *sucralose 2*: 50.3 ± 5 pmol/L vs. *baseline 2*: 25.2 ± 2.2 pmol/L, $p < 0.001$, $n = 6$, Figure 3c,d), which allowed us to test whether the sucralose-induced GLP-1 secretion could be inhibited by gurmarin.

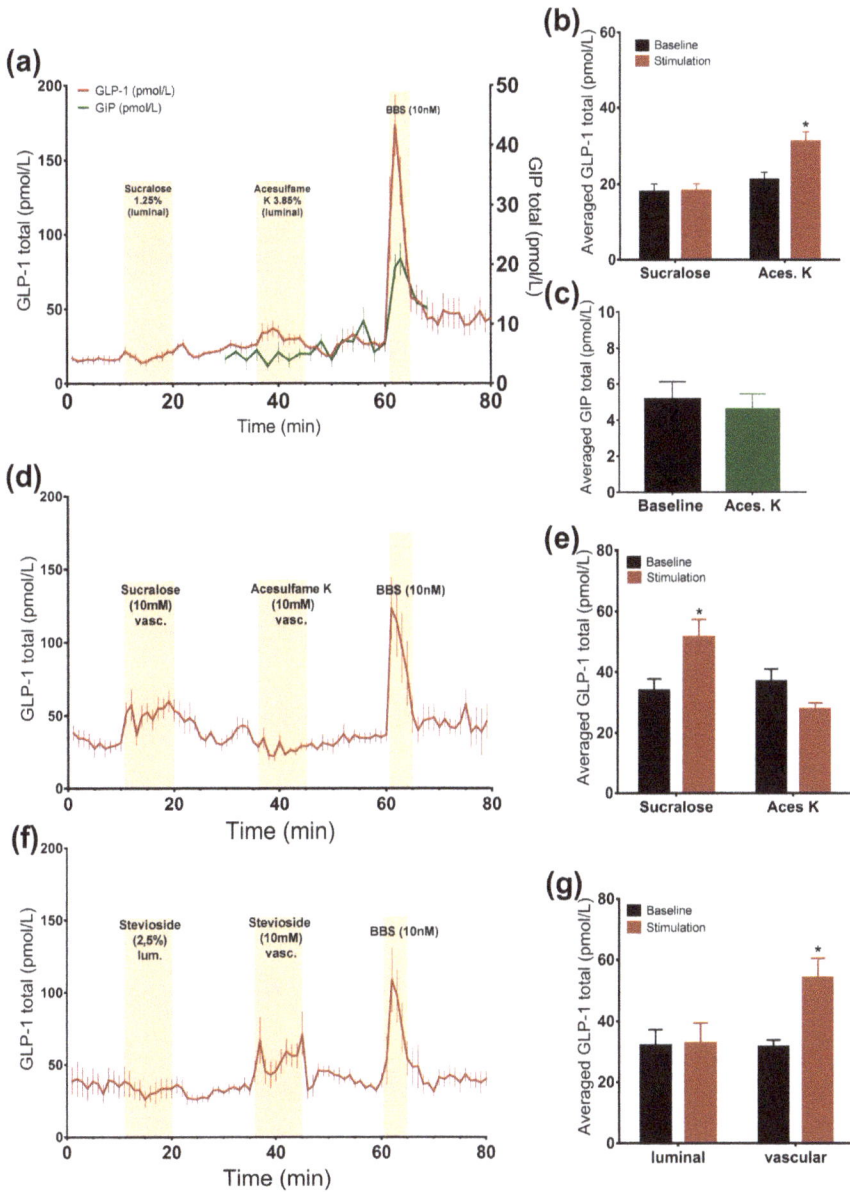

Figure 2. Effects of artificial sweeteners on incretin secretion. Data is shown as averaged mean values ± SEM (**a**) GLP-1 (red line) and GIP (green line) secretion in response to luminal sucralose and acesulfame K (**b**,**c**) Comparison between total GLP-1 or GIP output caused by luminal artificial sweeteners (stimulation) and saline (baseline) (**d**) GLP-1 secretion in response to vascular sucralose and acesulfame K (**e**) Comparison between the mean values of total GLP-1 secretion caused by vascular artificial sweeteners and saline (**f**) GLP-1 output in response to luminal and vascular stevioside administration (**g**) Comparison between the mean values of GLP-1 secretion upon liminal and vascular stevioside and saline * $p < 0.05$, ** $p < 0.01$, *** $p < 0.001$. BBS bombesin; GLP-1 glucagon-like peptide 1; GIP glucose-dependent insulinotropic peptide.

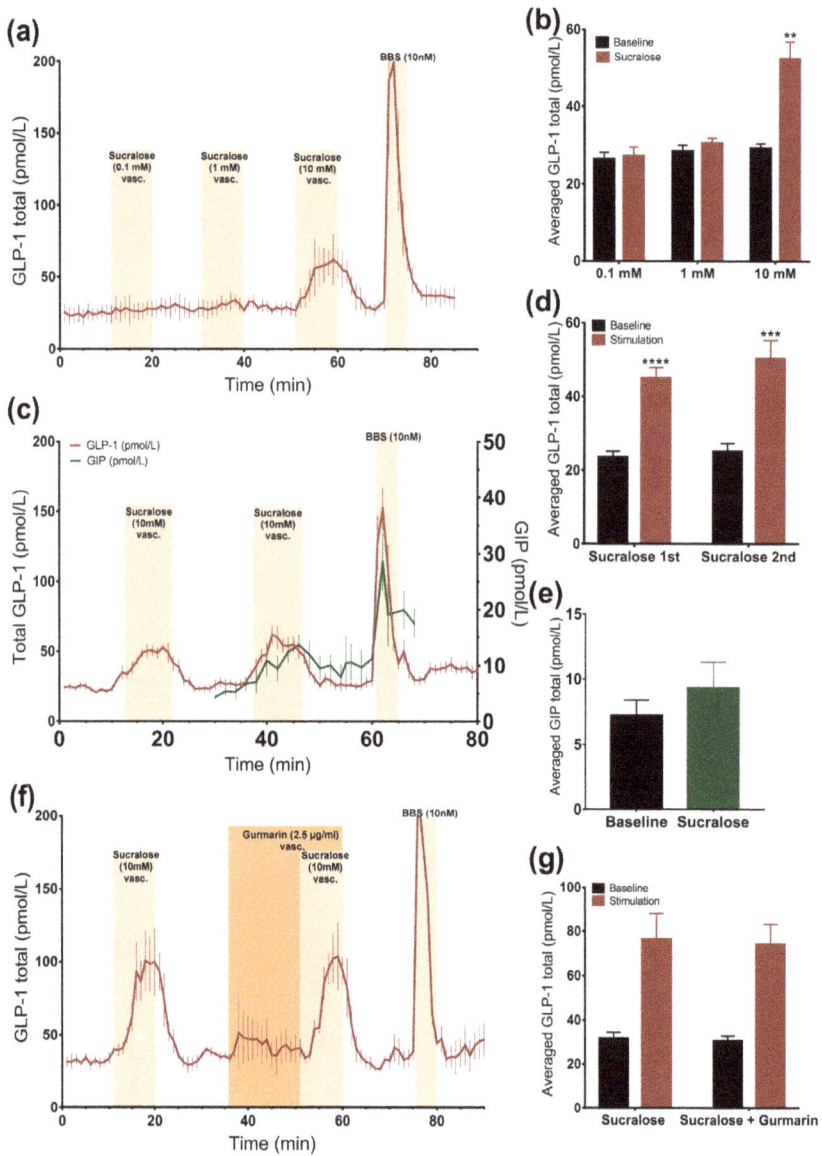

Figure 3. Effects of sucralose on the secretion of GLP-1 and GIP. Data is shown as averaged mean values ± SEM (**a**) GLP-1 secretion in response to vascular sucralose at 0.1 mM, 1 mM, and 10 mM concentrations (**b**) Comparison between the mean values of total GLP-1 output caused by vascular sucralose in increasing concentration (stimulation) and saline (baseline) (**c**) GLP-1 (red line) and GIP (green line) secretion in response to vascular administration of sucralose (**d,e**) Comparison between the mean values of total GLP-1 or GIP output caused by vascular sucralose and saline (**e**) GLP-1 secretion in response to vascular administration of sucralose ± gurmarin (**f,g**) Comparison between the mean values of GLP-1 output upon sucralose ± gurmarin * $p < 0.05$, ** $p < 0.01$, *** $p < 0.001$. BBS bombesin; GLP-1 glucagon-like peptide 1; GIP glucose-dependent insulinotropic peptide.

3.2.4. Inhibition of the Murine Sweet Taste Receptor Does Not Eliminate Sucralose-Induced GLP-1 secretion

The inhibition of the sweet taste receptor before and together with sucralose administration (10 mM) did not affect GLP-1 secretion compared to sucralose alone, as the baseline-subtracted responses were not significantly different, and sucralose increased GLP-1 levels by around two times, independently of gurmarin administration (*sucralose*: 76.4 ± 11.7 pmol/L vs. *baseline 1*: 31.6 ± 3 pmol/L, $p = 0.09$; *sucralose + gurmarin*: 74.2 ± 9.2 pmol/L vs. *baseline 2*: 30.6 ± 2.3 pmol/L, $p = 0.08$, $n = 3$, Figure 3f,g).

3.3. Inhibition of TRPM5-Channel Does Not Attenuate Glucose or Sucralose-Stimulated GLP-1 Secretion

3.3.1. Glucose-Induced GLP-1 Secretion Was not Reduced, but Increased, by Inhibition of TRPM5 Channels

The inhibition of the TRPM5 ion channel by TPPO did not lead to a sweet taste receptor mediated reduction in GLP-1 secretion, but on the contrary, led to a significant increase in glucose-stimulated GLP-1 secretion ($p = 0.04$). Due to an increase in basal secretion after the administration of TPPO, differences were assessed by a comparison between the baseline-subtracted responses. Glucose alone doubled GLP-1 secretion, whereas the addition of TPPO increased it even more (*glucose*: 62.3 ± 8.2 pmol/L vs. *baseline 1*: 31.8 ± 4.3 pmol/L, $p < 0.05$; *glucose + TPPO*: 99 ± 2.5 pmol/L vs. *baseline 2*: 44.7 ± 0.4 pmol/L, $p < 0.01$, $n = 3$, Figure 4a,b).

3.3.2. Sucralose-Induced GLP-1 Secretion Is not Changed by Inhibition of TRPM5 Channels

Sucralose-induced GLP-1 secretion was not reduced in the presence of the TRPM5 inhibitor TPPO. There was no significant difference between the responses to the administration of sucralose alone or sucralose concomitantly with TPPO, when comparing the baseline-subtracted responses ($p = 0.11$). Sucralose increased GLP-1 levels by around two times when infused alone or together with TPPO (*sucralose*: 35.4 ± 2.7 pmol/L vs. *baseline 1*: 20.7 ± 1.9 pmol/L, $p < 0.05$; *sucralose + TPPO*: 58 ± 11 pmol/L vs. *baseline 2*: 28.6 ± 2.3 pmol/L, $p = 0.07$, $n = 3$, Figure 4c,d). Interestingly, TPPO increased GLP-1 secretion when given alone (Figure 4).

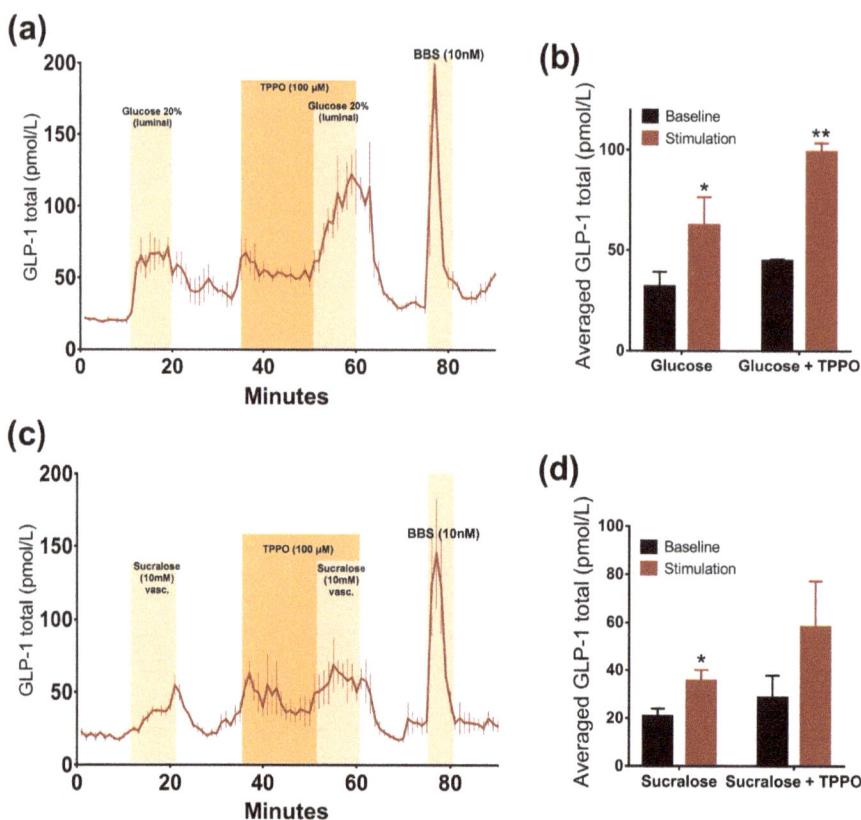

Figure 4. TRPM5 channel is not involved in glucose- and sucralose-stimulated GLP-1 secretion. Data is shown as averaged mean values values $\pm$ SEM (**a**) GLP-1 secretion in response to luminal glucose alone or in the presence of TPPO (**b**) Comparison between the mean values of total GLP-1 output caused by luminal glucose $\pm$ TPPO (stimulation) and saline (baseline) (**c**) GLP-1 secretion in response to vascular administration of sucralose alone or in presence of TPPO (**d**) Comparison between the mean values of total GLP-1 output caused by vascular sucralose $\pm$ TPPO and saline * $p < 0.05$, ** $p < 0.01$, *** $p < 0.001$. BBS bombesin; GLP-1 glucagon-like peptide 1; GIP glucose-dependent insulinotropic peptide.

4. Discussion

The involvement of the STR in glucose-stimulated GLP-1 and GIP secretion has been a matter of controversy during the last decade, with different studies suggesting that it may or may not be acutely involved in hormone secretion, glucose homeostasis, and appetite regulation [7,16,17,19,23–28,37]. This study shows that the ability of artificial sweeteners to stimulate GLP-1 secretion vascularly or luminally is sweetener-specific. Sucralose affected GLP-1 secretion when applied from the vascular side, whereas acesulfame K exclusively stimulated secretion when administrated in the intestinal lumen and only in pharmacological doses. This may explain why orally ingested artificial sweeteners do not trigger incretin hormones secretion in vivo [23–28], even though cell studies show the opposite [16,17].Vascular stimulation with sucralose in our perfusion model stimulated a secretory GLP-1 and GIP response, in agreement with the results from cell studies on GLUTag cells and NCI-H716 cells [16,17], but only at a concentration that must be considered to be pharmacological. However, as opposed to those studies, the secretory response in our model was not attenuated by STR inhibition with gurmarin. The fact that sucralose and stevioside triggered GLP-1 secretion when applied on the vascular side, but not on the luminal, suggests that the sweet taste receptor is either located on the basolateral membrane of the L-cells or that the response is triggered by other mechanisms. Nevertheless, we were not able to inhibit the sucralose-stimulated secretion by means of gurmarin or by inhibiting the TRPM5 channel, which is involved in the Gq-coupled taste sense and hormonal secretion [22]. Therefore, it seems that sucralose triggered hormone secretion by an STR-independent mechanism, which is consistent with our finding that sucralose at 0.1 and 1 mM did not affect secretion, albeit the sweetness of 1 mM is above the EC_{50}-value of sucralose (0.3 mM) [33]. It may be argued that sucralose could stimulate GLP-1 and GIP secretion by acting on the bitter receptors, but as TRPM5 is also involved in other taste signal pathways, like umami and bitter [22], it is unlikely that sucralose acts on the L-cells by activating one of these receptors. Nevertheless, TRPM5 expression on the L-cells is low [38] and may not be as important for taste receptor signaling in the small intestine as it is for the taste cells on the tongue. Sucralose in concentrations of 10 mM and 100 mM, seem to exert toxic effects on IP3 production in GLUTag cells, which express the STR subunits [39] (data not shown), suggesting that it stimulates the secretion by another signal pathway. One could argue that the response seen following the vascular administration of sucralose and stevioside is triggered by high osmolarity. However, this is unlikely as intra-arterial acesulfame K at 10 mM in this study, and intra-arterial glucose at concentrations of 5 to 25 mM in one of our previous studies [7], did not affect GLP-1 secretion.

Also, glucose-stimulated GLP-1 and GIP secretion was unaffected by gurmarin, standing in contrast to the finding from two human studies, where STR inhibtion (with lactisole—an inhibitor of the human STR) [19,37] attenuated glucose-stimulated GLP-1 secretion by about 50%. Surprisingly, the inhibition of the TRPM5 channel did not attenuate glucose-stimulated GLP-1 secretion, but even slightly increased it. This once again shows that it is probably not the STR-activated signal pathway that regulates secretion. As the IC_{50} of gurmarin on the STR was reported to be 0.62 µg/mL [40], and 0.5 µM gurmarin decreases the magnitude of sweet perception to sucralose by 70% on the taste buds in rats [41]. We anticipate that the lack of the effect of gurmarin in our experimental model is unlikely to be dose-related, as we applied the IC_{50} dose (2.5 µg/mL) four times, and this dose is comparable to the dose used by Margolskee and colleagues (3 µg/mL). Experiments with GLUTag cells showed that glucose increases intracellular calcium at a concentration of 100 mM, whereas gurmarin (5 µg/mL) attenuated glucose-stimulated intracellular calcium by around 10% (data not shown). This proves that gurmarin was bioactive. Nevertheless, we cannot exclude that the lack of an effect in our model is due to an unfavorable ratio between the inhibitor and the sweet-tasting agonists, as they were applied in high concentrations.

Our finding that sucralose and stevioside did not stimulate GLP-1 secretion when applied into the lumen, even in a very high concentration, is in agreement with the results from human studies showing no effect of artificial sweeteners on GLP-1 secretion [23–25,27] or in vivo studies in rats [28]. Interestingly, intra-luminal acesulfame K increased GLP-1 secretion by 1.5-fold, which is in contrast to the results of a previous study by our group [7], but may be explained by the fact that in this study a five-times higher concentration was applied. Along this notation, the reason why luminal acesulfame K, but not sucralose and stevioside, stimulated GLP-1 secretion may be explained by the fact that a given dose of acesulfame K is completely recovered in the urine [42]. Therefore, it may be absorbed by the enterocytes in non-metabolized form and acts on the basolateral side of the L-cells in contrast to sucralose and stevioside, which are either incompletely absorbed or are metabolized by the bacteria in the colon and then absorbed [43,44]. In this way, acesulfame K may stimulate GLP-1 secretion by mechanisms similar to vascularly applied sucralose and stevioside, as the dose applied in the lumen corresponds to 191 mM. On the other hand, the lack of a response to acesulfame K when applied vascularly may be explained by the fact that it is less potent in activating the sweet taste receptor compared to sucralose and stevioside, and the applied dose was, therefore, insufficient.

Our study further shows that GLP-1 and GIP have similar dynamics of secretion and are therefore probably triggered by similar mechanisms, presumably involving the SGLT1 transporter as indicated by a number of studies from different groups using different experimental models [7,8,12].

The proximal part of the small intestine was chosen as a model in the current study, as glucose is almost entirely absorbed in the duodenum and jejunum [45]. Therefore, studying the effects of glucose on hormone secretion in the proximal small intestine gives a more physiologically relevant picture. In particular, in relation to this study, the relevant anatomical area of the intestine was used, as the sweet taste receptor is predominantly expressed in the duodenum and jejunum [14–17]. However, it may be a limitation that the very proximal part of the small intestine (the duodenum and the most proximal segment of the jejunum) was not included for technical reasons.

The advantage of the isolated perfused organ model, over in vivo studies, is that the confounding effects of several whole body parameters can be excluded. These include the effect of gastric emptying, the breakdown of various substances by whole body metabolism, and the impact of other regulatory hormones, while the physiological impact of specific compounds can be studied locally in the preserved organ. This gives the opportunity to establish a cause and effect relationship between the studied agent and the outcome. The risk of having the results influenced by indirect factors is minimal, since all compounds entering the system are strictly controlled. Therefore, in the present study, it could be established that sucralose and stevioside stimulate GLP-1 secretion when infused vascularly, but not when infused luminally. Compared to isolated cell studies, an alternative controlled system for the study of hormonal secretion, the perfused model also has the benefit that the natural polarity, inter-cell connection, and neural communication are preserved [46].

Limitations of the study include the limited translatability of the findings to humans in respect to artificial sweeteners, as they were applied in doses in the toxic range for humans. However, this was justified by the aim of the study to use them as a tool to explore sweet taste receptor functions, rather than to explore their physiological relevance.

5. Conclusions

This study does not support the view that the activation of the gut sweet taste receptor plays a crucial role in the glucose-stimulated incretin secretion, as the inhibition of the receptor did not significantly reduce this secretion, suggesting that other mechanisms are fundamental for the GLP-1 secretion upon glucose administration. Our work suggests that the presence of pharmacological concentrations of sucralose and stevioside on the basolateral membrane may increase GLP-1 secretion. However, given the high concentrations needed to stimulate secretion, this finding is probably of limited clinical relevance. Future research should concentrate on compounds that target SGLT1- and GLUT2-mediated GLP-1 and GIP secretion, instead of compounds targeting the sweet taste receptor.

Acknowledgments: The authors thank Nicolai J. Wewer Albrechtsen (Novo Nordisk Foundation Center for Basic Metabolic Research, Department of Biomedical Sciences, the Panum Institute, University of Copenhagen) for reviewing the paper and Novo Nordisk A/S for supplying the gurmarin. The study was funded by the Novo Nordisk Center for Basic Metabolic Research (Novo Nordisk Foundation, Denmark) and European Union's Seventh Framework Programme for Research, Technological Development, and Demonstration Activities (Grant 266408). Funding agencies had no involvement in the study design and results interpretation.

Author Contributions: M.Y.S., R.E.K., J.J.H., and C.B.C. conceived and designed the study, and interpreted results. M.Y.S. performed the experiments, analyzed the data, prepared the figures, and drafted the manuscript. M.Y.S., R.E.K., C.B.C., R.E., K.W.C.-F., M.M.R. and J.J.H. approved the final version of the manuscript. R.E. and K.W.C.-F. produced and supplied gurmarin. M.M.R. tested the bioactivity of gurmarin in GLUTag cells. J.J.H. supervised the experimental work, and edited and revised the manuscript.

Conflicts of Interest: The authors declare no conflict of interest.

References

1.	Fowler, S.P.; Williams, K.; Resendez, R.G.; Hunt, K.J.; Hazuda, H.P.; Stern, M.P. Fueling the Obesity Epidemic? Artificially Sweetened Beverage Use and Long-term Weight Gain. *Obesity* **2008**, *16*, 1894–1900. [CrossRef] [PubMed]

2.   Nettleton, J.A.; Lutsey, P.L.; Wang, Y.; Lima, J.A.; Michos, E.D.; Jacobs, D.R. Diet soda intake and risk of incident metabolic syndrome and type 2 diabetes in the Multi-Ethnic Study of Atherosclerosis (MESA). *Diabetes Care* **2009**, *32*, 688–694. [CrossRef] [PubMed]

3.   Peters, J.C.; Beck, J.; Cardel, M.; Wyatt, H.R.; Foster, G.D.; Pan, Z.; Wojtanowski, A.C.; Vander Veur, S.S.; Herring, S.J.; Brill, C.; Hill, J.O. The effects of water and non-nutritive sweetened beverages on weight loss and weight maintenance: A randomized clinical trial. *Obesity (Silver Spring)* **2016**, *24*, 297–304. [CrossRef] [PubMed]

4.   Tate, D.F.; Turner-McGrievy, G.; Lyons, E.; Stevens, J.; Erickson, K.; Polzien, K.; Diamond, M.; Wang, X.; Popkin, B. Replacing caloric beverages with water or diet beverages for weight loss in adults: Main results of the Choose Healthy Options Consciously Everyday (CHOICE) randomized clinical trial. *Am. J. Clin. Nutr.* **2012**, *95*, 555–563. [CrossRef] [PubMed]

5.   Holst, J.J. On the physiology of GIP and GLP-1. *Horm. Metab. Res.* **2004**, *36*, 747–754. [CrossRef] [PubMed]

6.   Elliott, R.M.; Morgan, L.M.; Tredger, J.A.; Deacon, S.; Wright, J.; Marks, V. Glucagon-like peptide-1 (7–36)amide and glucose-dependent insulinotropic polypeptide secretion in response to nutrient ingestion in man: Acute post-prandial and 24-h secretion patterns. *J. Endocrinol.* **1993**, *138*, 159–166. [CrossRef] [PubMed]

7.   Kuhre, R.E.; Frost, C.R.; Svendsen, B.; Holst, J.J. Molecular mechanisms of glucose-stimulated GLP-1 secretion from perfused rat small intestine. *Diabetes* **2015**, *64*, 370–382. [CrossRef] [PubMed]

8.   Gorboulev, V.; Schürmann, A.; Vallon, V.; Kipp, H.; Jaschke, A.; Klessen, D.; Friedrich, A.; Scherneck, S.; Rieg, T.; Cunard, R.; et al. Na +-D-glucose cotransporter SGLT1 is pivotal for intestinal glucose absorption and glucose-dependent incretin secretion. *Diabetes* **2012**, *61*, 187–196. [CrossRef] [PubMed]

9.   Röder, P.V.; Geillinger, K.E.; Zietek, T.S.; Thorens, B.; Koepsell, H.; Daniel, H. The Role of SGLT1 and GLUT2 in Intestinal Glucose Transport and Sensing. *PLoS ONE* **2014**, *9*, e89977. [CrossRef] [PubMed]

10.   Parker, H.E.; Adriaenssens, A.; Rogers, G.; Richards, P.; Koepsell, H.; Reimann, F.; Gribble, F.M. Predominant role of active versus facilitative glucose transport for glucagon-like peptide-1 secretion. *Diabetologia* **2012**, *55*, 2445–2455. [CrossRef] [PubMed]

11.   Parker, H.E.; Habib, A.M.; Rogers, G.J.; Gribble, F.M.; Reimann, F. Nutrient-dependent secretion of glucose-dependent insulinotropic polypeptide from primary murine K cells. *Diabetologia* **2009**, *52*, 289–298. [CrossRef] [PubMed]

12.   Gribble, F.M.; Williams, L.; Simpson, A.K.; Reimann, F. A novel glucose-sensing mechanism contributing to glucagon-like peptide-1 secretion from the GLUTag cell line. *Diabetes* **2003**, *52*, 1147–1154. [CrossRef] [PubMed]

13.   Reimann, F.; Gribble, F.M. Glucose-sensing in glucagon-like peptide-1-secreting cells. *Diabetes* **2002**, *51*, 2757–2763. [CrossRef] [PubMed]

14.   Dyer, J.; Salmon, K.S. H.; Zibrik, L.; Shirazi-Beechey, S.P. Expression of sweet taste receptors of the T1R family in the intestinal tract and enteroendocrine cells. *Biochem. Soc. Trans.* **2005**, *33*, 302–305. [CrossRef] [PubMed]

15.   Höfer, D.; Püschel, B.; Drenckhahn, D. Taste receptor-like cells in the rat gut identified by expression of alpha-gustducin. *Proc. Natl. Acad. Sci. USA* **1996**, *93*, 6631–6634. [CrossRef] [PubMed]

16.   Jang, H.-J.; Kokrashvili, Z.; Theodorakis, M.J.; Carlson, O.D.; Kim, B.-J.; Zhou, J.; Kim, H.H.; Xu, X.; Chan, S.L.; Juhaszova, M.; et al. Gut-expressed gustducin and taste receptors regulate secretion of glucagon-like peptide-1. *Proc. Natl. Acad. Sci. USA* **2007**, *104*, 15069–15074. [CrossRef] [PubMed]

17.   Margolskee, R.F.; Dyer, J.; Kokrashvili, Z.; Salmon, K.S.H.; Ilegems, E.; Daly, K.; Maillet, E.L.; Ninomiya, Y.; Mosinger, B.; Shirazi-Beechey, S.P. T1R3 and gustducin in gut sense sugars to regulate expression of Na+-glucose cotransporter 1. *Proc. Natl. Acad. Sci. USA* **2007**, *104*, 15075–15080. [CrossRef] [PubMed]

18.   Li, X.; Staszewski, L.; Xu, H.; Durick, K.; Zoller, M.; Adler, E. Human receptors for sweet and umami taste. *Proc. Natl. Acad. Sci. USA* **2002**, *99*, 4692–4696. [CrossRef] [PubMed]

19.   Steinert, R.E.; Gerspach, A.C.; Gutmann, H.; Asarian, L.; Drewe, J.; Beglinger, C. The functional involvement of gut-expressed sweet taste receptors in glucose-stimulated secretion of glucagon-like peptide-1 (GLP-1) and peptide YY (PYY). *Clin. Nutr.* **2011**, *30*, 524–532. [CrossRef] [PubMed]

20.   Sutherland, K.; Young, R.L.; Cooper, N.J.; Horowitz, M.; Blackshaw, L.A. Phenotypic characterization of taste cells of the mouse small intestine. *Am. J. Physiol. Gastrointest. Liver Physiol.* **2007**, *292*, G1420–G1428. [CrossRef] [PubMed]

21.   Roper, S.D. Signal transduction and information processing in mammalian taste buds. *Pflugers Arch. Eur. J. Physiol.* **2007**, *454*, 759–776. [CrossRef] [PubMed]

22. Liu, D.; Liman, E.R. Intracellular Ca2+ and the phospholipid PIP2 regulate the taste transduction ion channel TRPM5. *Proc. Natl. Acad. Sci. USA* **2003**, *100*, 15160–15165. [CrossRef] [PubMed]
23. Ford, H.E.; Peters, V.; Martin, N.M.; Sleeth, M.L.; Ghatei, M.A.; Frost, G.S.; Bloom, S.R. Effects of oral ingestion of sucralose on gut hormone response and appetite in healthy normal-weight subjects. *Eur. J. Clin. Nutr.* **2011**, *65*, 508–513. [CrossRef] [PubMed]
24. Ma, J.; Bellon, M.; Wishart, J.M.; Young, R.; Blackshaw, L.A.; Jones, K.L.; Horowitz, M.; Rayner, C.K. Effect of the artificial sweetener, sucralose, on gastric emptying and incretin hormone release in healthy subjects. *Am. J. Physiol. Gastrointest. Liver Physiol.* **2009**, *296*, G735–G739. [CrossRef] [PubMed]
25. Maersk, M.; Belza, A.; Holst, J.; Fenger-Grøn, M.; Pedersen, S.; Astrup, A.; Richelsen, B. Satiety scores and satiety hormone response after sucrose-sweetened soft drink compared with isocaloric semi-skimmed milk and with non-caloric soft drink: A controlled trial. *Eur. J. Clin. Nutr.* **2012**, *66*, 523–529. [CrossRef] [PubMed]
26. Steinert, R.E.; Frey, F.; Töpfer, A.; Drewe, J.; Beglinger, C. Effects of carbohydrate sugars and artificial sweeteners on appetite and the secretion of gastrointestinal satiety peptides. *Br. J. Nutr.* **2011**, *105*, 1320–1328. [CrossRef] [PubMed]
27. Wu, T.; Zhao, B.R.; Bound, M.J.; Checklin, H.L.; Bellon, M.; Little, T.J.; Young, R.L.; Jones, K.L.; Horowitz, M.; Rayner, C.K. Effects of different sweet preloads on incretin hormone secretion, gastric emptying, and postprandial glycemia in healthy humans. *Am. J. Clin. Nutr.* **2012**, *95*, 78–83. [CrossRef] [PubMed]
28. Fujita, Y.; Wideman, R.D.; Speck, M.; Asadi, A.; King, D.S.; Webber, T.D.; Haneda, M.; Kieffer, T.J. Incretin release from gut is acutely enhanced by sugar but not by sweeteners in vivo. *Am. J. Physiol. Endocrinol. Metab.* **2009**, *296*, 473–479. [CrossRef] [PubMed]
29. Brown, R.J.; Walter, M.; Rother, K.I. Ingestion of diet soda before a glucose load augments glucagon-like peptide-1 secretion. *Diabetes Care* **2009**, *32*, 2184–2186. [CrossRef] [PubMed]
30. Sylvetsky, A.C.; Brown, R.J.; Blau, J.E.; Walter, M.; Rother, K.I. Hormonal responses to non-nutritive sweeteners in water and diet soda. *Nutr. Metab. (Lond.)* **2016**, *13*, 71. [CrossRef] [PubMed]
31. Shankar, P.; Ahuja, S.; Sriram, K. Non-nutritive sweeteners: Review and update. *Nutrition* **2013**, *29*, 1293–1299. [CrossRef] [PubMed]
32. De, S.; Mondal, S.; Banerjee, S. Introduction to stevioside. *Stevioside Technol. Appl. Heal.* **2013**. [CrossRef]
33. Fujiwara, S.; Imada, T.; Nakagita, T.; Okada, S.; Nammoku, T.; Abe, K.; Misaka, T. Sweeteners interacting with the transmembrane domain of the human sweet-taste receptor induce sweet-taste synergisms in binary mixtures. *Food Chem.* **2012**, *130*, 561–568. [CrossRef]
34. Imoto, T.; Miyasaka, A.; Ishima, R.; Akasaka, K. A novel peptide isolated from the leaves of gymnema sylvestre-i. Characterization and its suppressive effect on the neural responses to sweet taste stimuli in the rat. *Camp. Biochem. Physiot* **1991**, *100*, 309–314. [CrossRef]
35. Eliasen, R.; Andresen, T.L.; Conde-Frieboes, K.W. Handling a tricycle: Orthogonal versus random oxidation of the tricyclic inhibitor cystine knotted peptide gurmarin. *Peptides* **2012**, *37*, 144–149. [CrossRef] [PubMed]
36. Palmer, R.K.; Atwal, K.; Bakaj, I.; Carlucci-Derbyshire, S.; Buber, M.T.; Cerne, R.; Cortés, R.Y.; Devantier, H.R.; Jorgensen, V.; Pawlyk, A.; et al. Triphenylphosphine Oxide Is a Potent and Selective Inhibitor of the Transient Receptor Potential Melastatin-5 Ion Channel. *Assay Drug Dev. Technol.* **2010**, *8*, 703–713. [CrossRef] [PubMed]
37. Gerspach, A.C.; Steinert, R.E.; Schönenberger, L.; Beglinger, C. The role of the gut sweet taste receptor in regulating GLP-1, PYY, and CCK release in humans. *Am. J. Physiol. Endocrinol. Metab.* **2011**, *301*, 317–325. [CrossRef] [PubMed]
38. Emery, E.C.; Diakogiannaki, E.; Gentry, C.; Psichas, A.; Habib, A.M.; Bevan, S.; Fischer, M.J. M.; Reimann, F.; Gribble, F.M. Stimulation of GLP-1 Secretion Downstream of the Ligand-Gated Ion Channel TRPA1. *Diabetes* **2015**, *64*, 1202–1210. [CrossRef] [PubMed]
39. Reimann, F.; Habib, A.M.; Tolhurst, G.; Parker, H.E.; Rogers, G.J.; Gribble, F.M. Glucose Sensing in L Cells: A Primary Cell Study. *Cell Metab.* **2008**, *8*, 532–539. [CrossRef] [PubMed]
40. Jyotaki, M.; Sanematsu, K.; Shigemura, N.; Yoshida, R.; Ninomiya, Y. Leptin suppresses sweet taste responses of enteroendocrine STC-1 cells. *Neuroscience* **2016**, *332*, 76–87. [CrossRef] [PubMed]
41. Miyasaka, A.; Imoto, T. Electrophysiological characterization of the inhibitory effect of a novel peptide gurmarin on the sweet taste response in rats. *Brain Res.* **1995**, *676*, 63–68. [CrossRef]
42. Wilson, L.A.; Wilkinson, K.; Crews, H.M.; Davies, A.M.; Dick, C.S.; Dumsday, V.L. Urinary monitoring of saccharin and acesulfame-K as biomarkers of exposure to these additives. *Food Addit. Contam.* **1999**, *16*, 227–238. [CrossRef] [PubMed]

43. Schiffman, S.S.; Rother, K.I. Sucralose, A Synthetic Organochlorine Sweetener: Overview Of Biological Issues. *J. Toxicol. Environ. Health* **2013**, *17*, 399–451. [CrossRef] [PubMed]
44. Hutapea, M. Digestion of Stevioside, a Natural Sweetener, by Various Digestive Enzymes. *J. Clin. Biochem. Nutr.* **1997**, *1*, 177–186. [CrossRef]
45. Ferraris, R.P.; Yasharpour, S.; Lloyd, K.C.; Mirzayan, R.; Diamond, J.M. Luminal glucose concentrations in the gut under normal conditions. *Am. J. Physiol.* **1990**, *259*, G822–G837. [PubMed]
46. Svendsen, B.; Holst, J.J. Regulation of gut hormone secretion. Studies using isolated perfused intestines. *Peptides* **2016**, *77*, 47–53. [CrossRef] [PubMed]

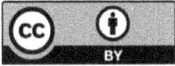

nutrients

Review

Sugars, Sweet Taste Receptors, and Brain Responses

Allen A. Lee [1] and Chung Owyang [2,*]

[1] 1500 East Medical Center Drive, Division of Gastroenterology, Department of Internal Medicine, Michigan Medicine, University of Michigan, Ann Arbor, MI 48109-5362, USA; allenlee@med.umcih.edu
[2] 3912 Taubman Center, SPC 5362, Ann Arbor, MI 48109-5362, USA
* Correspondence: cowyang@med.umich.edu; Tel.: +1-734-936-4785; Fax: +1-734-936-7392

Received: 10 April 2017; Accepted: 21 June 2017; Published: 24 June 2017

Abstract: Sweet taste receptors are composed of a heterodimer of taste 1 receptor member 2 (T1R2) and taste 1 receptor member 3 (T1R3). Accumulating evidence shows that sweet taste receptors are ubiquitous throughout the body, including in the gastrointestinal tract as well as the hypothalamus. These sweet taste receptors are heavily involved in nutrient sensing, monitoring changes in energy stores, and triggering metabolic and behavioral responses to maintain energy balance. Not surprisingly, these pathways are heavily regulated by external and internal factors. Dysfunction in one or more of these pathways may be important in the pathogenesis of common diseases, such as obesity and type 2 diabetes mellitus.

Keywords: sweet taste receptors; glucose sensing; nutrient sensing; leptin; hypothalamus

1. Chemosensory Cells in the Tongue

Humans can distinguish between five basic tastes, including sweet, salty, umami, bitter, and sour. Recently, lipid sensors have been identified on the tongue which suggests that fat can be considered as the sixth taste [1]. Taste processing is first achieved at the level of taste receptor cells (TRCs) which are clustered in taste buds on the tongue. When TRCs are activated by specific tastants, they transmit information via sensory afferent fibers to specific areas in the brain that are involved in taste perception. Four morphologic subtypes of TRCs have been identified. Type I glial-like cells detect salty taste. Type II cells express G-protein coupled receptors (GPCRs) to detect sweet, umami, and bitter tastes. Type III cells sense sour stimuli, while Type IV cells likely represent stem or progenitor taste cells [2]. Type II cells do not form traditional synapses with afferent nerve fibers. Rather, these cells release ATP through hemichannels, which can then activate purinergic receptors (P2N2 and P2X3) present on the cranial nerve fibers innervating each taste bud (Figure 1) [3–5].

Two classes of GPCRs have been identified, including taste 1 receptor family (T1R) and the taste 2 receptor family (T2R) [6]. Two subtypes of the T1R family, including T1R member 2 (T1R2) and T1R member 3 (T1R3), form heterodimers to act as sweet taste receptors [7,8].

Type I glial-like cell		Type II receptor cell		Type III presynaptic cell	
Neurotransmitter clearance		**Taste transduction**		**Surface glycoproteins, Ion channels**	
GLAST	Glutamate reuptake	T1Rs, T2Rs	Taste GPCRs	NCAM	Neuronal adhesion
NTPDase2	Ecto-ATPase	mGluRs	Taste GPCRs	PKD channels	Sour taste?
NET	Norepinephrine uptake	Gα-gus, Gγ13	G protein subunits		
		PLCβ2	Synthesis of IP3	**Neurotransmitter synthesis**	
Ion redistribution and transport		TRPM5	Depolarizing cation current	AADC	Biogenic amine synthesis
ROMK	K⁺ homeostasis			GAD67	GABA synthesis
		Excitation and transmitter release		5-HT	Neurotransmitter
Other		$Na_v1.7$, $Na_v1.3$	Action potential generation	Chromogranin	Vesicle packaging
OXTR	Oxytocin signaling?	Panx1	ATP release channel		
				Excitation, transmitter release	
				$Na_v1.2$	Action potential generation
				$Ca_v2.1$, $Ca_v1.2$	Voltage-gated Ca^{2+} current
				SNAP25	SNARE protein, exocytosis

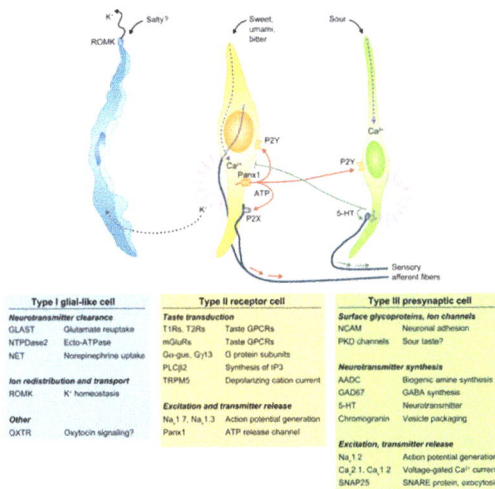

Figure 1. The four major classes of taste cells. This classification incorporates ultrastructural features, patterns of gene expression, and the functions of each Types I, II (receptor), III (presynaptic), and IV (progenitor, not depicted) taste cells. Type I cells (blue) degrade or absorb neurotransmitters. They also may clear extracellular K+ that accumulates after action potentials (shown as bursts) in receptor (yellow) and presynaptic (green) cells. K+ may be extruded through an apical K channel such as renal outer medullary potassium channel (ROMK). Salty taste may be transduced by some Type I cells, but this remains uncertain. Sweet, bitter, and umami taste compounds activate receptor cells, inducing them to release ATP through pannexin 1 (Panx1) hemichannels. The extracellular ATP excites ATP receptors (P2X, P2Y) on sensory nerve fibers and on taste cells. Presynaptic cells, in turn, release serotonin (5-HT), which inhibits receptor cells. Sour stimuli (and carbonation, not depicted) directly activate presynaptic cells. Only presynaptic cells form ultrastructurally identifiably synapses with nerves. Tables below the cells list some of the proteins that are expressed in a cell type-selective manner. AADC, aromatic L-amino acid decarboxylase; Ca, voltage-gated calcium channel; Gα-gus, alpha-gustducin; Gγ13, Gγ13 subunit; GAD, glutamate decarboxylase; GLAST, glutamate aspartate transporter; 5-HT, 5-hydroxytryptamine; mGluRs, metabotropic glutamate receptor; Na, voltage-gated sodium channel; NCAM, neural cell adhesion molecule; NET, norepinephrine transporter; NTPDase; nucleoside triphosphate diphosphohydrolase; OXTR, oxytoxin receptor; Panx1, pannexin 1; PKD, polycystic kidney disease-like channel; PLCβ2, phospholipase C β2; ROMK, renal outer medullary potassium channel; SNAP, synaptosomal-associated protein; T1R, taste 1 receptor family; T2R, taste 2 receptor family; TRPM5, transient receptor potential cation channel M5; Adapted with permission from [6].

2. Sweet Taste Signaling

Sweet taste receptors can be activated by a wide range of chemically different compounds, including sugars (glucose, fructose, sucrose, maltose), artificial sweeteners (e.g., saccharin, aspartame, cyclamate), sweet amino acids (D-tryptophan, D-phenylalanine, D-serine), and sweet proteins (monellin, brazzein, thaumatin) [9]. Binding of a ligand to the sweet taste receptor leads to activation of the heterotrimeric G-protein α-gustducin. Phospholipase C β2 is subsequently stimulated, leading to release of intracellular Ca^{2+} and activation of the transient receptor potential cation channel M5 (TRPM5). This sequence results in the release of ATP, which can then activate adjacent sensory afferent neurons that send signals to brain centers involved in taste perception (Figure 2) [10].

Taste cells also express bioactive peptides, including glucagon-like peptide-1 (GLP-1), glucagon, neuropeptide Y, peptide YY (PYY), cholecystokinin (CCK), vasoactive intestinal peptide, and ghrelin [11]. Although the function of these peptides in taste buds is still unknown, their presence suggests a role in the processing and modulation of taste information at the level of the taste bud.

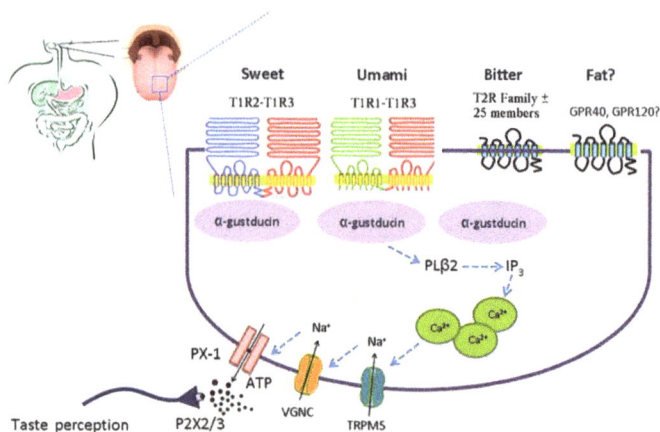

Figure 2. Simplified model of the taste GPCR signaling pathways involved in chemosensing by taste receptors of the tongue. Subtypes of the T1R family heterodimerize to detect sweet (T1R2-T1R3) and umami (T1R1-T1R3). Bitter is detected by the T2R family. Medium-chain and long-chain fatty acids are detected by FFAR1 and GPR120. Taste receptor binding leads to activation of gustatory G-proteins, release of intracellular Ca^{2+}, activation of TRPM5, depolarization, activation of voltage-gated Na^+ channels (VGNC), and release of ATP which activates purinergic receptors on afferent fibers leading to taste perception. ATP, adenosine triphosphate; FFAR1, free fatty acid receptor 1; GPCR, G-protein coupled receptor; PX-1, pannexin 1-hemichannel; T1R, taste receptor type 1; T1R1, taste receptor type 1 member 1; T1R2, taste receptor type 1 member 2; T1R3, taste receptor type 1 member 3; T2R, taste receptor type 2; TRPM5, transient receptor potential cation channel M5; VGNC, voltage-gated Na^+ channel. Reproduced with permission from [10].

3. Chemosensory Cells in the GI Tract

Although taste receptors were initially discovered in taste buds, a growing number of studies have demonstrated that sweet taste receptors are expressed throughout the body, including the nasal epithelium, respiratory system, pancreatic islet cells, and even in sperm and testes [12–14].

In the gut, sweet taste receptors are mainly concentrated on enteroendocrine cells. Although these cells represent a small proportion of the total number of epithelial cells in the gastrointestinal (GI) tract, collectively they form the largest endocrine organ in the body [15]. Over 20 different types of enteroendocrine cell types have been identified to date, each of which secretes one or more regulatory peptides or bioactive molecules (Table 1). These hormones can act locally on enteroendocrine cells, on immune cells, nerve endings, or organs at remote sites including pancreatic islets and the central nervous system (CNS). This results in changes in appetite and satiety, inhibition of gastric emptying, stimulation of gastric secretion, pancreatic exocrine and endocrine secretion, induction of nutrient transporters and digestive enzymes, an increase in intestinal barrier function, and modulation of immune responses and tissue growth [15–19].

Table 1. Enteroendocrine cells of the mammalian gastrointestinal tract. Adapted with permission from [15]. Several of the enteroendocrine cell types, notably A, K, and L cells, have subgroups or gradients along the intestine that contain different combinations of products; subgroups of I and L cells contain 5-HT.

Cell	Products	Luminal Receptors	Locations	Principal Effects
A (X-like) cells and subtypes	Ghrelin, nesfatin-1	T1R1-T1R3; T2Rs	Stomach	Appetite control, growth hormone release
Enterochromaffin cells [*,‡]	5-HT (5-HT is also contained in subgroups of I, K, and L cells)	FFARs 2, 3; TRPA1; toxin receptors; TLRs	Stomach, small and large intestine	Facilitation of intestinal motility reflexes and secretion; triggering of emesis and nausea in response to toxins
I cells	CCK (5-HT)	T2Rs; FFA1; GPR120; LPAR5; CaSR; TRPA1; TLRs	Proximal small intestine	Activation of gallbladder contraction and stimulation of pancreatic enzyme secretion
K cells, and subtypes	GIP	GPR119, GPR120; FFAR1	Proximal small intestine	Stimulation of insulin release
L cells, and subtypes [‡]	GLP-1, GLP-2, PYY, oxyntomodulin (5-HT)	T2Rs; T1R2–T1R3; FFARs 1–3; GPR119, LPAR5; GPR120; CaSR	Distal small intestine, colon	Stimulation of carbohydrate uptake, slowing of intestinal transit, appetite regulation, insulin release
P cells	Leptin	Nutrient receptors	Stomach	Appetite regulation, reduction of food intake

* ECL cells do not contact the lumen. ‡ Sweet taste receptor molecules have been identified within L cells and enterochromaffin (EC) cells. Abbreviations: T1R, taste 1 receptor family; T2R, taste 2 receptor family; 5-HT, serotonin; ECL, enterochromaffin-like; FFAR, free fatty acid receptor; TRP, transient receptor potential; TLR, Toll-like receptor; FFA, free fatty acid; FFARs, free fatty acid receptors; GPR, G protein-coupled receptor; LPAR, lysophosphatidic acid receptor; CaSR, calcium-sensing receptor; CCK, cholecystokinin; GIP, gastric inhibitory polypeptide; GLP, glucagon-like peptide; PYY, peptide YY.

The function of the sweet taste receptor system in the gastrointestinal tract is likely involved in nutrient sensing, glucose homeostasis, as well as secretion of GI peptides. The intestinal mucosa is highly expressed with taste receptor proteins, including T1R2 and T1R3 [20]. The Na$^+$/glucose cotransporter SGLT1 is the major route for transport of dietary sugars from the lumen of the intestine into enterocytes. Dietary sugar and artificial sweeteners increased SGLT1 expression in wild-type mice, but not in T1R3 or α-gustducin knockout mice [21]. Activation of sweet taste receptors on enteroendocrine cells led to increased GLP-1 and glucagon-like insulinotropic peptide (GIP) release, which in turn leads to upregulation of SGLT1 expression. Furthermore, there is a significant decrease in transcript levels of T1R2 following jejunal glucose perfusion in mice [22]. This suggests that sweet taste receptors function as gut luminal nutrient sensors which helps to regulate glucose balance and nutrient intake.

3.1. L Cells

Sweet taste receptors are expressed by L cells in the distal small intestine. L cells are distributed throughout the GI tract, with greatest density in the ileum and colon [23]. It has long been known that orally administered glucose triggers a much higher release of insulin compared with intravenous injection of glucose. However, the mechanism was largely unknown until Jang et al. demonstrated that human duodenal L cells express sweet taste receptors that act as glucose sensors in the gut [24]. Activation of L cells by glucose leads to release of hormones, including GLP-1 [25]. GLP-1 leads to increased satiety signals, stimulates insulin release, suppresses glucagon secretion, and slows gastric emptying [26,27]. Glucose-stimulated GLP-1 secretion (GSGS) is severely impaired in *T1R3*-knockout rodents but not in *T1R2*-knockout mice [28]. This suggests that T1R3 can mediate GSGS by itself in the absence of the full sweet taste receptor heterodimer. Furthermore, *SGLT-1*-knockout mice show an 80% reduction in GSGS [29]. These data taken collectively suggest that T1R3 and SGLT1 interact in L cells to produce GLP-1, which stimulates insulin production, regulates glucose absorption, and sends satiety signals to the brain.

3.2. K Cells

K cells in the proximal intestine secrete glucagon-like insulinotropic peptide (GIP) in the presence of glucose. GIP is released rapidly postprandially and leads to release of insulin as well as promotes lipid storage in adipocytes [30]. This process is also SGLT1-dependent but it is not currently known whether this process involves taste receptors.

3.3. Enterochromaffin Cells

Enterochromaffin (EC) cells are distributed throughout the GI tract; the EC cells secrete serotonin (5-HT) to mediate changes in motility and secretion as well as in transduction of visceral stimuli [31]. Sweet taste molecules have been reported in EC cells. Animal studies indicate intestinal EC cells express α-gustducin and T1R [32,33]. T1R3 and T2R have also been identified in human small intestinal EC cells which release 5-HT in response to stimulation with sucralose [34]. This suggests that one role for EC cells is nutrient sensing in the gut with subsequent release of 5-HT leading to a variety of downstream effects.

4. Glucose-Sensing by Gut Endocrine Cells

Glucose in the intestinal lumen leads to the release of several regulatory peptides, including the incretin hormones GIP, GLP-1, and GLP-2 as well as 5-HT [35,36]. Several different mechanisms may be involved in glucose-sensing by gut enteroendocrine cells. Evidence suggests that glucose is metabolized, leading to generation of ATP and the closing of K_{ATP} channels in the cell membrane, a process that is similar to insulin release from the pancreatic β cell [37,38].

There is likely an additional mechanism of glucose-sensing in the gut, as GLP-1 is secreted in response to non-metabolizable sugars. As described above, glucose and non-metabolizable sugars are transported via SGLT-1. In addition to serving as glucose co-transporters, SGLT-1 and SGLT-3 may also be involved in glucose-sensing with subsequent release of 5-HT and GLP-1 [39–41].

Taste receptors in the gut may also be responsible for glucose-sensing. Elements of the sweet taste transduction pathway, including T1R2, T1R3, and α-gustducin are co-expressed in mouse and human enteroendocrine cells [24,32,42,43]. T1Rs may also play a role in the upregulation of SGLT-1 and GLUT2 in the intestinal epithelium in response to glucose as well as in the regulation of GLP-1 secretion [21,24].

5. Neuroanatomy of Sweet Taste

Upon activation of sweet taste receptors, neural afferents of cranial nerves send gustatory information to the rostral division of the nucleus tractus solitarius (rNTS) of the medulla (Figure 3) [44]. In rodents, fibers then ascend ipsilaterally to the parabrachial nucleus (PBN) [45]. From the PBN, a dorsal pathway projects to the parvicellular part of the ventroposteromedial nucleus of the thalamus (VPMpc, the taste thalamic nucleus) and a ventral pathway to the amygdalar and lateral hypothalamic areas. Thalamic afferents then project to the primary gustatory cortex, which is defined as the VPMpc cortical target located within the insular cortex [46]. In primates and humans, rNTS projections bypass PBN and proceed directly to VPMpc [47].

Imaging studies have indicated that sweet, salty, bitter, and umami tastes activate distinct cortical fields in the mammalian primary gustatory cortex and suggest the existence of a gustotopic map in the brain [48]. A recent study demonstrated that direct activation of the cortical fields associated with sweet and bitter tastes elicits specific behavioral responses in mice using two different tasks [49]. In the first task, mice were placed into a two-chamber arena and a light stimulus was delivered to the relevant cortical field only when the animals entered a specific chamber. Mice expressing channelrhodopsin 2 (ChR2) in the sweet cortical field showed a preference for the chamber associated with light stimulation. Meanwhile, mice expressing ChR2 in the bitter cortical field demonstrated avoidance of that chamber. In the second task, mice were trained to lick from a water bottle on presentation of a cue. During licking, a light stimulus was applied to the relevant cortical field. Stimulation of the bitter cortical field in thirsty mice led to a marked reduction in licking. Conversely, light stimulation of the sweet cortical field led to an increase in licking. These findings demonstrate that activation of a specific taste cortical field can bring about specific behaviors that are characteristic of exposure to that taste.

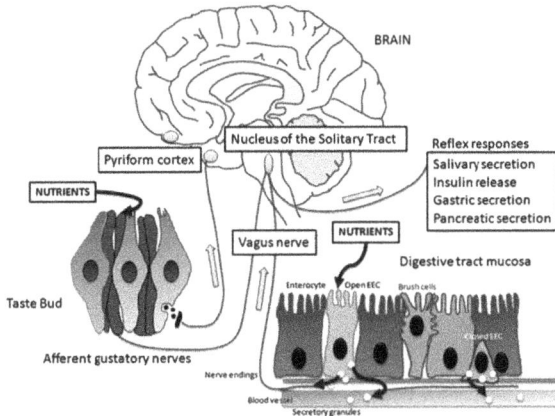

Figure 3. Schematic representation of the taste circuitry. The gustatory system is represented by taste cells in taste buds and their gustatory nerves. Corresponding to the gastrointestinal system, there are two enteroendocrine cells (EEC), one that is open to the lumen releasing cholecystokinin (CCK) and glucagon-like peptide 1 (GLP-1) in response to luminal nutrients and one that is closed. Vagal fibers are located underneath the GI mucosa in close contact with hormone secretions. The signals from the gustatory system reach the rostral nucleus of the solitary tract whereas visceral impulses terminate at the caudal nucleus of the solitary tract. From the nucleus of the solitary tract, gustatory and visceral information projects to several brain regions including the amygdala, the hypothalamus, and the ventral posterior nucleus of the thalamus. These regions are involved with ingestive motivation, physiological reflexes, and energy homeostasis. Reproduced with permission from [50].

6. Central Regulation of Food Intake and Energy Balance

Nutrient sensing initially occurs in the GI tract. Signals via vagal afferent neurons are sent directly to sympathetic neurons in hindbrain nuclei. These nuclei then project to forebrain areas such as the hypothalamus [51]. The gut thus sends signals to the rest of the body, including the brain, about current nutritional status by secreting hormones, such as ghrelin, GIP, PYY, CCK, and GLP-1, as well as neurotransmitters, such as 5-HT, that are important regulators of glucose and energy homeostasis [52].

These signals are then processed in different brain nuclei, including the melanocortin system. This system is composed of two peptide-expressing populations of neurons in the arcuate nucleus (ARC) and their downstream targets. One set of ARC neurons express the precursor peptide pro-opiomelanocortin (POMC), which is transformed into α-melanocyte-stimulating hormone and serves as an agonist for melanocortin receptor 4 (MC4R). Activation of POMC neurons results in anorexigenic effects, including decreased food intake and weight loss. The second set of neurons express neuropeptide Y (NPY) and the MC4R antagonist/inverse agonist agouti-related protein (AGRP). Activation of NPY-AGRP neurons results in increased food intake and weight gain [53,54].

Downstream sites for both neurons are located in the hypothalamus, including the paraventricular nucleus (PVN), ventromedial hypothalamus (VMH), and the lateral hypothalamic area [55].

The POMC and NPY-AGRP expressing neurons receive input from many different sources (Figure 4). Insulin and leptin may act as adiposity signals, as plasma levels are directly proportional to the amount of stored fuel in adipose tissue. Furthermore, insulin and leptin receptors are expressed throughout the hypothalamus, including on POMC and NPY-AGRP neurons in the ARC [56–59].

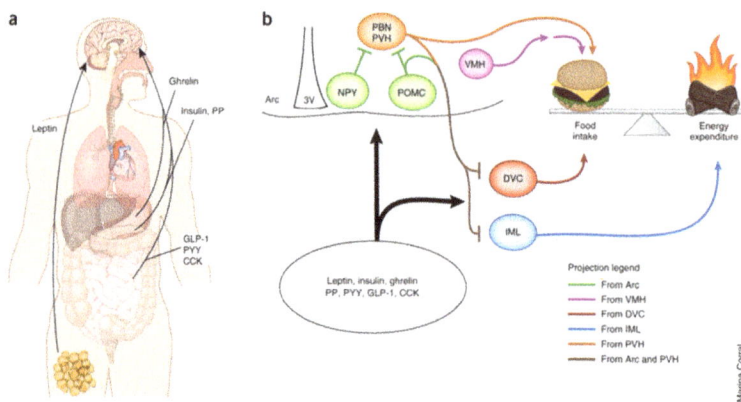

Figure 4. (**a**) Multiple peripheral factors have been shown to modify food intake and energy expenditure through direct effects on the central nervous system. Leptin, which likely acts on sweet taste receptor cells, is the primary regulator of energy balance and food intake in the hypothalamus. (**b**) Evidence suggests that melanocortin signaling regulates these physiological processes by means of distinct projection patterns originating from pro-opiomelanocortin (POMC) neurons in the arcuate nucleus (Arc). Sweet taste receptors likely act on neuropeptide Y (NPY) neurons in the hypothalamus to regulate energy homeostasis. Ultimately, MC4 receptor (MC4R)-expressing neurons downstream of POMC neurons act to suppress food intake and increase energy expenditure. Hypothalamic NPY/AgRP, paraventricular nucleus of the hypothalamus (PVH) and VMH neurons, as well as hindbrain dorsal vagal complex (DVC), parabrachial nucleus (PBN) and spinal cord intermediolateral cell column (IML) neurons, also regulate or counter-regulate these activities. PP, pancreatic polypeptide; PYY, peptide YY; 3V, third ventricle. Adapted with permission from [60].

Sweet taste receptors also play a role in nutrient sensing in the hypothalamus similar to mechanisms used in the periphery. Neurons containing T1R2 and T1R3 have been identified in the CNS, including the hypothalamus. Recent data suggest that the majority of sweet taste receptor activity occurs on non-POMC leptin-responding neurons in the hypothalamus [61].

7. Central Actions of Gut Hormones

7.1. Effect of Leptin

Leptin is an anorexigenic hormone that is primarily produced by adipocytes. Leptin is the primary mediator in the hypothalamus that regulates energy balance and food intake [62]. Leptin acts on a specific obese receptor (Ob-R) which is encoded by the db gene [63]. Ob-R is expressed in several hypothalamic nuclei and leads to increased expression of POMC as well as simultaneous reduction of NPY-AGRP expression [64,65]. Mutations in leptin (*ob/ob*) or its receptor (*db/db*) produce mice that are hyperphagic and severely obese [66–68].

7.2. Leptin and Sweet Taste in Mice

Leptin displays a sweet suppressive effect in studies with mutant mice containing a point mutation of the *db* gene (*db/db* mice) that lack a functional leptin receptor (Ob-Rb) [69]. Chorda tympani nerve responses to various taste stimuli were compared in *db/db* and lean control mice before and after intraperitoneal (i.p.) injection of recombinant leptin. The chorda tympani (CT) nerve transmits taste information from the anterior two-thirds of the tongue [64]. The *db/db* mice demonstrated greater CT nerve responses to sweet compounds compared to lean control mice. However, after i.p. injection of leptin, CT nerve responses to sweet substances were significantly suppressed in control mice but not in *db/db* mice. Other substances, such as NaCl, HCl, and quinine were not affected by leptin administration, which suggests that leptin selectively affects sweet taste sensitivity.

Leptin's target appears to be on sweet taste receptor cells. Studies using real-time polymerase chain reaction (RT-PCR), in situ hybridization, and immunohistochemistry show that the functional leptin receptor Ob-Rb is expressed on taste bud cells, with approximately 30–40% of T1R3 expressing cells co-expressing Ob-Rb (unpublished data) [64]. Further studies show that application of leptin to isolated taste cells leads to a reduction of cell excitability [69]. This suggests that leptin acting on Ob-Rb may suppress sweet taste sensitivity by decreasing responsiveness of sweet taste cells.

7.3. Leptin and Sweet Taste in Humans

Plasma leptin levels show a diurnal variation in humans, with levels peaking around midnight and lowest around noon to mid-afternoon [70]. A study of 91 non-obese subjects demonstrated a link between plasma leptin levels and sweet taste sensitivity in humans [71]. Recognition thresholds for sweet, salty, sour, bitter, and umami tastes were measured using different concentrations of sucrose, glucose, saccharin Na, NaCl, citric acid, quinine HCl, and monosodium glutamate. The authors demonstrated that recognition thresholds for sweet substances were tightly linked with circulating leptin levels. This was not seen with other taste stimuli.

7.4. Effect of Endocannabinoids

Cannabinoids, such as *Cannabis sativa* (marijuana), have long been known to have an appetite-stimulating effect. However, endogenous endocannabinoids, including anandamide (AEA) and 2-arachidonoyl glycerol (2-AG), and their specific receptors, cannabinoid receptor type 1 (CB1) and cannabinoid receptor 2 (CB2), were only discovered in the 1980s [72,73]. CB1 receptors, which are located in the hypothalamus as well as peripherally, are likely involved in the orexigenic effects of endocannabinoids [74,75]. Evidence of these effects are demonstrated by injection of endocannabinoids in the hypothalamus which stimulates food intake while CB1 deletion in animal models leads to a lean phenotype and resistance to diet-induced obesity [76,77].

The endocannabinoid system is normally tonically inactive and only becomes transiently activated when needed. Leptin likely plays an important counter regulatory role. Genetically obese mice deficient in leptin (*ob/ob*) who were given a single i.p. injection of rimonabant, a CB1 receptor antagonist, showed reduced food intake [76]. Subsequent experiments where *ob/ob* mice were then treated with leptin demonstrated significant decreases in levels of endocannabinoids in the hypothalamus, but not in the cerebellum.

Recently, the relationship between endocannabinoids and leptin was further clarified. Jo et al. demonstrated that neurons containing melanin-concentrating hormone (MCH) in the hypothalamus project to the mesolimbic ventral tegmental area [78]. Thus, the area of the brain controlling appetite is linked to the region devoted to pleasure and reward. These MCH neurons are tonically inhibited by γ-aminobutyric acid (GABA) and receive input from the endocannabinoid system as well as leptin. When these MCH neurons are stimulated, it leads to an increase in intracellular calcium and release of endocannabinoids. This subsequently leads to the activation of CB1 receptors on GABA interneurons, which suppresses GABA release, increases excitability of MCH-containing neurons, and results in increased food intake. Conversely, when leptin receptors on MCH neurons are activated, voltage-gated calcium channels are blocked, suppressing endocannabinoid release, and this leads to an appetite-suppressing effect of leptin.

7.5. Sweet Enhancing Effect of Endocannabinoids

Endocannabinoids also likely enhance taste cell responses to sweeteners. Intraperitoneal administration of endocannabinoids led to a dose-dependent increase in CT glossopharyngeal nerve responses to sweeteners in mice [79]. This was not observed for salty, sour, bitter, or umami compounds or in CB1 knockout mice. These effects were also blocked by administration of AM251, a CB1 receptor antagonist, but not by AM630, a CB2 receptor antagonist. The authors further demonstrated by immunohistochemistry that sweet taste cells expressing T1R3 also express CB1 receptors. These findings suggest that endocannabinoids may enhance sweet taste response in sweet taste cells expressing T1R3.

8. Conclusions

Sweet taste receptors and sweet taste molecules are involved in transduction of sweet taste in taste buds. Furthermore, it is clear that sweet taste pathways are present in the gut and in the CNS, including the appetite center in the hypothalamus. Accumulating data suggest that these pathways act as nutrient sensors in the gut and the brain. They also serve to regulate energy balance, glucose homeostasis, and food intake. Interactions between peripheral and central pathways are carefully regulated with input from peripheral mediators, such as leptin, ghrelin, insulin, GLP-1, and endocannabinoids. Further elucidation of these pathways may provide invaluable insight into the pathogenesis of common diseases, including obesity and type 2 diabetes mellitus.

Acknowledgments: This was work supported by the National Institute of Diabetes and Digestive and Kidney Diseases (NIDDK) Grants R01-DK048419 (C. Owyang) and P30-DK34933 (C. Owyang).

Conflicts of Interest: The authors declare no conflict of interest.

References

1. Laugerette, F.; Passilly-Degrace, P.; Patris, B.; Niot, I.; Febbraio, M.; Montmayeur, J.-P.; Besnard, P. CD36 involvement in orosensory detection of dietary lipids, spontaneous fat preference, and digestive secretions. *J. Clin. Investig.* **2005**, *115*, 3177–3184. [CrossRef] [PubMed]
2. Janssen, S.; Depoortere, I. Nutrient sensing in the gut: New roads to therapeutics? *Trends Endocrinol. Metab.* **2013**, *24*, 92–100.
3. Finger, T.E.; Danilova, V.; Barrows, J.; Bartel, D.L.; Vigers, A.J.; Stone, L.; Hellekant, G.; Kinnamon, S.C. Neuroscience: ATP signalling is crucial for communication from taste buds to gustatory nerves. *Science* **2005**, *310*, 1495–1499. [CrossRef] [PubMed]
4. Bo, X.; Alavi, A.; Xiang, Z.; Oglesby, I.; Ford, A.; Burnstock, G. Localization of ATP-gated P2X2 and P2X3 receptor immunoreactive nerves in rat taste buds. *NeuroReport* **1999**, *10*, 1107–1111. [CrossRef] [PubMed]
5. Yang, R.; Montoya, A.; Bond, A.; Walton, J.; Kinnamon, J.C. Immunocytochemical analysis of P2X2 in rat circumvallate taste buds. *BMC Neurosci.* **2012**, *13*, 51. [CrossRef] [PubMed]
6. Chaudhari, N.; Roper, S.D. The cell biology of taste. *J. Cell Biol.* **2010**, *190*, 285–296. [CrossRef] [PubMed]
7. Nelson, G.; Hoon, M.A.; Chandrashekar, J.; Zhang, Y.; Ryba, N.J.P.; Zuker, C.S. Mammalian sweet taste receptors. *Cell* **2001**, *106*, 381–390. [CrossRef]
8. Li, X.; Staszewski, L.; Xu, H.; Durick, K.; Zoller, M.; Adler, E. Human receptors for sweet and umami taste. *Proc. Natl. Acad. Sci. USA* **2002**, *99*, 4692–4696. [CrossRef] [PubMed]
9. Jiang, P.; Cui, M.; Zhao, B.; Snyder, L.A.; Benard, L.M.J.; Osman, R.; Max, M.; Margolskee, R.F. Identification of the Cyclamate Interaction Site within the Transmembrane Domain of the Human Sweet Taste Receptor Subunit T1R3. *J. Biol. Chem.* **2005**, *280*, 34296–34305. [CrossRef] [PubMed]
10. Depoortere, I. Taste receptors of the gut: Emerging roles in health and disease. *Gut* **2014**, *63*, 179–190. [CrossRef] [PubMed]

11. Dotson, C.D.; Geraedts, M.C.P.; Munger, S.D. Peptide regulators of peripheral taste function. *Semin. Cell Dev. Biol.* **2013**, *24*, 232–239. [CrossRef] [PubMed]

12. Kohno, D. Sweet taste receptor in the hypothalamus: A potential new player in glucose sensing in the hypothalamus. *J. Physiol. Sci.* **2017**, *67*, 459–465. [CrossRef] [PubMed]

13. Lee, R.J.; Cohen, N.A. Bitter and sweet taste receptors in the respiratory epithelium in health and disease. *J. Mol. Med. Berl. Ger.* **2014**, *92*, 1235–1244. [CrossRef] [PubMed]

14. Meyer, D.; Voigt, A.; Widmayer, P.; Borth, H.; Huebner, S.; Breit, A.; Marschall, S.; Hrabé de Angelis, M.; Boehm, U.; Meyerhof, W.; et al. Expression of Tas1 Taste Receptors in Mammalian Spermatozoa: Functional Role of Tas1r1 in Regulating Basal Ca^{2+} and cAMP Concentrations in Spermatozoa. *PLoS ONE* **2012**, *7*, e32354. [CrossRef] [PubMed]

15. Furness, J.B.; Rivera, L.R.; Cho, H.-J.; Bravo, D.M.; Callaghan, B. The gut as a sensory organ. *Nat. Rev. Gastroenterol. Hepatol.* **2013**, *10*, 729–740. [CrossRef] [PubMed]

16. Raybould, H.E. Nutrient Tasting and Signaling Mechanisms in the Gut. I. Sensing of lipid by the intestinal mucosa. *Am. J. Physiol.-Gastrointest. Liver Physiol.* **1999**, *277*, G751–G755.

17. Owyang, C.; Logsdon, C.D. New insights into neurohormonal regulation of pancreatic secretion. *Gastroenterology* **2004**, *127*, 957–969. [CrossRef] [PubMed]

18. Drucker, D.J. The role of gut hormones in glucose homeostasis. *J. Clin. Investig.* **2007**, *117*, 24–32. [CrossRef] [PubMed]

19. Strader, A.D.; Woods, S.C. Gastrointestinal hormones and food intake. *Gastroenterology* **2005**, *128*, 175–191. [CrossRef] [PubMed]

20. Bezençon, C.; le Coutre, J.; Damak, S. Taste-signaling proteins are coexpressed in solitary intestinal epithelial cells. *Chem. Senses* **2007**, *32*, 41–49. [CrossRef] [PubMed]

21. Margolskee, R.F.; Dyer, J.; Kokrashvili, Z.; Salmon, K.S.H.; Ilegems, E.; Daly, K.; Maillet, E.L.; Ninomiya, Y.; Mosinger, B.; Shirazi-Beechey, S.P. T1R3 and gustducin in gut sense sugars to regulate expression of Na^+-glucose cotransporter 1. *Proc. Natl. Acad. Sci. USA* **2007**, *104*, 15075–15080. [CrossRef] [PubMed]

22. Young, R.L.; Sutherland, K.; Pezos, N.; Brierley, S.M.; Horowitz, M.; Rayner, C.K.; Blackshaw, L.A. Expression of taste molecules in the upper gastrointestinal tract in humans with and without type 2 diabetes. *Gut* **2009**, *58*, 337–346. [CrossRef] [PubMed]

23. Young, R.L. Sensing via Intestinal Sweet Taste Pathways. *Front Neurosci.* **2011**, *5*, 23. [CrossRef] [PubMed]

24. Jang, H.-J.; Kokrashvili, Z.; Theodorakis, M.J.; Carlson, O.D.; Kim, B.-J.; Zhou, J.; Kim, H.H.; Xu, X.; Chan, S.L.; Juhaszova, M.; et al. Gut-expressed gustducin and taste receptors regulate secretion of glucagon-like peptide-1. *Proc. Natl. Acad. Sci. USA* **2007**, *104*, 15069–15074. [CrossRef] [PubMed]

25. Gerspach, A.C.; Steinert, R.E.; Schönenberger, L.; Graber-Maier, A.; Beglinger, C. The role of the gut sweet taste receptor in regulating GLP-1, PYY, and CCK release in humans. *Am. J. Physiol.-Endocrinol. Metab.* **2011**, *301*, E317–E325. [CrossRef] [PubMed]

26. Schirra, J.; Göke, B. The physiological role of GLP-1 in human: Incretin, ileal brake or more? *Regul. Pept.* **2005**, *128*, 109–115. [CrossRef] [PubMed]

27. Horowitz, M.; Nauck, M.A. To be or not to be—An incretin or enterogastrone? *Gut* **2006**, *55*, 148–150. [CrossRef] [PubMed]

28. Geraedts, M.C.P.; Takahashi, T.; Vigues, S.; Markwardt, M.L.; Nkobena, A.; Cockerham, R.E.; Hajnal, A.; Dotson, C.D.; Rizzo, M.A.; Munger, S.D. Transformation of postingestive glucose responses after deletion of sweet taste receptor subunits or gastric bypass surgery. *Am. J. Physiol.-Endocrinol. Metab.* **2012**, *303*, E464–E474. [CrossRef] [PubMed]

29. Gorboulev, V.; Schürmann, A.; Vallon, V.; Kipp, H.; Jaschke, A.; Klessen, D.; Friedrich, A.; Scherneck, S.; Rieg, T.; Cunard, R.; et al. Na(+)-D-glucose cotransporter SGLT1 is pivotal for intestinal glucose absorption and glucose-dependent incretin secretion. *Diabetes* **2012**, *61*, 187–196. [CrossRef] [PubMed]

30. Baggio, L.L.; Drucker, D.J. Biology of incretins: GLP-1 and GIP. *Gastroenterology* **2007**, *132*, 2131–2157. [CrossRef] [PubMed]

31. Mawe, G.M.; Hoffman, J.M. Serotonin signalling in the gut—Functions, dysfunctions and therapeutic targets. *Nat. Rev. Gastroenterol. Hepatol.* **2013**, *10*, 473–486. [CrossRef] [PubMed]

32. Sutherland, K.; Young, R.L.; Cooper, N.J.; Horowitz, M.; Blackshaw, L.A. Phenotypic characterization of taste cells of the mouse small intestine. *Am. J. Physiol.-Gastrointest. Liver Physiol.* **2007**, *292*, G1420–G1428. [CrossRef] [PubMed]

33. Moran, A.W.; Al-Rammahi, M.A.; Arora, D.K.; Batchelor, D.J.; Coulter, E.A.; Ionescu, C.; Bravo, D.; Shirazi-Beechey, S.P. Expression of Na$^+$/glucose co-transporter 1 (SGLT1) in the intestine of piglets weaned to different concentrations of dietary carbohydrate. *Br. J. Nutr.* **2010**, *104*, 647–655. [CrossRef] [PubMed]

34. Kidd, M.; Modlin, I.M.; Gustafsson, B.I.; Drozdov, I.; Hauso, O.; Pfragner, R. Luminal regulation of normal and neoplastic human EC cell serotonin release is mediated by bile salts, amines, tastants, and olfactants. *Am. J. Physiol. Gastrointest. Liver Physiol.* **2008**, *295*, G260–G272. [CrossRef] [PubMed]

35. Dubé, P.E.; Brubaker, P.L. Frontiers in glucagon-like peptide-2: Multiple actions, multiple mediators. *Am. J. Physiol.-Endocrinol. Metab.* **2007**, *293*, E460–E465. [CrossRef] [PubMed]

36. Raybould, H.E. Sensing of glucose in the gastrointestinal tract. *Auton. Neurosci. Basic. Clin.* **2007**, *133*, 86–90. [CrossRef] [PubMed]

37. Reimann, F.; Gribble, F.M. Glucose-Sensing in Glucagon-Like Peptide-1-Secreting Cells. *Diabetes* **2002**, *51*, 2757–2763. [CrossRef] [PubMed]

38. Schuit, F.C.; Huypens, P.; Heimberg, H.; Pipeleers, D.G. Glucose Sensing in Pancreatic β-Cells. *Diabetes* **2001**, *50*, 1–11. [CrossRef] [PubMed]

39. Gribble, F.M.; Williams, L.; Simpson, A.K.; Reimann, F. A novel glucose-sensing mechanism contributing to glucagon-like peptide-1 secretion from the GLUTag cell line. *Diabetes* **2003**, *52*, 1147–1154. [CrossRef] [PubMed]

40. Freeman, S.L.; Bohan, D.; Darcel, N.; Raybould, H.E. Luminal glucose sensing in the rat intestine has characteristics of a sodium-glucose cotransporter. *Am. J. Physiol.-Gastrointest. Liver Physiol.* **2006**, *291*, G439–G445. [CrossRef] [PubMed]

41. Raybould, H.E. Gut chemosensing: Interactions between gut endocrine cells and visceral afferents. *Auton. Neurosci.* **2010**, *153*, 41–46. [CrossRef] [PubMed]

42. Dyer, J.; Daly, K.; Salmon, K.S.H.; Arora, D.K.; Kokrashvili, Z.; Margolskee, R.F.; Shirazi-Beechey, S.P. Intestinal glucose sensing and regulation of intestinal glucose absorption. *Biochem. Soc. Trans.* **2007**, *35*, 1191–1194. [CrossRef] [PubMed]

43. Rozengurt, N.; Wu, S.V.; Chen, M.C.; Huang, C.; Sternini, C.; Rozengurt, E. Colocalization of the α-subunit of gustducin with PYY and GLP-1 in L cells of human colon. *Am. J. Physiol.-Gastrointest. Liver Physiol.* **2006**, *291*, G792–G802. [CrossRef] [PubMed]

44. Hamilton, R.B.; Norgren, R. Central projections of gustatory nerves in the rat. *J. Comp. Neurol.* **1984**, *222*, 560–577. [CrossRef] [PubMed]

45. Norgren, R.; Leonard, C.M. Taste Pathways in Rat Brainstem. *Science* **1971**, *173*, 1136–1139. [CrossRef] [PubMed]

46. Fernstrom, J.D.; Munger, S.D.; Sclafani, A.; de Araujo, I.E.; Roberts, A.; Molinary, S. Mechanisms for sweetness. *J. Nutr.* **2012**, *142*, 1134S–1141S. [CrossRef] [PubMed]

47. Scott, T.R.; Small, D.M. The Role of the Parabrachial Nucleus in Taste Processing and Feeding. *Ann. N. Y. Acad. Sci.* **2009**, *1170*, 372–377. [CrossRef] [PubMed]

48. Chen, X.; Gabitto, M.; Peng, Y.; Ryba, N.J.P.; Zuker, C.S. A gustotopic map of taste qualities in the mammalian brain. *Science* **2011**, *333*, 1262–1266. [CrossRef] [PubMed]

49. Peng, Y.; Gillis-Smith, S.; Jin, H.; Tränkner, D.; Ryba, N.J.P.; Zuker, C.S. Sweet and bitter taste in the brain of awake behaving animals. *Nature* **2015**, *527*, 512–515. [CrossRef] [PubMed]

50. San Gabriel, A.M. Taste receptors in the gastrointestinal system. *Flavour* **2015**, *4*, 14. [CrossRef]

51. DiRocco, R.J.; Grill, H.J. The forebrain is not essential for sympathoadrenal hyperglycemic response to glucoprivation. *Science* **1979**, *204*, 1112–1114. [CrossRef] [PubMed]

52. Perry, B.; Wang, Y. Appetite regulation and weight control: The role of gut hormones. *Nutr. Diabetes* **2012**, *2*, e26. [CrossRef] [PubMed]

53. Grayson, B.E.; Seeley, R.J.; Sandoval, D.A. Wired on sugar: The role of the CNS in the regulation of glucose homeostasis. *Nat. Rev. Neurosci.* **2013**, *14*, 24–37. [CrossRef] [PubMed]

54. Hahn, T.M.; Breininger, J.F.; Baskin, D.G.; Schwartz, M.W. Coexpression of Agrp and NPY in fasting-activated hypothalamic neurons. *Nat. Neurosci.* **1998**, *1*, 271–272. [PubMed]

55. Cone, R.D. Anatomy and regulation of the central melanocortin system. *Nat. Neurosci.* **2005**, *8*, 571–578. [CrossRef] [PubMed]

56. Brüning, J.C.; Gautam, D.; Burks, D.J.; Gillette, J.; Schubert, M.; Orban, P.C.; Klein, R.; Krone, W.; Müller-Wieland, D.; Kahn, C.R. Role of Brain Insulin Receptor in Control of Body Weight and Reproduction. *Science* **2000**, *289*, 2122–2125. [CrossRef] [PubMed]

57. Halaas, J.L.; Gajiwala, K.S.; Maffei, M.; Cohen, S.L.; Chait, B.T.; Rabinowitz, D.; Lallone, R.L.; Burley, S.K.; Friedman, J.M. Weight-reducing effects of the plasma protein encoded by the obese gene. *Science* **1995**, *269*, 543–546. [CrossRef] [PubMed]

58. Baskin, D.G.; Breininger, J.F.; Schwartz, M.W. Leptin receptor mRNA identifies a subpopulation of neuropeptide Y neurons activated by fasting in rat hypothalamus. *Diabetes* **1999**, *48*, 828–833. [CrossRef] [PubMed]

59. Baskin, D.G.; Figlewicz Lattemann, D.; Seeley, R.J.; Woods, S.C.; Porte, D., Jr.; Schwartz, M.W. Insulin and leptin: Dual adiposity signals to the brain for the regulation of food intake and body weight. *Brain Res.* **1999**, *848*, 114–123. [CrossRef]

60. Williams, K.W.; Elmquist, J.K. From neuroanatomy to behavior: Central integration of peripheral signals regulating feeding behavior. *Nat. Neurosci.* **2012**, *15*, 1350–1355. [CrossRef] [PubMed]

61. Kohno, D.; Koike, M.; Ninomiya, Y.; Kojima, I.; Kitamura, T.; Yada, T. Sweet Taste Receptor Serves to Activate Glucose-and Leptin-Responsive Neurons in the Hypothalamic Arcuate Nucleus and Participates in Glucose Responsiveness. *Front Neurosci.* **2016**, *10*, 502. [CrossRef] [PubMed]

62. Friedman, J.M.; Halaas, J.L. Leptin and the regulation of body weight in mammals. *Nature* **1998**, *395*, 763–770. [CrossRef] [PubMed]

63. Zhang, Y.; Proenca, R.; Maffei, M.; Barone, M.; Leopold, L.; Friedman, J.M. Positional cloning of the mouse obese gene and its human homologue. *Nature* **1994**, *372*, 425–432. [CrossRef] [PubMed]

64. Yoshida, R.; Niki, M.; Jyotaki, M.; Sanematsu, K.; Shigemura, N.; Ninomiya, Y. Modulation of sweet responses of taste receptor cells. *Semin. Cell Dev. Biol.* **2013**, *24*, 226–231. [CrossRef] [PubMed]

65. Woods, S.C.; Seeley, R.J.; Porte, D.; Schwartz, M.W. Signals That Regulate Food Intake and Energy Homeostasis. *Science* **1998**, *280*, 1378–1383. [CrossRef] [PubMed]

66. Chen, H.; Charlat, O.; Tartaglia, L.A.; Woolf, E.A.; Weng, X.; Ellis, S.J.; Lakey, N.D.; Culpepper, J.; Moore, K.J.; Breitbart, R.E.; et al. Evidence that the diabetes gene encodes the leptin receptor: Identification of a mutation in the leptin receptor gene in db/db mice. *Cell* **1996**, *84*, 491–495. [CrossRef]

67. Lee, G.H.; Proenca, R.; Montez, J.M.; Carroll, K.M.; Darvishzadeh, J.G.; Lee, J.I. Abnormal splicing of the leptin receptor in diabetic mice. *Nature* **1996**, *379*, 632–635. [CrossRef] [PubMed]

68. Berglund, E.D.; Vianna, C.R.; Donato, J.; Kim, M.H.; Chuang, J.-C.; Lee, C.E.; Friedman, J.M. Direct leptin action on POMC neurons regulates glucose homeostasis and hepatic insulin sensitivity in mice. *J. Clin. Investig.* **2012**, *122*, 1000–1009. [CrossRef] [PubMed]

69. Kawai, K.; Sugimoto, K.; Nakashima, K.; Miura, H.; Ninomiya, Y. Leptin as a modulator of sweet taste sensitivities in mice. *Proc. Natl. Acad. Sci. USA* **2000**, *97*, 11044–11049. [CrossRef] [PubMed]

70. Sinha, M.K.; Sturis, J.; Ohannesian, J.; Magosin, S.; Stephens, T.; Heiman, M.L.; Polonsky, K.S.; Caro, J.F. Ultradian oscillations of leptin secretion in humans. *Biochem. Biophys. Res. Commun.* **1996**, *228*, 733–738. [CrossRef] [PubMed]

71. Nakamura, Y.; Sanematsu, K.; Ohta, R.; Shirosaki, S.; Koyano, K.; Nonaka, K.; Shigemura, N.; Ninomiya, Y. Diurnal variation of human sweet taste recognition thresholds is correlated with plasma leptin levels. *Diabetes* **2008**, *57*, 2661–2665. [CrossRef] [PubMed]

72. Matsuda, L.A.; Lolait, S.J.; Brownstein, M.J.; Young, A.C.; Bonner, T.I. Structure of a cannabinoid receptor and functional expression of the cloned cDNA. *Nature* **1990**, *346*, 561–564. [CrossRef] [PubMed]

73. Munro, S.; Thomas, K.L.; Abu-Shaar, M. Molecular characterization of a peripheral receptor for cannabinoids. *Nature* **1993**, *365*, 61–65. [CrossRef] [PubMed]

74. Cota, D.; Marsicano, G.; Tschöp, M.; Grübler, Y.; Flachskamm, C.; Schubert, M.; Auer, D.; Yassouridis, A.; Thöne-Reineke, C.; Ortmann, S.; et al. The endogenous cannabinoid system affects energy balance via central orexigenic drive and peripheral lipogenesis. *J. Clin. Investig.* **2003**, *112*, 423–431. [CrossRef] [PubMed]

75. Jamshidi, N.; Taylor, D.A. Anandamide administration into the ventromedial hypothalamus stimulates appetite in rats. *Br. J. Pharmacol.* **2001**, *134*, 1151–1154. [CrossRef] [PubMed]

76. Di Marzo, V.; Goparaju, S.K.; Wang, L.; Liu, J.; Bátkai, S.; Járai, Z.; Fezza, F.; Miura, G.I.; Palmiter, R.D.; Sugiura, T.; et al. Leptin-regulated endocannabinoids are involved in maintaining food intake. *Nature* **2001**, *410*, 822–825. [CrossRef] [PubMed]

77. Ravinet Trillou, C.; Delgorge, C.; Menet, C.; Arnone, M.; Soubrié, P. CB1 cannabinoid receptor knockout in mice leads to leanness, resistance to diet-induced obesity and enhanced leptin sensitivity. *Int. J. Obes.* **2004**, *28*, 640–648. [CrossRef] [PubMed]

78. Jo, Y.-H.; Chen, Y.-J.J.; Chua, J.; Talmage, D.A.; Role, L.W. Integration of endocannabinoid and leptin signaling in an appetite-related neural circuit. *Neuron* **2005**, *48*, 1055–1066. [CrossRef] [PubMed]

79. Yoshida, R.; Ohkuri, T.; Jyotaki, M.; Yasuo, T.; Horio, N.; Yasumatsu, K.; Sanematsu, K.; Shigemura, N.; Yamamoto, T.; Margolskee, R.F.; et al. Endocannabinoids selectively enhance sweet taste. *Proc. Natl. Acad. Sci. USA* **2010**, *107*, 935–939. [CrossRef] [PubMed]

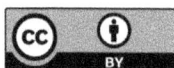

nutrients

MDPI

Review

Early Life Fructose Exposure and Its Implications for Long-Term Cardiometabolic Health in Offspring

Jia Zheng [1], Qianyun Feng [2], Qian Zhang [1], Tong Wang [1] and Xinhua Xiao [1,*]

[1] Department of Endocrinology, Key Laboratory of Endocrinology, Ministry of Health, Peking Union Medical College Hospital, Diabetes Research Center of Chinese Academy of Medical Sciences & Peking Union Medical College, Beijing 100730, China; zhengjiapumc@163.com (J.Z.); rubiacordifolia@yahoo.com (Q.Z.); tongtong0716@sina.com (T.W.)

[2] Department of Pediatrics, The Second Teaching Hospital of Tianjin University of Traditional Chinese Medicine, Tianjin 300193, China; fengqianyun@yahoo.com

* Correspondence: xiaoxinhua@medmail.com.cn; Tel./Fax: +86-10-6915-5073

Received: 17 September 2016; Accepted: 24 October 2016; Published: 1 November 2016

Abstract: It has become increasingly clear that maternal nutrition can strongly influence the susceptibility of adult offspring to cardiometabolic disease. For decades, it has been thought that excessive intake of fructose, such as sugar-sweetened beverages and foods, has been linked to increased risk of obesity, type 2 diabetes, and cardiovascular disease in various populations. These deleterious effects of excess fructose consumption in adults are well researched, but limited data are available on the long-term effects of high fructose exposure during gestation, lactation, and infancy. This review aims to examine the evidence linking early life fructose exposure during critical periods of development and its implications for long-term cardiometabolic health in offspring.

Keywords: early life; fructose; sugar-sweetened beverages; cardiometabolic health; offspring

1. Introduction

The prevalence of obesity and type 2 diabetes are increasing dramatically throughout the world, now considered a pandemic non-communicable disease. In 2015, the International Diabetes Federation estimated that 415 million people worldwide have diabetes, and the number will rise to 642 million by 2040, implying that one in eleven adults will have diabetes. Moreover, one in seven births is affected by gestational diabetes [1]. As such, type 2 diabetes yields enormous tolls at individual, public health, and economic levels.

In recent years, it has become increasingly clear that susceptibility to obesity and type 2 diabetes is strongly influenced by exposure to an adverse early life development environment during pregnancy and postnatal life. A combination of human epidemiology studies and rodent studies has clearly established that maternal environment—especially nutrition during pregnancy and the postnatal period—are critical factors influencing the development of cardiometabolic disease, such as obesity, type 2 diabetes, and cardiovascular diseases in offspring [2–4]. Growing numbers of clinical and animal studies suggest that maternal consumption of a diet high in fat and other potential nutrients promotes obesity and increased metabolic risk in offspring. However, little is known about the effects of fructose exposure during early life development.

2. An Overview of Fructose

2.1. Consumption of Fructose Is Increasing

Fructose, or fruit sugar, is a simple ketonic monosaccharide found in many plants. It is one of the three dietary monosaccharides, and can be absorbed directly into the bloodstream. Fructose is widely used commercially in foods and beverages, due to its low cost and high relative sweetness. Fructose is the sweetest of all naturally-occurring carbohydrates; however, we rarely consume fructose in isolation. The major source of fructose in the diet comes from fructose-containing sugars, such as sucrose and high fructose corn syrup (HFCS) [5]. A national survey in the United States showed that the mean intake of total fructose increased from 8.1% in 1978 to 9.1% in 2004 as a percentage of total energy. It is important to note that this increase was greater in adolescents and young adults [6]. The intake of refined sugar—particularly HFCS—has increased from a yearly estimate of 8.1 kg/person at the beginning of the nineteenth century to a current estimate of 65 kg/person [7]. Sugar-sweetened beverages (SSBs) are the greatest source of fructose-containing sugars in the diet, and the consumption of SSBs shows a steady increase in both children and adults [8]. The National Health and Nutrition Examination Survey showed that one-half of the population consumes SSBs on any given day, and 25% consumes at least 200 kcal in United States [9]. It is noticeable that fructose was primarily from artificially sweetened beverages and SSBs, but not from naturally occurring fructose in fruits.

2.2. Adverse Metabolic Effects of Fructose

The consumption of fructose has become a hot topic, due to its multiple metabolic effects [10]. For decades, it has been thought that excessive intake of fructose from SSBs and foods has been linked to increased risk of obesity, type 2 diabetes, and cardiovascular disease in various populations [11]. One large clinical study showed a close parallel between the rise in HFCS intake and the obesity and diabetes epidemics in the United States [12]. Excess fructose consumption has been demonstrated to be a risk factor of insulin resistance [13], elevated low-density lipoprotein cholesterol (LDL-c), and triglycerides [14], leading to obesity, type 2 diabetes, and cardiovascular disease [15]. The Nurses' Health Study cohort study showed that women consuming one or more sugar-sweetened soft drinks per day had an 83% greater risk of developing type 2 diabetes mellitus over the course of eight years compared with those who consumed less than one of these beverages per month [16]. It also indicated that a higher level of SSB intake was found to increase the risk of developing nonfatal myocardial infarction and fatal coronary heart disease, and women who consumed ≥2 SSBs per day had a 35% greater risk of coronary heart disease, compared to infrequent consumers [17]. One recent meta-analysis of nine prospective cohort studies with 308,420 participants, conducted in the USA, Japan, Sweden, and Singapore found a greater risk of myocardial infarction and stroke with incremental increase in the consumption of SSBs [18]. Therefore, widespread increase in dietary fructose consumption is associated with the development of chronic cardiometabolic disorders.

3. Early Life Fructose Exposure and Long-Term Cardiometabolic Health

3.1. Implications of Human Studies

The deleterious effects of excess fructose consumption in adults are well researched, but limited data are available on the long-term effects of high fructose exposure during gestation, lactation, and infancy. More importantly, emerging research suggests that fructose consumption by both mothers and their offspring during these stages of early life can lead to persistent metabolic dysfunction. It is common sense that fresh fruit and vegetable intake during pregnancy has multiple benefits to the mothers and babies. One clinical cohort study of pregnant women conducted by the Norwegian Institute of Public Health found that intakes of foods high in natural sugars (such as fresh and dried fruits) are associated with decreased risk of preeclampsia [19,20]. However, because fructose was mainly from artificially sweetened beverages and SSBs and not from natural fruit, most pregnant women are exposed to the same artificially sweetened foods and beverages as the general non-pregnant population. It reported that added sugar represents 14% of the energy intake in diets consumed by pregnant women [21]. Little clinical research exists addressing the effect of excessive fructose during pregnancy. One large prospective cohort study of 60,761 pregnant women showed that high intake of both artificially sweetened beverages and SSBs during pregnancy were associated with increased risks of preterm delivery [22]. Therefore, high intake of fructose from artificially sweetened beverages and SSBs will impact pregnancy outcomes.

3.2. Implications of Rodent Experiments

Some rodent experiments have also demonstrated that excessive fructose consumption during early development can increase the incidence of metabolic disorders Studies in rats have shown that the adult male offspring suckled by mothers consuming an iso-caloric fructose-rich diet during lactation displayed increased body weight and food intake, enhanced leptinemia, and impaired insulin sensitivity, with decreased hypothalamic ob-Rb gene expression and STAT-3 phosphorylation [23]. In rats, dams fed a high fructose (20%) solution during pregnancy and lactation displayed sex-specific effects on placental growth and fetal and neonatal metabolic profiles [24]. Maternal fructose intake significantly elevated circulating plasma fructose and leptin levels in female fetuses. By postnatal day 10, both male and female neonates born to fructose-fed mothers showed high circulating fructose and insulin levels, as well as increased leptin content [24]. Additional studies showed that dams with fed 100 g/L fructose ate more food and drank less water. Moreover, the offspring of fructose-fed dams had almost double the fasting insulin levels at weaning compared with the offspring of glucose-fed dams [25].

Further experiments revealed that a maternal 60% fructose diet led to increased serum triglycerides, free fatty acids, and insulin in offspring at 23 weeks old. This was concomitant with elevated increased expression of carnitine palmitoyltransferase (CPT1a) and acetyl-coenzyme A carboxylase beta (ACC2), and decreased expression of peroxisome proliferatoractivated receptor-α (PPARα) and PPAR-gamma coactivator 1-α (PGC1-α) [26]. A recent study showed that maternal consumption of a high-fructose diet leads to the developmental programming of adverse cardiometabolic health in offspring at 1 year of age, including obesity, hypertension, insulin resistance, increased liver fat infiltrates, and visceral adipose tissue [27]. Another recent study found that male offspring exposed to a maternal fructose-rich diet during pregnancy developed severe hyperglycemia, hypertriglyceridemia, hyperleptinemia, and augmented adipose tissue mass with hypertrophic adipocytes [28]. Gray et al. showed that excess fructose consumption before and during pregnancy lead to a marked skew in the secondary sex ratio and reduced fertility, reflected as a 50% reduction in preimplantation and term litter size [29]. They further found that increased fructose in the maternal diet had lasting effects on offspring cardiovascular function, including hypertension, heart rate, and relative non-dipping of nocturnal pressure that was sex-dependent and related to the offspring's stress–response axis. Up-regulation of vasoconstrictor, anti-natriuretic, or diminished vasodilatory pathways may be causal [30]. Tain et al. found that maternal high-fructose diet caused increases in blood pressure in the 12-week-old offspring, and melatonin therapy blunted the high-fructose-induced programmed hypertension and increased nitric oxide level in the kidney [31]. They further showed that aliskiren administration prevented high-fructose-induced programmed hypertension in both sexes of adult offspring, which increased angiotensin-converting enzyme 2 and angiotensin (1–7) receptor (MAS) protein levels in female kidneys [32]. Together, the above studies (summarized in Table 1) suggest that excessive fructose exposure during fetal and early postnatal development increases the susceptibility to hypertension, hypertriglyceridemia, insulin resistance, and possibly other metabolic disturbances later in life.

Table 1. Summary of early life fructose exposure and cardiometabolic health in rodents.

Fructose Exposure	Species	Age	Metabolic Disorders	Potential Mechanism	Reference
Maternal iso-caloric 10% fructose rich diet during lactation	Sprague Dawley rats	Between 49–60 days	Increased body weight and food intake, enhanced leptinemia, and impaired insulin sensitivity	Disrupted hypothalamic activity: decreased hypothalamic ob-Rb gene expression and STAT-3 phosphorylation	Alzamendi et al. [23]
Maternal 20% of caloric intake from fructose from day 1 of pregnancy until postnatal day 10	Wistar rats	Embryonic day 21 and postnatal day 10	Elevated circulating plasma fructose, insulin, and leptin levels	Placental fructose sensitivity and transfer: glucose transporter 5 and IGF-1	Vickers et al. [24]
Maternal 100 g/L fructose water during pregnancy	Sprague Dawley rats	Postweaning day 5	Hyperglycemia and hyperinsulinemia	Elevated phosphoenolpyruvate carboxykinase	Rawana et al. [25]
Maternal 60% fructose throughout pregnancy and lactation	Sprague Dawley rats	14–23 weeks old	Increased serum triglycerides, free fatty acids, and insulin	Increased expression of ACC2 and CPT1α, and decreased expression of PPARα and PGC1-α	Ching et al. [26]
Maternal 10% fructose during pregnancy	C57BL/6J mouse	1 year old	Hypertension, insulin resistance, and obesity	Increased expression of PTP1B and JNK	Saad et al. [27]
Maternal 10% fructose during pregnancy	Sprague Dawley rats	60 days	Hyperglycemia, hypertriglyceridemia, and hyperleptinemia	Reduced adipocyte precursor cells number	Alzamendi et al. [28]
Maternal 10% fructose during before conception and during the mating period	Sprague Dawley rats	At day 20 gestation	Growth, fertility, sex ratio, and birth order	Glycolyzable monosaccharide on the maternal ovary and/or ovulated oocyte	Gray et al. [29]
Maternal 10% fructose before and during gestation and through lactation	Sprague Dawley rats	9 to 14 weeks of age	Hypertension	Vasoconstrictor, anti-natriuretic, or diminished vasodilatory pathways	Gray et al. [30]
60% fructose throughout pregnancy and lactation	Sprague Dawley rats	12 weeks of age	Hypertension	Nitric oxide and arachidonic acid metabolites	Tain et al. [31]
60% fructose throughout pregnancy and lactation	Sprague Dawley rats	12 weeks of age	Hypertension	ACE and MAS	Hsu et al. [32]

STAT-3: signal transducer and activator of transcription-3; IGF-1: insulin-like growth factors-1; ACC2: acetyl-coenzyme A carboxylase beta; CPT1a: carnitine palmitoyltransferase; PPARα: peroxisome proliferatoractivated receptor-α; PGC1-α: PPAR-gamma coactivator 1-α; PTP1B: protein tyrosine phosphatase 1B; JNK: phosphorylation of c-Jun *N*-terminal kinase; ACE: angiotensin-converting enzyme; MAS: angiotensin (1–7) receptor.

3.3. Potential Mechanisms of Early Life Fructose Exposure and Cardiometabolic Health

Gestation and early postnatal life is a critical time window that can affect the growth and development of offspring. It is widely accepted that maternal and postnatal nutrition status is a key determinant of offspring health. The Developmental Origins of Health and Disease (DOHaD) hypothesis proposes that exposures during early life play a critical role in determining the risk of developing metabolic diseases in adulthood, and is also known as the "fetal programming hypothesis" [33]. Although little information is available about the mechanisms between early life fructose exposure and cardiometabolic health, we speculate that "metabolic programming" is the underlying mechanism, because it can link maternal nutrition and metabolic health in offspring.

Several potential points could explain the adverse effects of high fructose exposure during these periods, which are summarized in Figure 1. First, fructose can bypass the main rate-limiting step of glycolysis at the level of phosphofructokinase and provide lipogenic substrates for conversion to fatty acids and triglycerides as well as transcription factors and enzymes involved in lipogenesis, including acetyl-coenzyme A carboxylase and sterol regulatory element binding protein 1c; thus, it can lead to increased hepatic de novo lipogenesis [5]. Second, a rodent study showed that a maternal fructose-rich diet during lactation decreased hypothalamic sensitivity to exogenous leptin, enhanced food intake, and decreased several anorexigenic signals (e.g., corticotropin-releasing hormone, thyrotropin-releasing hormone, cocaine- and amphetamine-regulated transcript, proopiomelanocortin) in offspring [23]. Third, fructose is transported passively across membranes by a member of the facilitative glucose transporter (GLUT) family, named GLUT5 [34]. David et al. showed that GLUT5 expression and function in weaning and post-weaning rats can be markedly enhanced in vivo by the consumption of high-fructose diets [35]. However, it is still unclear whether the impacts on the offspring are the direct effects of fructose transfer through the placenta or the mother's milk, or due to adaptive responses to altered maternal metabolism. Thus, further studies are urgently warranted to clarify the underlying mechanisms.

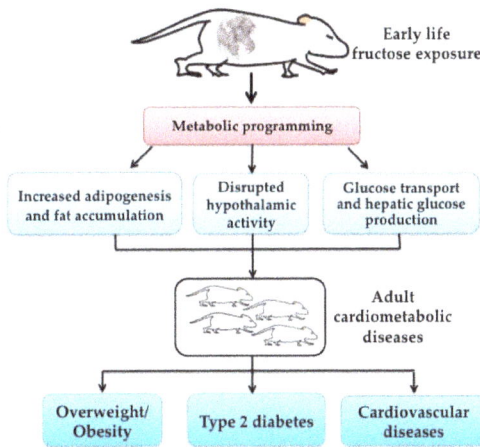

Figure 1. Early life fructose exposure and long-term cardiometabolic health.

4. Conclusions

In summary, pregnancy and early postnatal life are the critical periods of growth and development, and are sensitive to the environment. One important point that should be taken into consideration is that early life fructose exposure may determine the susceptibility of long-term metabolic diseases in offspring. However, limited data suggest that the offspring would be protected from these well-known adverse effects during early life. More intervention studies are necessary to explore the beneficial measures. Moreover, little information is available regarding which period is more critical to determine the risks of cardiometabolic diseases in offspring. Further investigations are imperative to determine the effects of excess fructose consumption during critical periods of gestation, lactation, and early postnatal period. The increasing rates of obesity, prediabetes, and diabetes in individuals of reproductive age can initiate a vicious cycle, propagating risk to subsequent generations. A better understanding of the role and mechanism of early life fructose exposure and metabolic health can provide critical implications for the early prevention of obesity and type 2 diabetes, and ensure a healthier future for subsequent generations.

Acknowledgments: This work was supported by the National Natural Science Foundation of China (No. 81570715), National Key Research and Development Program of China (No. 2016YFA0101002) and National Natural Science Foundation for Young Scholars of China (No. 81300649).

Author Contributions: Z.J. and X.H.H. have made substantial contributions to ideas, conception and design of the review. F.Q.Y. and Y.M. have been involved in drafting the manuscript and revising it critically for important intellectual content. Q.Z. and T.W. reviewed and edited the manuscript. X.H.X. contributed to the design and reviewed and edited the manuscript.

Conflicts of Interest: The authors declare no conflict of interest.

References

1. International Diabetes Federation (IDF). *IDF Diabetes Atlas*, 7th ed.; IDF: Brussels, Belgium, 2015.
2. Pinhas-Hamiel, O.; Zeitler, P. The global spread of type 2 diabetes mellitus in children and adolescents. *J. Pediatr.* **2005**, *146*, 693–700. [CrossRef] [PubMed]
3. Rando, O.J.; Simmons, R.A. I'm eating for two: Parental dietary effects on offspring metabolism. *Cell* **2015**, *161*, 93–105. [CrossRef] [PubMed]
4. Patel, N.; Pasupathy, D.; Poston, L. Determining the consequences of maternal obesity for offspring health. *Exp. Physiol.* **2015**, *100*, 1421–1428. [CrossRef] [PubMed]
5. Malik, V.S.; Hu, F.B. Fructose and cardiometabolic health: What the evidence from sugar-sweetened beverages tells us. *J. Am. Coll. Cardiol.* **2015**, *66*, 1615–1624. [CrossRef] [PubMed]
6. Marriott, B.P.; Cole, N.; Lee, E. National estimates of dietary fructose intake increased from 1977 to 2004 in the United States. *J. Nutr.* **2009**, *139*, 1228s–1235s. [CrossRef] [PubMed]
7. Stephan, B.C.; Wells, J.C.; Brayne, C.; Albanese, E.; Siervo, M. Increased fructose intake as a risk factor for dementia. *J. Gerontol. Ser. A Biol. Sci. Méd. Sci.* **2010**, *65*, 809–814. [CrossRef] [PubMed]
8. Hu, F.B.; Malik, V.S. Sugar-sweetened beverages and risk of obesity and type 2 diabetes: Epidemiologic evidence. *Physiol. Behav.* **2010**, *100*, 47–54. [CrossRef] [PubMed]
9. Ogden, C.L.; Kit, B.K.; Carroll, M.D.; Park, S. Consumption of sugar drinks in the United States, 2005–2008. *NCHS Data Brief* **2011**, *71*, 1–8.
10. Rosset, R.; Surowska, A.; Tappy, L. Pathogenesis of cardiovascular and metabolic diseases: Are fructose-containing sugars more involved than other dietary calories? *Curr. Hypertens. Rep.* **2016**, *18*, 44. [CrossRef] [PubMed]
11. Goran, M.I.; Dumke, K.; Bouret, S.G.; Kayser, B.; Walker, R.W.; Blumberg, B. The obesogenic effect of high fructose exposure during early development. *Nat. Rev. Endocrinol.* **2013**, *9*, 494–500. [CrossRef] [PubMed]
12. Bray, G.A.; Nielsen, S.J.; Popkin, B.M. Consumption of high-fructose corn syrup in beverages may play a role in the epidemic of obesity. *Am. J. Clin. Nutr.* **2004**, *79*, 537–543. [PubMed]
13. Elliott, S.S.; Keim, N.L.; Stern, J.S.; Teff, K.; Havel, P.J. Fructose, weight gain, and the insulin resistance syndrome. *Am. J. Clin. Nutr.* **2002**, *76*, 911–922. [PubMed]
14. Basciano, H.; Federico, L.; Adeli, K. Fructose, insulin resistance, and metabolic dyslipidemia. *Nutr. Metab.* **2005**, *2*, 5. [CrossRef] [PubMed]
15. Rippe, J.M.; Angelopoulos, T.J. Fructose-containing sugars and cardiovascular disease. *Adv. Nutr.* **2015**, *6*, 430–439. [CrossRef] [PubMed]
16. Schulze, M.B.; Manson, J.E.; Ludwig, D.S.; Colditz, G.A.; Stampfer, M.J.; Willett, W.C.; Hu, F.B. Sugar-sweetened beverages, weight gain, and incidence of type 2 diabetes in young and middle-aged women. *JAMA* **2004**, *292*, 927–934. [CrossRef] [PubMed]

17. Fung, T.T.; Malik, V.; Rexrode, K.M.; Manson, J.E.; Willett, W.C.; Hu, F.B. Sweetened beverage consumption and risk of coronary heart disease in women. *Am. J. Clin. Nutr.* **2009**, *89*, 1037–1042. [CrossRef] [PubMed]

18. Narain, A.; Kwok, C.S.; Mamas, M.A. Soft drinks and sweetened beverages and the risk of cardiovascular disease and mortality: A systematic review and meta-analysis. *Int. J. Clin. Pract.* **2016**, *70*, 791–805. [CrossRef] [PubMed]

19. Brantsaeter, A.L.; Haugen, M.; Samuelsen, S.O.; Torjusen, H.; Trogstad, L.; Alexander, J.; Magnus, P.; Meltzer, H.M. A dietary pattern characterized by high intake of vegetables, fruits, and vegetable oils is associated with reduced risk of preeclampsia in nulliparous pregnant Norwegian women. *J. Nutr.* **2009**, *139*, 1162–1168. [CrossRef] [PubMed]

20. Borgen, I.; Aamodt, G.; Harsem, N.; Haugen, M.; Meltzer, H.M.; Brantsaeter, A.L. Maternal sugar consumption and risk of preeclampsia in nulliparous Norwegian women. *Eur. J. Clin. Nutr.* **2012**, *66*, 920–925. [CrossRef] [PubMed]

21. George, G.C.; Hanss-Nuss, H.; Milani, T.J.; Freeland-Graves, J.H. Food choices of low-income women during pregnancy and postpartum. *J. Am. Diet. Assoc.* **2005**, *105*, 899–907. [CrossRef] [PubMed]

22. Englund-Ogge, L.; Brantsaeter, A.L.; Haugen, M.; Sengpiel, V.; Khatibi, A.; Myhre, R.; Myking, S.; Meltzer, H.M.; Kacerovsky, M.; Nilsen, R.M.; et al. Association between intake of artificially sweetened and sugar-sweetened beverages and preterm delivery: A large prospective cohort study. *Am. J. Clin. Nutr.* **2012**, *96*, 552–559. [CrossRef] [PubMed]

23. Alzamendi, A.; Castrogiovanni, D.; Gaillard, R.C.; Spinedi, E.; Giovambattista, A. Increased male offspring's risk of metabolic-neuroendocrine dysfunction and overweight after fructose-rich diet intake by the lactating mother. *Endocrinology* **2010**, *151*, 4214–4223. [CrossRef] [PubMed]

24. Vickers, M.H.; Clayton, Z.E.; Yap, C.; Sloboda, D.M. Maternal fructose intake during pregnancy and lactation alters placental growth and leads to sex-specific changes in fetal and neonatal endocrine function. *Endocrinology* **2011**, *152*, 1378–1387. [CrossRef] [PubMed]

25. Rawana, S.; Clark, K.; Zhong, S.; Buison, A.; Chackunkal, S.; Jen, K.L. Low dose fructose ingestion during gestation and lactation affects carbohydrate metabolism in rat dams and their offspring. *J. Nutr.* **1993**, *123*, 2158–2165. [PubMed]

26. Ching, R.H.; Yeung, L.O.; Tse, I.M.; Sit, W.H.; Li, E.T. Supplementation of bitter melon to rats fed a high-fructose diet during gestation and lactation ameliorates fructose-induced dyslipidemia and hepatic oxidative stress in male offspring. *J. Nutr.* **2011**, *141*, 1664–1672. [CrossRef] [PubMed]

27. Saad, A.F.; Dickerson, J.; Kechichian, T.B.; Yin, H.; Gamble, P.; Salazar, A.; Patrikeev, I.; Motamedi, M.; Saade, G.R.; Costantine, M.M. High-fructose diet in pregnancy leads to fetal programming of hypertension, insulin resistance, and obesity in adult offspring. *Am. J. Obstet. Gynecol.* **2016**, *215*, 378. [CrossRef] [PubMed]

28. Alzamendi, A.; Zubiria, G.; Moreno, G.; Portales, A.; Spinedi, E.; Giovambattista, A. High risk of metabolic and adipose tissue dysfunctions in adult male progeny, due to prenatal and adulthood malnutrition induced by fructose rich diet. *Nutrients* **2016**, *8*, 178. [CrossRef] [PubMed]

29. Gray, C.; Long, S.; Green, C.; Gardiner, S.M.; Craigon, J.; Gardner, D.S. Maternal fructose and/or salt intake and reproductive outcome in the rat: Effects on growth, fertility, sex ratio, and birth order. *Biol. Reprod.* **2013**, *89*, 51. [CrossRef] [PubMed]

30. Gray, C.; Gardiner, S.M.; Elmes, M.; Gardner, D.S. Excess maternal salt or fructose intake programmes sex-specific, stress- and fructose-sensitive hypertension in the offspring. *Br. J. Nutr.* **2016**, *115*, 594–604. [CrossRef] [PubMed]

31. Tain, Y.L.; Leu, S.; Wu, K.L.; Lee, W.C.; Chan, J.Y. Melatonin prevents maternal fructose intake-induced programmed hypertension in the offspring: Roles of nitric oxide and arachidonic acid metabolites. *J. Pineal Res.* **2014**, *57*, 80–89. [CrossRef] [PubMed]

32. Hsu, C.N.; Wu, K.L.; Lee, W.C.; Leu, S.; Chan, J.Y.; Tain, Y.L. Aliskiren administration during early postnatal life sex-specifically alleviates hypertension programmed by maternal high fructose consumption. *Front. Physiol.* **2016**, *7*, 299. [CrossRef] [PubMed]

33. Wallack, L.; Thornburg, K. Developmental origins, epigenetics, and equity: Moving upstream. *Matern. Child Health J.* **2016**, *20*, 935–940. [CrossRef] [PubMed]

34. Douard, V.; Ferraris, R.P. Regulation of the fructose transporter GLUT5 in health and disease. *Am. J. Physiol. Endocrinol. Metab.* **2008**, *295*, E227–E237. [CrossRef] [PubMed]
35. David, E.S.; Cingari, D.S.; Ferraris, R.P. Dietary induction of intestinal fructose absorption in weaning rats. *Pediatr. Res.* **1995**, *37*, 777–782. [CrossRef] [PubMed]

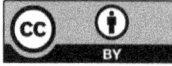

nutrients

MDPI

Review

Maternal Fructose Intake Affects Transcriptome Changes and Programmed Hypertension in Offspring in Later Life

You-Lin Tain [1,2], Julie Y. H. Chan [2] and Chien-Ning Hsu [3,4,*]

1   Department of Pediatrics, Kaohsiung Chang Gung Memorial Hospital, Chang Gung University College of Medicine, Kaohsiung 833, Taiwan; tainyl@hotmail.com
2   Institute for Translational Research in Biomedicine, Kaohsiung Chang Gung Memorial Hospital, Chang Gung University College of Medicine, Kaohsiung 833, Taiwan; jchan@cgmh.org.tw
3   Department of Pharmacy, Kaohsiung Chang Gung Memorial Hospital, Kaohsiung 833, Taiwan
4   School of Pharmacy, Kaohsiung Medical University, Kaohsiung 807, Taiwan
*   Correspondence: chien_ning_hsu@hotmail.com; Tel.: +886-975-368-975; Fax: +886-7733-8009

Received: 8 October 2016; Accepted: 21 November 2016; Published: 25 November 2016

Abstract: Hypertension originates from early-life insults by so-called "developmental origins of health and disease" (DOHaD). Studies performed in the previous few decades indicate that fructose consumption is associated with an increase in hypertension rate. It is emerging field that tends to unfold the nutrient–gene interactions of maternal high-fructose (HF) intake on the offspring which links renal programming to programmed hypertension. Reprogramming interventions counteract disturbed nutrient–gene interactions induced by maternal HF intake and exert protective effects against developmentally programmed hypertension. Here, we review the key themes on the effect of maternal HF consumption on renal transcriptome changes and programmed hypertension. We have particularly focused on the following areas: metabolic effects of fructose on hypertension and kidney disease; effects of maternal HF consumption on hypertension development in adult offspring; effects of maternal HF consumption on renal transcriptome changes; and application of reprogramming interventions to prevent maternal HF consumption-induced programmed hypertension in animal models. Provision of personalized nutrition is still a faraway goal. Therefore, there is an urgent need to understand early-life nutrient–gene interactions and to develop effective reprogramming strategies for treating hypertension and other HF consumption-related diseases.

Keywords: developmental programming; developmental origins of health and disease (DOHaD); fructose; hypertension; kidney; next-generation sequencing; reprogramming; transcriptome

1. Introduction

Fructose consumption has grown over the past several decades and its growth has been paralleled by an increase in hypertension [1–3]. Nutrition during pregnancy and lactation exerts long-term effects on the health of offspring. Developmental origins of health and disease (DOHaD) is an emerging branch of science that assesses the effects of these early insults on the health of offspring [4]. Adult-onset hypertension develops from nutritional insults in early life [5]. Because the developing kidney is particularly vulnerable to insults of programming in early life, renal programming plays an essential role in the developmental programming of hypertension [6]. The DOHaD concept offers a novel approach to prevent programmed hypertension through reprogramming [7].

This review provides an overview of maternal high-fructose (HF) consumption-induced gene–diet interactions in the offspring kidneys that affect programmed hypertension, with an emphasis on the following areas: metabolic effects of fructose on hypertension and the kidney; effects of maternal HF consumption on programmed hypertension; effects of maternal HF consumption on renal transcriptome changes; and application of reprogramming interventions to prevent maternal HF-induced programmed hypertension.

2. Metabolic Effects of Fructose on Renal Biology and Hypertension

Fructose is a monosaccharide naturally present in honey, fruits, and vegetables. In our body, fructose is endogenously produced from glucose through aldose reductase pathway and is also obtained through exogenous supply [8]. Because the food industry refines fructose and adds it to various processed foods, our fructose consumption has increased dramatically in the past few decades [2]. Most of our daily fructose comes from HF corn syrup and refined sugar (e.g., table sugar). Fructose is absorbed in the intestine through specific glucose transporters such as glucose transporter 5 (Glut 5) and Glut 2. The liver is the major site of fructose metabolism. Fructose is converted into glucose, lactate, and fatty acids [8]. Fructose metabolism differs markedly from glucose metabolism because these two sugars require different enzymes in the initial steps of metabolism. Fructose is oxidized to CO_2 and is then converted to lactate and glucose; moreover, fructose leads to ATP depletion and uric acid production and does not induce insulin release [8].

Limited epidemiological data indicate that fructose exerts pressor effects, thus increasing blood pressure (BP) [9,10]. Although human experimental studies have reported the acute effects of dietary fructose on BP [11–13], its chronic effects have not been established to date. Moreover, although the kidneys are particularly sensitive to the effects of fructose, only a few epidemiological studies have examined the relationship between fructose consumption and renal disease [11]. Thus, human studies have not yet established the direct cause-and-effect relationship between excessive fructose consumption and hypertension and kidney disease. HF diets have been used to generate animal models of hypertension and kidney disease [14–16]. Similar to the results of human studies [17,18], results of animal studies indicate that rats fed HF diet develop various features of metabolic syndrome, including hypertriglyceridemia, insulin resistance, obesity, hyperinsulinemia, and hypertension [16,19]. Adverse effects of fructose feeding depend on the amount and duration of fructose consumption. Because rats express uricase (which degrades uric acid) and because they develop early phenotypes after exposure to high fructose concentrations, most studies on rats have been performed using diets containing 50%–60% fructose [16]. Although most studies on fructose-induced hypertension have used fructose doses amounting to ~60% of the total energy requirement [16], evidence indicates that 20% fructose diet significantly increases BP in rats after 8 months [20]. Fructose induces renal hypertrophy and tubulointerstitial disease in the rat kidneys [21]. Numerous pathways have been proposed to induce fructose-induced hypertension, including oxidative stress, increased sodium absorption, endothelial dysfunction, nitric oxide (NO) deficiency, renin-angiotensin system (RAS) activation, and sympathetic nervous system stimulation [16,22]. Fructose increases the reabsorption of salt and water in the kidneys; thus, a combination of fructose and salt exerts synergistic effect on hypertension development [23].

3. Effect of Maternal Fructose Consumption on Programmed Hypertension

Although numerous studies have assessed the effect of fructose on adult metabolism, limited studies have explored the effects of maternal fructose consumption on fetus and disease risk in offspring. Thus far, only a limited number of human studies have shown an association between excessive sweetened food and beverage consumption and poor pregnancy outcome [24]. Animal studies have shown that fructose alone alters fetal and offspring metabolism [24]. However, several animal studies have often used fructose as a part of diet along with sucrose, fat, and salt.

Several studies have shown that HF diet induces hypertension in adult rats, which have been well reviewed elsewhere [16,22,25]. However, limited data are available at present on the effects of maternal fructose consumption on the BP of adult offspring. Studies listed in Table 1 indicate that consumption of HF alone or as a part of diet by rodent mothers induces programmed hypertension in adult offspring [26–33]. We found that adult offspring of mothers exposed to 60% HF diet during pregnancy and lactation developed hypertension [26], which is consistent with the results of earlier studies involving fructose-fed adult rats [16,19]. "Western diet" is characterized by the high intake of high-sugar drinks, high-fat products, and excess salt. Therefore, it is important to consider the potential interactions and programmed processes between fructose, fat, and salt. Animal studies examining the combined effects of maternal fructose consumption and other key components of the Western diet (e.g., high fat and high salt) have shown their synergistic effects on the elevation of BP in adult offspring [29,30].

Table 1. Maternal high-fructose (HF) consumption exerts programming effects on blood pressure (BP) in rodent models.

Types of Fructose Intake	Strain	Programming Effects	Age at Which the Effects Were Measured	References
10% w/v fructose plus 4% NaCl in drinking water 28 days before conception and throughout gestation and lactation	Male Sprague–Dawley rats	↑ systolic BP, ↑ mean arterial BP	At 9 weeks of age	[26]
60% HF diet throughout pregnancy and lactation	Male Sprague–Dawley rats	↑ systolic BP, ↑ mean arterial BP	At 12 weeks of age	[27–29]
60% HF diet throughout pregnancy and lactation	Male and female Sprague–Dawley rats	↑ systolic BP	At 12 weeks of age	[30]
60% HF diet throughout pregnancy and lactation plus 1% NaCl in drinking water from weaning to 3 months of age	Male Sprague–Dawley rats	↑ systolic BP, ↑ mean arterial BP; postnatal high-salt aggravates prenatal HF-induced programmed hypertension	At 12 weeks of age	[31]
56.7% HF/high-fat diet throughout pregnancy and lactation	Male Sprague–Dawley rats	↑ mean arterial BP	At 16 weeks of age	[32]
10% w/v fructose in drinking water throughout pregnancy and lactation	C57BL/6J mice	↑ mean arterial BP, obesity, metabolic dysfunction	At 12 months of age	[33]

Studies have been tabulated according to the age at which the effects were measured.

In adult rats, HF intake for >8 weeks induces renal damage [16]. However, our recent data indicate that rats receiving HF diet do not develop renal damage until 3 months of age. Unlike fructose-induced uric acid generation that induces oxidative stress and NO deficiency in adult rats [14,16,22], maternal HF consumption-induced programmed hypertension does not induce these abnormalities in adult offspring [27]. These data suggest that mechanisms underlying maternal HF consumption-induced programmed hypertension in offspring are different from those underlying fructose feeding-induced programmed hypertension adult rats.

4. HF Consumption Induces Renal Transcriptome Changes

Notably, almost entire oral fructose consumed by pregnant mother rats is converted to glucose, glycogen, fat, and lactate in the liver and is released into circulation [8]. Because fructose can be transported across the human placenta [34] and because human placenta generates endogenous fructose [35], it can be suggested that the key fetal programming process is driven by both fructose and its metabolites. Nutrigenomics has been introduced to understand existing reciprocal interactions between genes and nutrients [36]. Among different molecular nutrition approaches, transcriptomics provides information on mechanisms and physiological signals of a particular diet at a molecular level [36]. Recent advances in next-generation sequencing (NGS) allow us to monitor gene-diet interactions at a genome-wide level. The nutrigenomics approach indicates that fructose consumption leads to significant transcriptome changes in the brain of rats [37]. However, only limited studies have analyzed the transcriptome of the kidneys isolated from rodent models of maternal fructose consumption. We performed NGS by using RNA isolated from a 1-day-old offspring to analyze transcriptome changes in response to maternal HF consumption [28,38]. We found that in addition to genes associated with fructose metabolism, genes associated with other metabolic pathways such as glycolysis/gluconeogenesis, fatty acid metabolism, and insulin signaling were differential expressed (Table 2). Expression of genes encoding liver-type 6-phosphofructokinase (*Pfkl*), peroxisome proliferator-activated receptor gamma coactivator 1-α (*Ppargc1a*), glucose transporter 1 (*Slc2a1*), insulin receptor substrate 2 (*Irs2*), lactate dehydrogenase A (*Ldha*), and sterol regulatory element-binding transcription factor 1 (*Srebf1*) was upregulated in the kidneys. We also examined major organs that control BP, including the heart and brain, and observed that maternal HF consumption increased the mRNA levels of *Pfkl*, hexokinase 2 (*Hk2*), 6-phosphofructo-2-kinase/fructose-2,6-biphosphatase 3 (*Pfkfb3*), suppressor of cytokine signaling 3 (*Socs3*), NFκB inhibitor α (*Nfkbia*), *Ppargc1a*, liver glycogen phosphorylase (*Pygl*), and forkhead box protein O1 (*Foxo1*) in the heart. However, mRNA expression of only *Slc2a1* and short/branched chain specific acyl-CoA dehydrogenase (*Acadsb*) was upregulated, whereas that of *Socs3* was downregulated in the brain. Moreover, in contrast to the tightly regulated glucose metabolism in the brain, insulin signaling was perturbed in the kidneys and heart. Thus, our data suggest that different organs react differently to developmental programming, leading to organ-specific transcriptional modification of gene cascades.

Table 2. Changes in the expression of shared differential expressed genes (DEGs) associated with fructose metabolism in the kidneys, brain, and heart of offspring exposed to maternal HF diet at 1 day of age.

Gene ID	Symbol	Kidney	Brain	Heart
Fructose and mannose metabolism				
ENSRNOG00000001214	*Pfkl*	**2.3**	1.5	**2.2**
ENSRNOG00000006116	*Hk2*	1.8	ND	**2.1**
ENSRNOG00000018911	*Pfkfb3*	1.8	ND	**4.5**
Adipocytokine signaling pathway				
ENSRNOG00000002946	*Socs3*	1.6	**0.5**	**3.9**
ENSRNOG00000007390	*Nfkbia*	1.9	1.9	**3.5**
ENSRNOG00000004473	*Ppargc1a*	**2.3**	1.6	**2.7**
ENSRNOG00000007284	*Slc2a1*	**3.0**	**2.3**	ND
ENSRNOG00000023509	*Irs2*	**2.1**	ND	1.6
Glycolysis/Gluconeogenesis				
ENSRNOG00000001214	*Pfkl*	**2.3**	1.5	**2.2**
ENSRNOG00000006116	*Hk2*	1.8	ND	**2.1**
ENSRNOG00000013009	*Ldha*	**2.2**	ND	1.6
Fatty acid metabolism				
ENSRNOG00000020624	*Acadsb*	1.9	**2.0**	ND
Insulin signaling pathway				
ENSRNOG00000002946	*Socs3*	1.6	**0.5**	**3.9**
ENSRNOG00000004473	*Ppargc1a*	**2.3**	1.6	**2.7**
ENSRNOG00000006388	*Pygl*	1.9	ND	**3.2**
ENSRNOG00000006116	*Hk2*	1.8	ND	**2.1**
ENSRNOG00000023509	*Irs2*	**2.1**	ND	1.6
ENSRNOG00000003463	*Srebf1*	**2.1**	ND	1.6
ENSRNOG00000013397	*Foxo1*	1.8	ND	**2.2**

Gene expression was quantified as reads per kilobase of exon per million mapped reads (RPKM). Genes that changed by RPKM of >0.3 and ≥2-fold differences between HF vs. control. Significant results are highlighted in bold. ND, not detectable.

Our data showed that maternal HF consumption elicited different metabolic pathways in the developing kidney and heart. A schematic representation of maternal HF consumption-induced transcriptome changes in fructose metabolism, glycolysis/gluconeogenesis, fatty acid metabolism, and insulin signaling is shown in Figure 1. Fructose and related sugars, amino acids, and fatty acids are important cellular nutrients. Specific nutrients function as signaling molecules that transmit and translate dietary signals into changes in gene expression through appropriate sensing mechanisms (also known as nutrient-sensing pathway) [39]. Transcription factors are the main agents through which nutrients influence gene expression. Nuclear receptor superfamily of transcription factors is the most important group of nutrient sensors. For example, peroxisome proliferator-activated receptors (PPARs) interact with other nutrient-sensing signals to trigger renal programming and hypertension in response to maternal nutritional insults [40]. Our NGS data suggest that the nutrient-sensing pathway is crucial for the response of different organs of offspring to maternal HF consumption for programming differential phenotypes of metabolic syndrome, including hypertension.

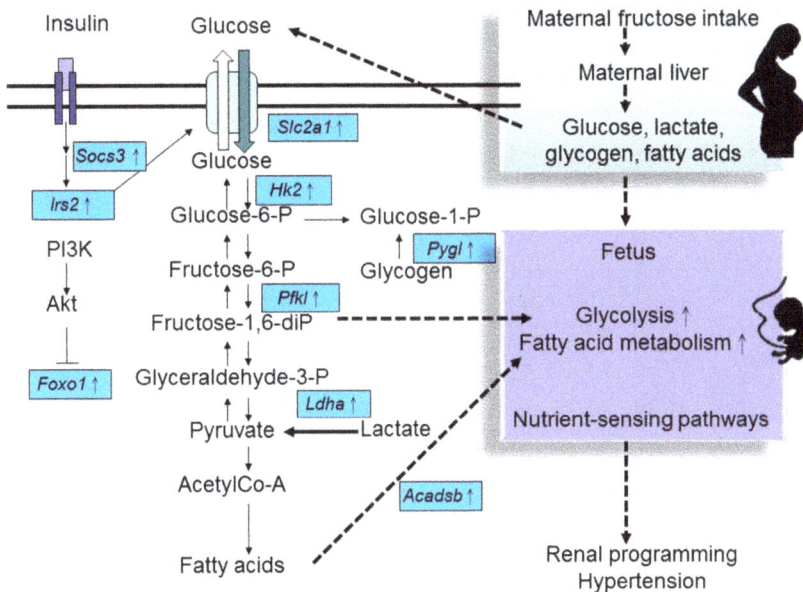

Figure 1. Schematic representation of changes in the expression of genes regulating glucose metabolism, fatty acid metabolism, and insulin signaling in the kidneys of offspring exposed to maternal HF diet. Solid lines with arrowheads indicate known signaling events and interactions between glucose metabolism, fatty acid metabolism, and insulin signaling. Dashed lines with arrowheads denote proposed mechanisms contributing to maternal HF consumption-induced programmed hypertension. Solid square boxes indicate DEGs identified by next-generation sequencing (NGS).

Our NGS data identified 10 significantly related Kyoto Encyclopedia of Genes and Genomes (KEGG) pathways shared by 3 different developmental windows in the kidneys of offspring exposed to maternal HF diet [28]. These KEGG pathways include complement and coagulation cascades; PPAR signaling; hematopoietic cell lineage; circadian rhythm; fatty acid metabolism; valine, leucine and isoleucine degradation; cell adhesion molecules; adipocytokine signaling pathway; arachidonic acid metabolism; and butanoate metabolism. Of these, the complement and coagulation cascade pathway is significantly regulated by maternal HF consumption, which is consistent with the results of a previous study involving a rat model of intrauterine growth retardation [41]. Arachidonic acid metabolism is another significant maternal HF consumption-related KEGG pathway. Arachidonic acid is metabolized by cytochrome P450, cyclooxygenase, or lipoxygenase to prostaglandins and related compounds [42]. We recently reported that arachidonic acid metabolites are the key components involved in hypertension development in various animal models [43].

In total, 20 DEGs in the kidneys of 1-day-old offspring exposed to maternal HF diet are associated with BP regulation [24]. Of these, *Adra2b*, *Bdkrb2*, *Col1a2*, *Hmox1*, *Ptgs2*, and *Tbxa2r* are associated with endothelium-derived hyperpolarizing factors (EDHFs). Because EDHFs play a crucial role in maintaining maternal and fetal circulation, our data suggest that early-life fructose exposure prevents interrelated EDHFs from adapting during nephrogenesis, leading to programmed hypertension in later life. Furthermore, our NGS data suggest that nutrigenomics approach can identify renal programming-associated genes and pathways that can be used as potential therapeutic targets for prevent maternal HF consumption-induced programmed hypertension in adult offspring.

Epigenetic regulation may induce programmed hypertension [6,7]. We used a maternal HF consumption model to analyze five groups of epigenetic regulators in the kidneys of 1-day-old offspring. Of these, expression of seven genes, namely, *Dnmt3l*, *Hdac9*, *Hdac11*, *Chd2*, *Brdt*, *Brwd1*, and *Myst2*, were found to be significantly regulated [28]. However, additional nutrigenomics studies are needed to determine whether fructose-induced epigenetic regulation, including DNA methylation, histone acetylation, and microRNA interference, is involved in maternal HF consumption-induced programmed hypertension.

5. Reprogramming Strategy to Prevent Maternal HF Consumption-Induced Programmed Hypertension

Several intervention strategies, including taurine, arginine, resveratrol, grape-derived polyphenols, sardine protein, vitamin E, and α-lipoic acid, have been used to prevent the adverse metabolic effects of excess fructose consumption in adults [44]. However, none of these strategies has been examined as a candidate reprogramming strategy for preventing maternal HF consumption-induced programmed hypertension.

Our data suggest that programmed processes promoting maternal HF consumption-induced programmed hypertension are different from those promoting fructose feeding-induced programmed hypertension in adult rats. Different mechanisms have been proposed to induce programmed hypertension, such as epigenetic regulation, glucocorticoid effects, RAS and sodium transporter alterations, oxidative stress, and nephron number reduction; these mechanisms can serve as potential targets for preventing maternal HF consumption-induced programmed hypertension [7,45]. The renal transcriptome is greatly altered in the adult offspring of various models of programmed hypertension [39,40]. We prevented hypertension development in adult offspring exposed to maternal HF diet by using three deprogramming approaches, namely, melatonin [27], soluble epoxide hydrolase (SEH) inhibitor [28], and renin inhibitor aliskiren.

Most reprogramming strategies have focused on restoring the balance of NO and reactive oxygen species (ROS) to prevent hypertension [7]. Melatonin is an endogenously produced indoleamine that exerts pleiotropic effects, including antioxidant effects [46]. We observed that maternal melatonin treatment prevented HF consumption-induced programmed hypertension and increased NO levels in the offspring kidneys [27]. Thus, reprogramming strategies that restore the NO–ROS balance can be applied in a broad range of prohypertensive developmental conditions.

Our NGS data indicate that the arachidonic acid metabolism pathway is involved in maternal HF consumption-induced renal programming and programmed hypertension [27,28]. Analysis by using two models of programmed hypertension indicated *Ephx2* expression and SEH (encoded by *Ephx2*) activity played a direct role in renal programming [43]. Our recent studies indicate that early postnatal treatment targeting the arachidonic acid metabolism pathway by using an SEH inhibitor 12-(3-adamantan-1-yl-ureido)-dodecanoic acid (AUDA) ameliorates hypertension in both maternal HF consumption-induced and prenatal dexamethasone-induced hypertension models [29,47]. Moreover, AUDA is effective in reprogramming BP in female spontaneously hypertensive rats (SHRs) but not in male SHRs [48]. Thus, reprogramming interventions for preventing hypertension may affect pathways that are common to nutrition and genetic models. However, it would be interesting to see whether SEH inhibition also prevents programmed hypertension in other models of nutritional programming.

RAS plays an essential role in BP control and nephrogenesis. Blockade of RAS with an angiotensin-converting enzyme inhibitor captopril, angiotensin receptor blocker losartan, or renin inhibitor aliskiren in young offspring from age 2 to 4 weeks of various animal models of hypertension counteracts programming effects [49–51]. We recently found that aliskiren administration during early postnatal life prevented maternal HF consumption-induced programmed hypertension in adult offspring of both the sexes [30]. We also observed that maternal HF consumption induced higher changes in the renal transcriptome of female rats than in that of male rats at 1 week of age [29]. Because sex differences exist in experimental models and human studies of hypertension [52], future studies should be aimed at identifying fundamental sex-specific mechanisms to provide a novel reprogramming strategy for achieving maximal optimization in both the sexes.

6. Conclusions

Diet is a major environmental factor in gene–environment interactions underlying the DOHaD concept. Maternal nutrition and its association with nutrient–gene interactions remains a challenging area of research. Although results obtained using animal models indicate that maternal HF consumption plays a role in the developmental programming of hypertension, early-life fructose–gene interactions in humans might be more complex and multifactorial. However, results of animal studies indicate that downstream pathways are largely reprogrammable irrespective of their upstream stimuli. This is fortunate because identification of upstream stimuli is often difficult in humans with programmed hypertension. Applications of newly developed high-throughput tools in nutrigenomics will allow us to identify genes or metabolites that are altered during prehypertension and will help in characterizing pathways regulated by dietary fructose. These tools can also help in developing early diagnostic methods and effective reprogramming strategies for treating HF diet-related diseases such as hypertension and metabolic syndrome. These new findings should be confirmed in further studies to develop personalized nutrition for health promotion and disease prevention.

Acknowledgments: This work was supported by a Grant MOST 104-2314-B-182-056-MY3 from the Ministry of Science and Technology, Taiwan, and Grants CMRPG8D0271 and CMRPG8F0021 from Chang Gung Memorial Hospital, Kaohsiung, Taiwan.

Author Contributions: You-Lin Tain: concept generation, data interpretation, manuscript drafting, critical manuscript revision, and article approval; Julie Y. H. Chan: concept generation, data interpretation, manuscript drafting, critical manuscript revision, and article approval; Chien-Ning Hsu: concept generation, data interpretation, critical manuscript revision, and article approval.

Conflicts of Interest: The authors declare no conflict of interest.

References

1. Johnson, R.J.; Segal, M.S.; Sautin, Y.; Nakagawa, T.; Feig, D.I.; Kang, D.H.; Gersch, M.S.; Benner, S.; Sánchez-Lozada, L.G. Potential role of sugar (fructose) in the epidemic of hypertension, obesity and the metabolic syndrome, diabetes, kidney disease, and cardiovascular disease. *Am. J. Clin. Nutr.* **2007**, *86*, 899–906. [PubMed]

2. Marriott, B.P.; Cole, N.; Lee, E. National estimates of dietary fructose intake increased from 1977 to 2004 in the United States. *J. Nutr.* **2009**, *139*, 1228S–1235S. [CrossRef] [PubMed]

3. Egan, B.M.; Zhao, Y.; Axon, R.N. US trends in prevalence, awareness, treatment, and control of hypertension, 1988–2008. *JAMA* **2010**, *303*, 2043–2050. [CrossRef] [PubMed]

4. Haugen, A.C.; Schug, T.T.; Collman, G.; Heindel, J.J. Evolution of DOHaD: The impact of environmental health sciences. *J. Dev. Orig. Health Dis.* **2015**, *6*, 55–64. [CrossRef] [PubMed]

5. Bagby, S.P. Maternal nutrition, low nephron number, and hypertension in later life: Pathways of nutritional programming. *J. Nutr.* **2007**, *137*, 1066–1072. [PubMed]

6. Kett, M.M.; Denton, K.M. Renal programming: Cause for concern? *Am. J. Physiol. Regul. Integr. Comp. Physiol.* **2011**, *300*, R791–R803. [CrossRef] [PubMed]

7. Tain, Y.L.; Joles, J.A. Reprogramming: A preventive strategy in hypertension focusing on the kidney. *Int. J. Mol. Sci.* **2015**, *17*, E23. [CrossRef] [PubMed]
8. Tappy, L.; Lê, K.A. Metabolic effects of fructose and the worldwide increase in obesity. *Physiol. Rev.* **2010**, *90*, 23–46. [CrossRef] [PubMed]
9. Chen, L.; Caballero, B.; Mitchell, D.C.; Loria, C.; Lin, P.H.; Champagne, C.M.; Elmer, P.J.; Ard, J.D.; Batch, B.C.; Anderson, C.A.; et al. Reducing consumption of sugar-sweetened beverages is associated with reduced blood pressure: A prospective study among United States adults. *Circulation* **2010**, *121*, 2398–2406. [CrossRef] [PubMed]
10. Brown, I.J.; Stamler, J.; van Horn, L.; Robertson, C.E.; Chan, Q.; Dyer, A.R.; Huang, C.C.; Rodriguez, B.L.; Zhao, L.; Daviglus, M.L.; et al. Sugar-sweetened beverage, sugar intake of individuals, and their blood pressure: International study of macro/micronutrients and blood pressure. *Hypertension* **2011**, *57*, 695–701. [CrossRef] [PubMed]
11. Brown, C.M.; Dulloo, A.G.; Yepuri, G.; Montani, J.P. Fructose ingestion acutely elevates blood pressure in healthy young humans. *Am. J. Physiol. Regul. Integr. Comp. Physiol.* **2008**, *294*, R730–R737. [CrossRef] [PubMed]
12. Perez-Pozo, S.E.; Schold, J.; Nakagawa, T.; Sánchez-Lozada, L.G.; Johnson, R.J.; Lillo, J.L. Excessive fructose intake induces the features of metabolic syndrome in healthy adult men: Role of uric acid in the hypertensive response. *Int. J. Obes.* **2010**, *34*, 454–461. [CrossRef] [PubMed]
13. Le, M.T.; Frye, R.F.; Rivard, C.J.; Cheng, J.; McFann, K.K.; Segal, M.S.; Johnson, R.J.; Johnson, J.A. Effects of high-fructose corn syrup and sucrose on the pharmacokinetics of fructose and acute metabolic and hemodynamic responses in healthy subjects. *Metabolism* **2012**, *61*, 641–651. [CrossRef] [PubMed]
14. Johnson, R.J.; Sanchez-Lozada, L.G.; Nakagawa, T. The effect of fructose on renal biology and disease. *J. Am. Soc. Nephrol.* **2010**, *21*, 2036–2039. [CrossRef] [PubMed]
15. Karalius, V.P.; Shoham, D.A. Dietary sugar and artificial sweetener intake and chronic kidney disease: A review. *Adv. Chronic Kidney Dis.* **2013**, *20*, 157–164. [CrossRef] [PubMed]
16. Tran, L.T.; Yuen, V.G.; McNeill, J.H. The fructose-fed rat: A review on the mechanisms of fructose-induced insulin resistance and hypertension. *Mol. Cell Biochem.* **2009**, *332*, 145–159. [CrossRef] [PubMed]
17. Kelishadi, R.; Mansourian, M.; Heidari-Beni, M. Association of fructose consumption and components of metabolic syndrome in human studies: A systematic review and meta-analysis. *Nutrition* **2014**, *30*, 503–510. [CrossRef] [PubMed]
18. Jayalath, V.H.; de Souza, R.J.; Ha, V.; Mirrahimi, A.; Blanco-Mejia, S.; Di Buono, M.; Jenkins, A.L.; Leiter, L.A.; Wolever, T.M.; Beyene, J.; et al. Sugar-sweetened beverage consumption and incident hypertension: A systematic review and meta-analysis of prospective cohorts. *Am. J. Clin. Nutr.* **2015**, *102*, 914–921. [CrossRef] [PubMed]
19. Toop, C.R.; Gentili, S. Fructose beverage consumption induces a metabolic syndrome phenotype in the rat: A systematic review and meta-analysis. *Nutrients* **2016**, *8*, E577. [CrossRef] [PubMed]
20. Glushakova, O.; Kosugi, T.; Roncal, C.; Mu, W.; Heinig, M.; Cirillo, P.; Sánchez-Lozada, L.G.; Johnson, R.J.; Nakagawa, T. Fructose induces the inflammatory molecule ICAM-1 in endothelial cells. *J. Am. Soc. Nephrol.* **2008**, *19*, 1712–1720. [CrossRef] [PubMed]
21. Sánchez-Lozada, L.G.; Tapia, E.; Jiménez, A.; Bautista, P.; Cristóbal, M.; Nepomuceno, T.; Soto, V.; Avila-Casado, C.; Nakagawa, T.; Johnson, R.J.; et al. Fructose-induced metabolic syndrome is associated with glomerular hypertension and renal microvascular damage in rats. *Am. J. Physiol. Ren. Physiol.* **2007**, *292*, F423–F429. [CrossRef] [PubMed]
22. Klein, A.V.; Kiat, H. The mechanisms underlying fructose-induced hypertension: A review. *J. Hypertens.* **2015**, *33*, 912–920. [CrossRef] [PubMed]
23. Madero, M.; Perez-Pozo, S.E.; Jalal, D.; Johnson, R.J.; Sánchez-Lozada, L.G. Dietary fructose and hypertension. *Curr. Hypertens. Rep.* **2011**, *13*, 29–35. [CrossRef] [PubMed]
24. Regnault, T.R.; Gentili, S.; Sarr, O.; Toop, C.R.; Sloboda, D.M. Fructose, pregnancy and later life impacts. *Clin. Exp. Pharmacol. Physiol.* **2013**, *40*, 824–837. [CrossRef] [PubMed]
25. Dornas, W.C.; de Lima, W.G.; Pedrosa, M.L.; Silva, M.E. Health implications of high-fructose intake and current research. *Adv. Nutr.* **2015**, *6*, 729–737. [CrossRef] [PubMed]

26. Gray, C.; Gardiner, S.M.; Elmes, M.; Gardner, D.S. Excess maternal salt or fructose intake programmes sex-specific, stress- and fructose-sensitive hypertension in the offspring. *Br. J. Nutr.* **2016**, *115*, 594–604. [CrossRef] [PubMed]

27. Tain, Y.L.; Leu, S.; Wu, K.L.; Lee, W.C.; Chan, J.Y. Melatonin prevents maternal fructose intake-induced programmed hypertension in the offspring: Roles of nitric oxide and arachidonic acid metabolites. *J. Pineal Res.* **2014**, *57*, 80–89. [CrossRef] [PubMed]

28. Tain, Y.L.; Wu, K.L.; Lee, W.C.; Leu, S.; Chan, J.Y. Maternal fructose-intake-induced renal programming in adult male offspring. *J. Nutr. Biochem.* **2015**, *26*, 642–650. [CrossRef] [PubMed]

29. Tain, Y.L.; Lee, W.C.; Wu, K.L.; Leu, S.; Chan, J.Y. Targeting arachidonic acid pathway to prevent programmed hypertension in maternal fructose-fed male adult rat offspring. *J. Nutr. Biochem.* **2016**, *38*, 86–92. [CrossRef] [PubMed]

30. Hsu, C.N.; Wu, K.L.; Lee, W.C.; Leu, S.; Chan, J.Y.; Tain, Y.L. Aliskiren administration during early postnatal life sex-specifically alleviates hypertension programmed by maternal high fructose consumption. *Front. Physiol.* **2016**, *7*, 299. [CrossRef] [PubMed]

31. Yamada-Obara, N.; Yamagishi, S.I.; Taguchi, K.; Kaida, Y.; Yokoro, M.; Nakayama, Y.; Ando, R.; Asanuma, K.; Matsui, T.; Ueda, S.; et al. Maternal exposure to high-fat and high-fructose diet evokes hypoadiponectinemia and kidney injury in rat offspring. *Clin. Exp. Nephrol.* **2016**, in press. [CrossRef] [PubMed]

32. Tain, Y.L.; Lee, W.C.; Leu, S.; Wu, K.; Chan, J. High salt exacerbates programmed hypertension in maternal fructose-fed male offspring. *Nutr. Metab. Cardiovasc. Dis.* **2015**, *25*, 1146–1151. [CrossRef] [PubMed]

33. Saad, A.F.; Dickerson, J.; Kechichian, T.B.; Yin, H.; Gamble, P.; Salazar, A.; Patrikeev, I.; Motamedi, M.; Saade, G.R.; Costantine, M.M. High-fructose diet in pregnancy leads to fetal programming of hypertension, insulin resistance, and obesity in adult offspring. *Am. J. Obstet. Gynecol.* **2016**, *215*, e1–e6. [CrossRef] [PubMed]

34. Holmberg, N.G.; Kaplan, B.; Karvonen, M.J.; Lind, J.; Malm, M. Permeability of human placenta to glucose, fructose, and xylose. *Acta Physiol. Scand.* **1956**, *36*, 291–299. [CrossRef] [PubMed]

35. Hagerman, D.D.; Roux, J.; Villee, C.A. Studies of the mechanism of fructose production by human placenta. *J. Physiol.* **1959**, *146*, 98–104. [CrossRef] [PubMed]

36. Norheim, F.; Gjelstad, I.M.; Hjorth, M.; Vinknes, K.J.; Langleite, T.M.; Holen, T.; Jensen, J.; Dalen, K.T.; Karlsen, A.S.; Kielland, A.; et al. Molecular nutrition research: The modern way of performing nutritional science. *Nutrients* **2012**, *4*, 1898–1944. [CrossRef] [PubMed]

37. Meng, Q.; Ying, Z.; Noble, E.; Zhao, Y.; Agrawal, R.; Mikhail, A.; Zhuang, Y.; Tyagi, E.; Zhang, Q.; Lee, J.H.; et al. Systems nutrigenomics reveals brain gene networks linking metabolic and brain disorders. *EBioMedicine* **2016**, *7*, 157–166. [CrossRef] [PubMed]

38. Chao, Y.M.; Tain, Y.L.; Leu, S.; Wu, K.L.; Lee, W.C.; Chan, J.Y. Developmental programming of the metabolic syndrome: Next-generation sequencing analysis of transcriptome expression in a rat model of maternal high fructose intake. *Sheng Li Xue Bao* **2016**, *68*, 557–567. [PubMed]

39. Efeyan, A.; Comb, W.C.; Sabatini, D.M. Nutrient-sensing mechanisms and pathways. *Nature* **2015**, *517*, 302–310. [CrossRef] [PubMed]

40. Tain, Y.L.; Hsu, C.N.; Chan, J.Y. PPARs link early life nutritional insults to later programmed hypertension and metabolic syndrome. *Int. J. Mol. Sci.* **2015**, *17*, E20. [CrossRef] [PubMed]

41. Buffat, C.; Boubred, F.; Mondon, F.; Chelbi, S.T.; Feuerstein, J.M.; Lelièvre-Pégorier, M.; Vaiman, D.; Simeoni, U. Kidney gene expression analysis in a rat model of intrauterine growth restriction reveals massive alterations of coagulation genes. *Endocrinology* **2007**, *148*, 5549–5557. [CrossRef] [PubMed]

42. Campbell, W.B.; Falck, J.R. Arachidonic acid metabolites as endothelium-derived hyperpolarizing factors. *Hypertension* **2007**, *49*, 590–596. [CrossRef] [PubMed]

43. Tain, Y.L.; Huang, L.T.; Chan, J.Y.; Lee, C.T. Transcriptome analysis in rat kidneys: Importance of genes involved in programmed hypertension. *Int. J. Mol. Sci.* **2015**, *16*, 4744–4758. [CrossRef] [PubMed]

44. Sloboda, D.M.; Li, M.; Patel, R.; Clayton, Z.E.; Yap, C.; Vickers, M.H. Early life exposure to fructose and offspring phenotype: Implications for long term metabolic homeostasis. *J. Obes.* **2014**, *2014*, 203474. [CrossRef] [PubMed]

45. Paixão, A.D.; Alexander, B.T. How the kidney is impacted by the perinatal maternal environment to develop hypertension. *Biol. Reprod.* **2013**, *89*, 1–10. [CrossRef] [PubMed]

46. Tain, Y.L.; Huang, L.T.; Chan, J.Y. Transcriptional regulation of programmed hypertension by melatonin: An epigenetic perspective. *Int. J. Mol. Sci.* **2014**, *15*, 18484–18495. [CrossRef] [PubMed]

47. Lu, P.C.; Sheen, J.M.; Yu, H.R.; Lin, Y.J.; Chen, C.C.; Tiao, M.M.; Tsai, C.C.; Huang, L.T.; Tain, Y.L. Early postnatal treatment with soluble epoxide hydrolase inhibitor or 15-deoxy-Δ(12,14)-prostagandin J2 prevents prenatal dexamethasone and postnatal high saturated fat diet induced programmed hypertension in adult rat offspring. *Prostaglandins Other Lipid Mediat.* **2016**, *124*, 1–8. [CrossRef] [PubMed]

48. Koeners, M.P.; Wesseling, S.; Ulu, A.; Sepúlveda, R.L.; Morisseau, C.; Braam, B.; Hammock, B.D.; Joles, J.A. Soluble epoxide hydrolase in the generation and maintenance of high blood pressure in spontaneously hypertensive rats. *Am. J. Physiol. Endocrinol. Metab.* **2011**, *300*, E691–E698. [CrossRef] [PubMed]

49. Sherman, R.C.; Langley-Evans, S.C. Early administration of angiotensin-converting enzyme inhibitor captopril, prevents the development of hypertension programmed by intrauterine exposure to a maternal low-protein diet in the rat. *Clin. Sci.* **1998**, *94*, 373–381. [CrossRef] [PubMed]

50. Sherman, R.C.; Langley-Evans, S.C. Antihypertensive treatment in early postnatal life modulates prenatal dietary influences upon blood pressure in the rat. *Clin. Sci.* **2000**, *98*, 269–275. [CrossRef] [PubMed]

51. Hsu, C.N.; Lee, C.T.; Huang, L.T.; Tain, Y.L. Aliskiren in early postnatal life prevents hypertension and reduces asymmetric dimethylarginine in offspring exposed to maternal caloric restriction. *J. Renin Angiotensin Aldosterone Syst.* **2015**, *16*, 506–513. [CrossRef] [PubMed]

52. Sandberg, K.; Ji, H. Sex differences in primary hypertension. *Biol. Sex Differ.* **2012**, *3*, 7. [CrossRef] [PubMed]

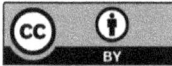

nutrients

MDPI

Article

High Dietary Fructose Intake on Cardiovascular Disease Related Parameters in Growing Rats

SooYeon Yoo [1], Hyejin Ahn [1] and Yoo Kyoung Park [1,2,*]

[1]   Department of Medical Nutrition, Kyung Hee University, 1732 Deogyeong-daero, Giheung-gu, Yongin 17104, Korea; sooyeon928@hanmail.net (S.Y.Y.); hjahn@khu.ac.kr (H.A.)
[2]   Research Institute of Medical Nutrition, Kyung Hee University, 26, Kyungheedae-ro, Dongdaemun-gu, Seoul 02447, Korea
*   Correspondence: ypark@khu.ac.kr; Tel.: +82-31-201-3816; Fax: +82-31-203-3816

Received: 29 October 2016; Accepted: 15 December 2016; Published: 26 December 2016

Abstract: The objective of this study was to determine the effects of a high-fructose diet on cardiovascular disease (CVD)-related parameters in growing rats. Three-week-old female Sprague Dawley rats were randomly assigned to four experimental groups; a regular diet group (RD: fed regular diet based on AIN-93G, $n = 8$), a high-fructose diet group (30Frc: fed regular diet with 30% fructose, $n = 8$), a high-fat diet group (45Fat: fed regular diet with 45 kcal% fat, $n = 8$) or a high fructose with high-fat diet group (30Frc + 45Fat, fed diet 30% fructose with 45 kcal% fat, $n = 8$). After an eight-week treatment period, the body weight, total-fat weight, serum glucose, insulin, lipid profiles and pro-inflammatory cytokines, abdominal aortic wall thickness, and expressions of eNOS and ET-1 mRNA were analyzed. The result showed that total-fat weight was higher in the 30Frc, 45Fat, and 30Frc + 45Fat groups compared to the RD group ($p < 0.05$). Serum triglyceride (TG) levels were highest in the 30Frc group than the other groups ($p < 0.05$). The abdominal aorta of 30Frc, 45Fat, and 30Frc + 45Fat groups had higher wall thickness than the RD group ($p < 0.05$). Abdominal aortic eNOS mRNA level was decreased in 30Frc, 45Fat, and 30Frc + 45Fat groups compared to the RD group ($p < 0.05$), and also 45Fat and 30Frc + 45Fat groups had decreased mRNA expression of eNOS compared to the 30Frc group ($p < 0.05$). ET-1 mRNA level was higher in 30Frc, 45Fat, and 30Frc + 45Fat groups than the RD group ($p < 0.05$). Both high fructose consumption and high fat consumption in growing rats had similar negative effects on CVD-related parameters.

Keywords: high fructose diet; cardiovascular disease (CVD); growing rat

1. Introduction

Sugar-sweetened beverages and processed foods are the main source of fructose [1]. According to The Korea National Health and Nutrition Examination Survey (KNHNES) [2], consumption of beverage products increased 3.7 folds from 1998 (45.5 ± 2.0 g) to 2014 (167.4 ± 5.2 g). Based on data collected from a 2010 study from The Korea Health Industry Development Institute (KHIDI) [3], consumption of sugar-sweetened beverages and processed foods in adolescents were higher than in the adult group.

Recently, a considerable volume of research was performed in both animals and humans dedicated to clarify the link between dietary fructose and health risk markers such as obesity and cardiovascular disease. Consumption of sugar-sweetened beverages has a positive correlation with body weight gain [4,5] in human, and in animals [6–8]. Bocarsly et al. [9] reported that rats fed with water containing high fructose corn syrup for eight weeks had increased body weight and body fat, and Crescenzo et al. [10] showed significant increases in body fat in rats that consumed fructose for eight weeks, with no significant difference in body weight. These observations are particularly important because accumulation of body fats leads to an increase of pro-inflammatory cytokines (TNF-α, IL-6, PAI-1) [11].

In addition, a high fructose diet is known to lead hypertension and insulin resistance in animals [12,13]. Insulin resistance has been proposed as an underlying mechanism that links endothelial dysfunction factors such as endothelial nitric oxide synthase (eNOS) and Endothelin-1 (ET-1) [14]. Also, chronic exposure of dyslipidemia has a major effect on cardiovascular disease (CVD) [15]. De Castro et al. [16] reported that rats fed with a high fructose diet had significantly increased levels of in serum total-cholesterol and triglyceride. These changes are significantly associated with an increased incidence of cardiovascular disease [17].

Changes of CVD-related parameters in childhood is correlated with development into CVD which affects CVD risks later in life [18]. Although high-fructose affects CVD-related parameters in adult human and animals, these effects have not been investigated in adolescent or growing animals. Therefore, this study investigates the effects of a high-fructose diet and compares the results with a high-fat diet on CVD-related parameters in growing rats.

2. Materials and Methods

2.1. Experimental Design and Diet

The experimental protocol was approved by the Animal Care Use Review Committee of Kyung Hee University (IACUC, protocol number: KHP-2014-01-1). Three-week-old female Sprague-Dawley rats ($n = 32$) were provided by SLC, Inc. (Shizuoka, Japan). Rats were housed individually in polycarbonate cages in temperature-controlled rooms (22 ± 2 °C) with a relative humidity of 55% $\pm$ 5%, and a 12-h light/dark cycle. The rats were fed a pellet chow diet, and given water ad libitum for an adaptation period of 10 days. All rats were weighed weekly, and food intake was measured daily. After a 10-day adaption period, animals were randomized selected into the four different groups: regular diet group (RD) ($n = 8$) rats were fed an AIN-93G (D10012G, Research Diets Inc., New Brunswick, NJ, USA) diet, high fructose diet group (30Frc) ($n = 8$) rats were fed a 30% fructose (D14010101, Research Diets Inc.) diet, high fat diet group (45Fat) ($n = 8$) rats were fed a 45 kcal% fat as soy bean oil and lard (D14010102, Research Diets Inc.) diet, and high fat diet with high fructose diet group (30Frc + 45Fat) ($n = 8$) rats were fed a diet with 30% fructose and 45 kcal% fat (D14010103, Research Diets Inc.). All animals were maintained on these diets ad libitum for eight weeks. Composition of experimental diets is shown in Table 1.

Table 1. Ingredient composition of experimental diets.

%	RD		30Frc		45Fat		30Frc + 45Fat	
	g	kcal	g	kcal	g	kcal	g	kcal
Protein	20	20	20	20	24	20	24	20
Carbohydrate	64	64	64	64	41	35	41	35
Fat	7	16	7	16	24	45	24	45
Total		100		100		100		100
kcal/gm	4.0		4.0		4.8		4.8	
Ingredient	**g**	**kcal**	**g**	**kcal**	**g**	**kcal**	**g**	**kcal**
Casein, 80 Mesh	200	800	200	800	200	800	200	800
L-Cystine	3	12	3	12	3	12	3	12
Corn Starch	397.5	1590	229.5	918	137	548	0	0
Maltodextrin 10	132	528	100	400	100	400	37	148
Sucrose	100	400	0	0	100	400	0	0
Fructose	0	0	300	1200	0	0	300	1200
Cellulose	50	0	50	0	50	0	50	0
Soybean Oil	70	630	70	630	26	234	26	234
t-Butylhydroquinone	0.014	0	0.014	0	0.014	0	0.014	0
Lard	0	0	0	0	174	1566	174	1566
Mineral Mix	35	0	35	0	35	0	35	0
Vitamin Mix	10	40	10	40	10	40	10	40
Choline Bitartrate	2.5	0	2.5	0	2.5	0	2.5	0
Total	1000	4000	1000	4000	837.5	4000	837.5	4000

RD: rats received a regular diet based on AIN-93G (4.0 kcal/g diet); 30Frc: rats received a 30% fructose-diet based on regular diet (4.0 kcal/g diet); 45Fat: rats received a 45 kcal% fat-diet (4.8 kcal/g diet); 30Frc + 45Fat: rats received a 45 kcal% fat -diet with 30% fructose (4.8 kcal/g diet).

2.2. Body Weight, Food Consumption, and Fat Mass

Body weights and food consumption were measured weekly and daily, respectively. The food efficiency ratio (FER) was calculated using the following formula: (weight gain (g)/week)/(food consumed (kcal)/week). At the end of the eight-week experimental period, total fat was removed and weighed immediately after killing. The total fat was measured by combining the weight of subcutaneous fat and visceral fat.

2.3. Analysis of Blood Parameters

Blood was collected at the end of experiment, following a 12-h overnight fast. Rats were anesthetized with a small amount of ethyl ether, and blood samples were taken by heart puncture. Blood samples were immediately collected into serum-separating tubes (SST) and were centrifuged at 3000 rpm for 15 min at 4 °C. Serum was stored at -70 °C until used in assays. Serum triglyceride (TG), Total cholesterol (T-Chol), HDL-cholesterol (HDL-C), and glucose levels were determined using commercial kits (Asan Co. Ltd., Seoul, Korea). Atherogenic Index (AI) was calculated using the following formula: AI = (total cholesterol $-$ HDL-cholesterol)/HDL-cholesterol. Serum Insulin concentrations were determined using an ELISA rat/mouse insulin kit (ALPCO Diagnostics, Salem, NH, USA). Insulin resistance was calculated by a homeostasis assessment model (HOMA-IR) and calculated from fasting insulin and glucose concentration according to the formula: (fasting insulin (ng/mL) × fasting glucose (mg/dL))/22.5. Quantitative insulin sensitivity check index (QUICKI) was also calculated using the following formula: QUICKI = 1/(log fasting insulin (mg/dL) + log fasting glucose(mg/dL)). Pro-inflammatory cytokines (TNF-α, IL-6, and PAI-1) were measured in duplicate using Milipore's MILLIPLEX rat CVD cytokine panel (Millipore, Billerica, MA, USA).

2.4. Analysis of Abdominal Aorta

Abdominal aorta samples were obtained after rats were sacrificed at the end of experiment. The abdominal aortas were fixed in a 4% formalin solution, followed by sequential dehydration (70% ethanol, 100% ethanol, and acetone), xylene clearance, and paraffin embedding. The paraffin-embedded aortas were cut into 5-micron slices with a microtome (820 II; Reichert-Jung, Bensheim, Germany). Then the sliced aortas were stained with Harris hematoxylin and eosinY (H & E). Wall thickness and lumen diameter of abdominal aortas were determined on five isotropic uniform random sections per animal at a magnification of 500:1 and phase contrast. All sections were photographed using a microscope (model Axiovert S100, Zeiss, Oberkochen, Germany) connected to a camera (model AxioCam, Zeiss) and MetaMorph software (Molecular Devices, Sunnyvale, CA, USA). Wall thickness and lumen diameter were determined as the mean of the minimal and maximal value.

2.5. Quantitative Real-Time Polymerase Chain Reaction (PCR)

Total RNA was extracted from abdominal aorta using an RNeasy mini kit (Qiagen, Gaithersburg, MD, USA) according to the manufacturer's instructions. Real-time quantitative PCR was performed using an Applied Bio-systems (Applied Bio-systems, Foster City, CA, USA); 1 μL with 100 nM of each primer (forward and reverse) reaction consisted of 10 μL of the SYBR Green Super-mix (iQ SYBR Green Super-mix, Bio-Rad Laboratories Inc. Hercules, CA, USA), according to the manufacturer's instructions. Thermal cycling was initiated by denaturation at 95 °C for 10 min, followed by 40 cycles of 95 °C for 15 s and 60 °C for 30 s, then an annealing step was performed at adequate temperature in function of the primers and 72 °C for 30 s for extension. After the final cycle, melting curves were monitored from 55 to 65 °C (0.05 °C/s). The primer sequences were: rat eNOS, 5′-CAACAAACCGAGGCAATCTTC-3′ (forward), 5′-CCCGGCCAGCGTAGCT-3′ (reverse), and rat ET-1, 5′-TGGACATCATCTGGGTCAACA-3′ (forward), 5′-GCTTAGACCTAGAAGGGCTTCCTAGT-3′ (reverse), and rat glyceraldehyde

3′-phosphate dehydrogenase (GAPDH), 5′-TGGCCTCCAAGGAGTAAGAAAC-3′ (forward), 5′-GGCCTCTCTCTTGCTCTCAGTATC-3′ (reverse). The detected genes were eNOS and ET-1.

2.6. Statistical Analysis

All measurements were performed in duplicate, and statistical calculations were performed with Statistical Package for the social Sciences (SPSS, version 20.0, IBM Corp., Armonk, NY, USA) software. All data were presented as mean ± SD. Differences in measured parameters among the experimental groups were analyzed by the one-way ANOVA and Duncan's multiple range tests. The respective effects of operation and diet were analyzed by two-way ANOVA. The differences were considered to be significant when the *p* value was less than 0.05.

3. Results

3.1. Body Weights, Food Intakes, Calorie Intakes, and Food Efficiency Ratios

The effect of the diet on body weight, body weight gain, food intake, calorie intake, and food efficiency ratio is shown in Table 2.

Table 2. Body weights, food intakes, calorie intakes, and food efficiency ratio.

	RD (n = 8)	30Frc (n = 8)	45Fat (n = 8)	30Frc + 45Fat (n = 8)
Initial body weight (g)	74.6 ± 2.6	74.9 ± 5.0	74.5 ± 4.71	74.4 ± 4.1
Final body weight (g)	251.3 ± 9.6 [b]	263.3 ± 15.0 [a,b]	278.1 ± 22.1 [a]	277.2 ± 16.6 [a]
Weight gain (g)	177.2 ± 9.8 [b]	188.0 ± 13.4 [a,b]	204.3 ± 22.6 [a]	201.9 ± 17.7 [a]
Food intake (g/day)	12.5 ± 0.8 [a]	13.2 ± 0.9 [a]	11.3 ± 0.9 [b]	11.5 ± 0.8 [b]
Calorie intake (kcal/day)	49.8 ± 2.9	52.4 ± 4.4	53.8 ± 4.6	54.7 ± 4.7
Food efficiency ratio	0.05 ± 0.00	0.05 ± 0.00	0.05 ± 0.01	0.05 ± 0.00

All values are presented as means ± standard deviation (SD). RD: rats received a regular diet based on AIN-93G (4.0 kcal/g diet); 30Frc: rats received a 30% fructose-diet based on control-diet (4.0 kcal/g diet); 45Fat: rats received a 45 kcal% fat-diet (4.8 kcal/g diet); 30Frc + 45Fat: rats received a 45 kcal% fat-diet with 30% fructose (4.8 kcal/g diet); Food efficiency ratio = (weight gain (g)/week)/(food consumed (kcal)/week). Statistical differences between the experimental groups were based on one-way ANOVA and Duncan's multiple range tests at $p < 0.05$. Means with different alphabetical superscripts are significantly different ($p < 0.05$).

The initial body weights were not significantly different among the experimental groups. Feeding of high fat diet groups (45Fat, 30Frc + 45Fat) resulted in a significantly higher body weight than the RD and 45Fat groups (278.1 ± 22.1 g, 277.2 ± 16.6 g vs. 251.3 ± 9.6 g, 263.3 ± 15.0 g, $p < 0.05$). The food intake was significantly higher in the RD (12.5 ± 0.8 g/day) and 30Frc (13.2 ± 1.0 g/day) groups compared to that of 45Fat (11.3 ± 0.9 g/day) and 30Frc + 45Fat (11.5 ± 0.8 g/day) groups ($p < 0.05$). However, total calorie intakes and food efficiency ratios were not significantly different among the experimental groups. Total calorie was calculated from food intake (g) × calorie density (kcal/g).

3.2. Total-Fat Weights

The total-fat weights of the experimental groups are shown in Figure 1.

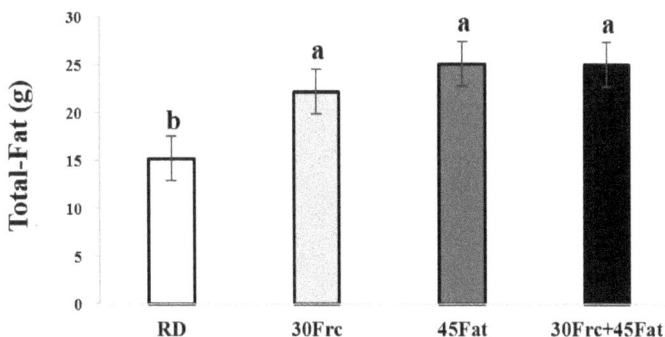

Figure 1. Total-fat weight in the experimental groups. RD: rats received a regular diet based on AIN-93G (4.0 kcal/g diet); 30Frc: rats received a 30% fructose-diet based on control-diet (4.0 kcal/g diet); 45Fat: rats a received 45 kcal% fat-diet (4.8 kcal/g diet); 30Frc + 45Fat: rats received a 45 kcal% fat-diet with 30% fructose (4.8 kcal/g diet). Statistical differences between the experimental groups were based on one-way ANOVA and Duncan's multiple range tests at $p < 0.05$. Means with different alphabetical letters are significantly different ($p < 0.05$).

The average total-fat weights were 15.2 ± 3.6, 22.2 ± 3.8, 25.1 ± 3.5, and 25.0 ± 2.4 g in the RD, 30Frc, 45Fat, and 30Frc + 45Fat groups. The total-fat weights were significantly higher in 30Frc, 45Fat, and 30Frc + 45Fat groups than the RD group ($p < 0.05$).

3.3. Serum Levels of Glucose and Insulin, HOMA-IR, and QUICKI

The blood glucose and insulin levels, HOMA-IR, and QUICKI are shown in Table 3. The serum glucose and insulin levels did not differ among the experimental groups. Also, no differences were observed in HOMA-IR and QUICKI among groups.

Table 3. Serum levels of glucose and insulin.

	RD (*n* = 8)	30Frc (*n* = 8)	45Fat (*n* = 8)	30Frc + 45Fat (*n* = 8)
Glucose (mg/dL)	143.6 ± 10.3	142.0 ± 9.2	141.4 ± 14.9	136.6 ± 15.8
Insulin (ng/mL)	1.2 ± 1.4	2.2 ± 1.7	0.9 ± 0.3	1.3 ± 0.9
HOMA-IR	8.1 ± 9.1	12.7 ± 11.7	5.9 ± 2.4	8.3 ± 6.2
QUICKI	0.5 ± 0.07	0.4 ± 0.07	0.5 ± 0.05	0.5 ± 0.07

All values are presented as means ± standard deviation (SD). RD: rats received a regular diet based on AIN-93G (4.0 kcal/g diet); 30Frc: rats received a 30% fructose-diet based on control-diet (4.0 kcal/g diet); 45Fat: rats received a 45 kcal% fat-diet (4.8 kcal/g diet); 30Frc + 45Fat: rats received a 45 kcal% fat-diet with 30% fructose (4.8 kcal/g diet), HOMA-IR: homoeostasis model assessment of insulin resistance was calculated by (fasting insulin (ng/mL); QUICKI: 1/(log(fasting insulin ng/mL) + log(fasting glucose mg/dL)) × fasting glucose (mg/dL))/22.5. There were no significant differences among groups according to ANOVA and Duncan's multiple range tests.

3.4. Serum Levels of Lipid Profiles

The serum lipid profile levels are shown in Table 4. Serum Total-C, HDL-C, and atherogenic index were not different among groups. However, the serum TG levels in the 30Frc group (108.6 ± 25.2 mg/dL) were significantly higher than the RD, 45Fat, and 30Frc + 45Fat groups (71.4 ± 19.8, 88.6 ± 26.9, and 93.9 ± 24.1 mg/dL, respectively) ($p < 0.05$).

Table 4. Serum levels of lipid profiles.

	RD (*n* = 8)	30Frc (*n* = 8)	45Fat (*n* = 8)	30Frc + 45Fat (*n* = 8)
TG (mg/dL)	71.4 ± 19.8 [b]	108.6 ± 25.2 [a]	88.6 ± 26.9 [a,b]	93.9 ± 24.1 [a,b]
Total-C (mg/dL)	107.9 ± 19.7	114.6 ± 17.5	97.8 ± 15.4	96.3 ± 18.4
HDL-C (mg/dL)	98.1 ± 12.4	103.8 ± 10.9	92.1 ± 13.4	91.8 ± 14.7
AI	0.09 ± 0.07	0.10 ± 0.05	0.06 ± 0.03	0.05 ± 0.05

All values are presented as means ± standard deviation (SD). RD: rats received a regular diet based on AIN-93G (4.0 kcal/g diet); 30Frc: rats received a 30% fructose-diet based on control-diet (4.0 kcal/g diet); 45Fat: rats received a 45 kcal% fat-diet (4.8 kcal/g diet); 30Frc + 45Fat: rats received a 45 kcal% fat-diet with 30% fructose (4.8 kcal/g diet); TG: Triglyceride; Total-C: Total cholesterol; AI: Atherogenic index = (total cholesterol − HDL-cholesterol)/HDL-cholesterol. Statistical difference between the experimental groups were based on one-way ANOVA and Duncan's multiple range tests at $p < 0.05$. Means with different alphabetical superscripts are significantly different ($p < 0.05$).

3.5. Serum Levels of Pro-Inflammatory Cytokines

The serum pro-inflammatory cytokines levels are shown in Table 5. The mean levels of serum pro-inflammatory cytokines levels (TNF-α, IL-6, PAI-1) did not differ among the experimental groups.

Table 5. Serum levels of pro-inflammatory cytokines.

	RD (*n* = 8)	30Frc (*n* = 8)	45Fat (*n* = 8)	30Frc + 45Fat (*n* = 8)
TNF-α (pg/mL)	55.1 ± 4.9	51.5 ± 5.5	47.0 ± 4.8	48.3 ± 10.9
IL-6 (pg/mL)	11.6 ± 4.2	18.2 ± 11.6	12.6 ± 4.0	15.5 ± 8.3
PAI-1 (pg/mL)	100.8 ± 13.3	101.5 ± 9.4	96.0 ± 4.8	99.4 ± 20.5

All values are presented as means ± standard deviation (SD). RD: rats received a regular diet based on AIN-93G (4.0 kcal/g diet); 30Frc: rats received a 30% fructose-diet based on control-diet (4.0 kcal/g diet); 45Fat: rats received a 45 kcal% fat-diet (4.8 kcal/g diet); 30Frc + 45Fat: rats received a 45 kcal% fat-diet with 30% fructose (4.8 kcal/g diet); TNF-α: Tumor Necrosis α; IL-6: Interleukin-6; PAI-1: Plasminogen activator inhibitor-1. There were no significant differences among groups according to ANOVA and Duncan's multiple range tests.

3.6. Analysis of Abdominal Aorta Wall Thickness and Lumen Diameter

The abdominal aorta wall thickness and lumen diameter are shown in Table 6 and Figure 2. The aorta wall thickness was significantly increased in 30Frc, 45Fat, and 30Frc + 45Fat groups (23.6 ± 0.9 μm, 23.7 ± 2.8 μm, and 22.5 ± 2.2 μm, respectively, $p < 0.05$) than the RD group (18.5 ± 0.5 μm). The lumen diameter was not different among the groups. The wall thickness:lumen ratio was increased in 30Frc, 45Fat and 30Frc + 45Fat groups (0.096 ± 0.001 μm, 0.098 ± 0.014 μm, and 0.085 ± 0.005 μm, respectively, $p < 0.05$) than the RD group (0.061 ± 0.009 μm).

Table 6. Abdominal aorta wall thickness and lumen diameter.

	RD (*n* = 8)	30Frc (*n* = 8)	45Fat (*n* = 8)	30Frc + 45Fat (*n* = 8)
Wall thickness (μm)	18.5 ± 0.5 [b]	23.6 ± 0.9 [a]	23.7 ± 2.8 [a]	22.5 ± 2.2 [a]
Lumen diameter (μm)	306.8 ± 54.4	248.4 ± 25.1	243.9 ± 29.4	266.9 ± 29.0
Wall thickness/ Lumen ratio (μm/μm)	0.061 ± 0.009 [b]	0.096 ± 0.001 [a]	0.098 ± 0.014 [a]	0.085 ± 0.005 [a]

All values are presented as means ± standard deviation (SD). RD: rats received a regular diet based on AIN-93G (4.0 kcal/g diet); 30Frc: rats received a 30% fructose-diet based on control-diet (4.0 kcal/g diet); 45Fat: rats received a 45 kcal% fat-diet (4.8 kcal/g diet); 30Frc + 45Fat: rats received a 45 kcal% fat-diet with 30% fructose (4.8 kcal/g diet). Statistical differences between the experimental groups were based on one-way ANOVA and Duncan's multiple range tests at $p < 0.05$. Means with different alphabetical superscripts are significantly different ($p < 0.05$).

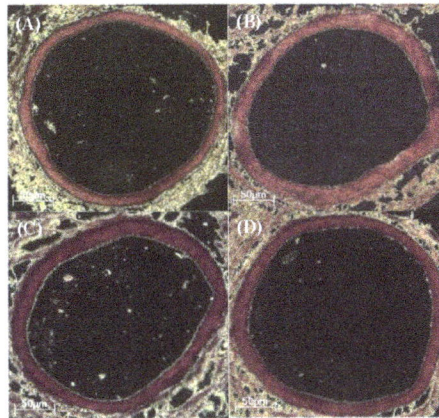

Figure 2. Abdominal aortic wall thickness and lumen diameter taken at eight weeks, pertaining to the respective groups (**A**) RD; (**B**) 30Frc; (**C**) 45Fat; (**D**) 30Frc + 45Fat. Hematoxylin and eosin (H & E) stained abdominal aorta × 500. Magnification bars 50 μm. RD: rats received a regular diet based on AIN-93G (4.0 kcal/g diet); 30Frc: rats received a 30% fructose-diet based on control-diet (4.0 kcal/g diet); 45Fat: rats received a 45 kcal% fat-diet (4.8 kcal/g diet); 30Frc + 45Fat: rats received a 45 kcal% fat-diet with 30% fructose (4.8 kcal/g diet).

3.7. Abdominal Aortic eNOS and ET-1 mRNA Expression Measured by qRTPC

The abdominal aortic eNOS and ET-1 mRNA expression of the experimental groups are shown in Figures 3 and 4. The aortic eNOS mRNA expression was significantly decreased in 45Fat and 30Frc + 45Fat groups (0.3 ± 0.06 and 0.4 ± 0.07, respectively, $p < 0.05$) compared to the RD and 30Frc groups (1.0 ± 0.00 and 0.7 ± 0.05, respectively). Also, for the 30Frc group that was fed the high fructose diet constantly, the aortic eNOS mRNA expression was significantly decreased compared to the RD group ($p < 0.05$). The aortic ET-1 mRNA expression of the 30Frc + 45Fat group was the highest among the four groups (10.3 ± 1.8 vs. 1.0 ± 0.4, 3.3 ± 0.3, and 7.4 ± 0.7, respectively, for the RD, 30Frc, and 45Fat groups, $p < 0.05$).

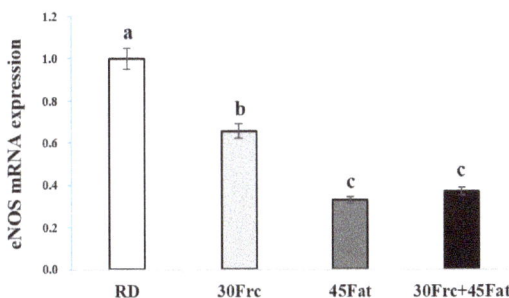

Figure 3. Aortic eNOS mRNA expression measured by quantitative real-time polymerase chain reaction (qRTPCR). RD: rats received a regular diet based on AIN-93G (4.0 kcal/g diet); 30Frc: rats received a 30% fructose-diet based on control-diet (4.0 kcal/g diet); 45Fat: rats received a 45 kcal% fat-diet (4.8 kcal/g diet); 30Frc + 45Fat: rats received a 45 kcal% fat-diet with 30% fructose (4.8 kcal/g diet). Statistical differences between the experimental groups were based on one-way ANOVA and Duncan's multiple range tests at $p < 0.05$. Means with different alphabetical letters are significantly different ($p < 0.05$).

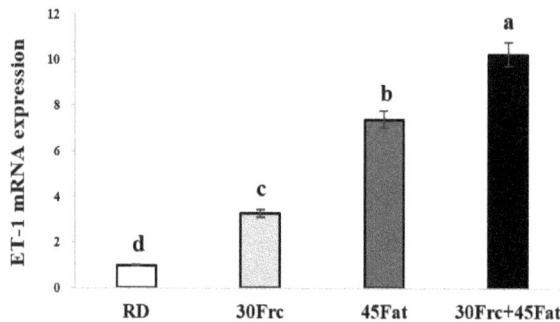

Figure 4. Aortic ET-1 mRNA expression measured by qRTPCR. RD: rats received a regular diet based on AIN-93G (4.0 kcal/g diet); 30Frc: rats received a 30% fructose-diet based on control-diet (4.0 kcal/g diet); 45Fat: rats received a 45 kcal% fat-diet (4.8 kcal/g diet); 30Frc + 45Fat: rats received a 45 kcal% fat-diet with 30% fructose (4.8 kcal/g diet). Statistical differences between the experimental groups were based on one-way ANOVA and Duncan's multiple range tests at $p < 0.05$. Means with different alphabetical letters are significantly different ($p < 0.05$).

4. Discussion

The purpose of this study was to determine the effects of a high-fructose diet on cardiovascular disease (CVD)-related parameters in growing rats.

It was known that rats fed high-fat diets increased body weight and body fat [19,20]. The present study showed that the consumption of a high-fat diet (45Fat, 30Frc + 45Fat) in growing rats significantly increased body weight and body fat compared to regular diet and high-fructose diet groups. The high-fructose diet did not affect the body weight, whereas it significantly increased the weight of body fat compared to the regular diet fed group. The previous study reported that rats fed with the high-fructose diet (60%) for 10 weeks increased body weight [7]. However, Crescenzo et al. [10] showed increased white adipose tissue (WAT) in rats fed fructose (60%), despite no difference in body weight gain. An increase in body weight alone does not necessarily indicate obesity, it has to be considered along with other factors, such as changes in body composition [21]. The increase in body fat reflected the obesogenic property. This suggests that obesity can be induced by high-fructose diet, as well as high-fat diet.

Dyslipidemia, especially hypertriglyceridemia and insulin resistance are major factors associated with CVD in rats fed a high-fructose diet (60%) [22,23]. Our data showed that the 30Frc group had significantly increased serum TG levels compared to the other groups. In the liver, fructose is divided into glyceraldehyde and dihydroxyacetone phosphate, ultimately becoming triglyceride [24]. Therefore, exposure to high fructose levels to rapidly increased levels of triglyceride synthesis. We consider that excessive fructose consumption can lead to dyslipidemia and obesity; these changes are caused CVD.

Insulin resistance is closely linked to dyslipimenia [25]. Many previous studies have reported that the high-fructose diet can induce hyperglycemia (35%, 66%) [26,27]. However, this study showed no difference in serum glucose and insulin levels. The previous study suggested that although fructose does not appear to acutely increase insulin levels, chronic exposure seems to indirectly cause insulin resistance and obesity through other mechanisms, such as GLUT5 fructose transporters and inflammation [28]. Iida et al. [29] reported that rats fed 40% fructose for eight weeks displayed no difference in serum insulin levels. Another study showed that rats fed with 66% fructose for two weeks increased plasma TG, even though there was no change in plasma glucose, insulin, and body weight [30]. Increased triglyceride levels in response to high-fructose diet could have resulted in insulin resistance by reducing the insulin signaling pathway [27]. Our data, together with the previously established literature showed, suggest that chronic exposure to a high-fructose diet can result in hypertriglycemia, and that this change could cause insulin resistance.

Enlarged body fat induces the expression of pro-inflammatory cytokines [11]. A previous study reported that a high fructose diet can increase hepatic mRNA expression of TNF-α, IL-6, and the weight of epididymal fat pads in rats [31]. However, the present study had shown that rats fed a high-fructose diet significantly increased the total body fat, but the serum pro-inflammatory cytokines (TNF-α, IL-6, PAI-1) did not change in between groups. Chronic inflammation is an important pathogenic factor in the development of CVD [32,33]. Large amounts of markers for inflammatory cytokines can be released from the adipose tissue [34]. Yudkin et al. [35] reported that adipose tissue can also synthesize pro-inflammatory cytokines such as TNF-α and IL-6. In this way, increased body fat itself promotes inflammation. According to this hypothesis, high fructose consumption leads to increased body fat and obesity, which can cause changes to inflammatory cytokines. In the present study we showed that rats fed a high-fructose diet significantly increased their total-fat weight, although the serum pro-inflammatory cytokines did not change.

Changes in the aorta wall thickness is significantly associated with serum lipid profiles and hypertension, which begins in childhood and may develop into cardiovascular disease [35–38]. According to a previous study, the tunica intima-media layer was increased in the high-fructose diet group [31]. Autopsy studies have reported that the first atherosclerotic lesions actually begin to develop in the abdominal aorta [39]. Therefore, we chose the abdominal aorta to conduct the present experiment. In the present study we showed that the abdominal aorta of high-fructose diet and high fat diet rats were thicker in comparison to the regular diet group. We consider that high-fructose consumption as well as high-fat consumption, can have a significant effect on abdominal aorta wall thickness in the growing rats. These early changes can possibly lead to endothelial dysfunction.

Endothelial dysfunction is a systemic disorder in the pathogenesis of atherosclerosis [40], which plays an important role in hypertension [41] and CVD [42]. The endothelium maintains the balance between vasoconstriction and vasodilation, but when this balance is disrupted, endothelial dysfunction occurs which can be lead to CVD [43]. A major vasodilator NO is synthesized by nitric oxide synthases [44]. Endothelial dysfunction may occur as a result of decreased eNOS activity or reduced bioavailability of NO [14]. The endothelium also produces vasoconstrictors, such as endothelin and angiotension II. Endothelin is the most potent endogenous vasoconstrictor [43]. As such, in this study, we analyzed vasodilator eNOS and vasoconstrictor ET-1. A previous study showed that NO synthesis inhibited rats had elevated blood pressure [45]. Endemann et al. [14] reported that the eNOS activity of rats fed high-fructose diet decreased in the aorta. In the present study, mRNA expression of eNOS in the abdominal aorta in 45Fat and 30Frc + 45Fat groups was significantly decreased in comparison to those of the other groups. Additionally, the 30Frc group had significantly decreased mRNA expression of eNOS compared to the RD group. ET-1 is an important vasoconstrictor produced by endothelial cells that contributes to enhanced blood pressure [43,46]. A previous study reported that rats fed a high-fructose diet for nine weeks had increased ET-1 levels [47]. Similarly, our study showed that the abdominal aortic ET-1 mRNA expression in 30Frc, 45Fat, and 30Frc + 45Fat groups were significantly higher than the RD group. Our data, together with the previously established literature, suggest that high-fructose diet, as well as the high-fat diet, negatively affected endothelium-derived relaxing and contracting factors. These changes are important factors for the development of hypertension and vascular dysfunction.

5. Conclusions

Collectively, the high-fructose diets increased the total-fat weight and serum TG levels in growing rats. Additionally, it had negative effects on abdominal aortic thickness and eNOS, ET-1 mRNA expression.

The strength of our study is that we fed 30% fructose-diets to the animals. Numerous animal studies have used extreme doses of ~60% fructose, which, as White [48] suggested, show results that

Nutrients **2017**, *9*, 11

are not physiological, and likely cause abnormal metabolism, and therefore cannot be depended on to assess human risk. In the present study we were able to show that 30% fructose can induce total-fat weight gain, increase aorta wall thickness, and affect eNOS and ET-1 mRNA expression, which are related to CVD risk factors. One potential limitation in the present study was that the sample size was small, which may lessen the significance of the results.

In conclusion, we confirmed high fructose consumption, as well as high fat consumption, in growing rats had negative effects on CVD-related parameters, such as total-fat weight, serum TG, aorta wall thickness, and eNOS, ET-1 mRNA expression of abdominal aorta.

Acknowledgments: This work was supported by Korea Institute of Planning and Evaluation for Technology in Food, Agriculture, Forestry and Fisheries (IPET), funded by Ministry of Agriculture, Food and Rural Affairs (MAFRA) (316055-3).

Author Contributions: The authors' responsibilities were as follows: S.Y. and H.A. designed animal model; S.Y. and H.A. conducted research; S.Y. and Y.K.P. analyzed data; S.Y., H.A., and Y.K.P. drafted and revised the paper; all authors read and approved the final manuscript.

Conflicts of Interest: The authors declare no conflict of interest.

References

1. Kim, S.D.; Moon, H.; Park, J.S.; Lee, Y.C.; Shin, G.Y.; Jo, H.B.; Kim, B.S.; Kim, J.H.; Chae, Y.Z. Macromineral intake in non-alcoholic beverages for children and adolescents: Using the fourth Korea national health and nutrition examination survey (KNHANES IV, 2007–2009). *Korean J. Nutr.* **2013**, *46*, 50–60. [CrossRef]

2. The Korea National Health and Nutrition Examination Survey (KNHNES). *Dietary Intake Survey of Infant, Children and Adolescents*; The Korea National Health and Nutrition Examination Survey: Cheongju, Korea, 2011.

3. Korea Health Industry Development Institute (KHIDI). *In-Depth Analysis on the Dietary Intake Survey of Infant, Children and Adolescents (II)*; Korea Health Industry Development Institute: Cheongju, Korea, 2010.

4. Bandini, L.G.; Vu, D.; Must, A.; Cyr, H.; Goldberg, A.; Dietz, W.H. Comparison of high-calorie, low-nutrient-dense food consumption among obese and non-obese adolescents. *Obes. Res.* **1999**, *7*, 438–443. [CrossRef] [PubMed]

5. Berkey, C.S.; Rockett, H.R.; Field, A.E.; Gillman, M.W.; Colditz, G.A. Sugar-added beverages and adolescent weight change. *Obes. Res.* **2004**, *12*, 778–788. [CrossRef] [PubMed]

6. Nakagawa, T.; Hu, H.; Zharikov, S.; Tuttle, K.R.; Short, R.A.; Glushakova, O.; Ouyang, X.; Feig, D.I.; Block, E.R.; Herrera-Acosta, J.; et al. A causal role for uric acid in fructose-induced metabolic syndrome. *Am. J. Physiol. Ren. Physiol.* **2006**, *290*, F625–F631. [CrossRef] [PubMed]

7. Mohamed, S.S.; Nallasamy, P.; Muniyandi, P.; Periyasami, V.; Carani, V.A. Genistein improves liver function and attenuates non-alcoholic fatty liver disease in a rat model of insulin resistance. *J. Diabetes* **2009**, *1*, 278–287. [CrossRef] [PubMed]

8. Shih, C.; Lin, C.; Lin, W.; Wu, J. *Momordica charantia* extract on insulin resistance and the skeletal muscle GLUT4 protein in fructose-fed rats. *J. Ethnopharmacol.* **2009**, *123*, 82–90. [CrossRef] [PubMed]

9. Bocarsly, M.E.; Powell, E.S.; Avena, N.M.; Hoebel, B.G. High-fructose corn syrup causes characteristics of obesity in rats: Increased body weight, body fat and triglyceride levels. *Pharmacol. Biochem. Behav.* **2010**, *97*, 101–106. [CrossRef] [PubMed]

10. Crescenzo, R.; Bianco, F.; Coppola, P.; Mazzoli, A.; Valiante, S.; Liverini, G.; Iossa, S. Adipose tissue remodeling in rats exhibiting fructose-induced obesity. *Eur. J. Nutr.* **2014**, *53*, 413–419. [CrossRef] [PubMed]

11. Muniyappa, R.; Montagnani, M.; Koh, K.K.; Quon, M.J. Cardiovascular actions of insulin. *Endocr. Rev.* **2007**, *28*, 463–491. [CrossRef] [PubMed]

12. Song, D.; Arikawa, E.; Galipeau, D.; Battell, M.; McNeill, J.H. Androgens are necessary for the development of fructose-induced hypertension. *Hypertension* **2004**, *43*, 667–672. [CrossRef] [PubMed]

13. Behr-Roussel, D.; Oudot, A.; Compagnie, S.; Gorny, D.; Le Coz, O.; Bernabe, J.; Wayman, C.; Alexandre, L.; Giuliano, F. Impact of a long-term sildenafil treatment on pressor response in conscious rats with insulin resistance and hypertriglyceridemia. *Am. J. Hypertens.* **2008**, *21*, 1258–1263. [CrossRef] [PubMed]

14. Endemann, D.H.; Schiffrin, E.L. Endothelial dysfunction. *J. Am. Soc. Nephrol.* **2004**, *15*, 1983–1992. [CrossRef] [PubMed]

15. Austin, M.A.; King, M.C.; Vranizan, K.M.; Krauss, R.M. Atherogenic lipoprotein phenotype: A proposed genetic marker for coronary heart disease risk. *Circulation* **1990**, *82*, 495–506. [CrossRef] [PubMed]

16. De Castro, U.G.; dos Santos, R.A.; Silva, M.E.; de Lima, W.G.; Campagnole-Santos, M.J.; Alzamora, A.C. Age-dependent effect of high-fructose and high-fat diets on lipid metabolism and lipid accumulation in liver and kidney of rats. *Lipids Health Dis.* **2013**, *12*. [CrossRef] [PubMed]

17. Yamauchi, T.; Kadowaki, T. Physiological and pathophysiological roles of adiponectin and adiponectin receptors in the integrated regulation of metabolic and cardiovascular diseases. *Int. J. Obes.* **2008**, *32*, S13–S18. [CrossRef] [PubMed]

18. Ross, R. The pathogenesis of atherosclerosis: A perspective for the 1990s. *Nature* **1993**, *362*, 801–809. [CrossRef] [PubMed]

19. Sinitskaya, N.; Gourmelen, S.; Schuster-Klein, C.; Guardiola-Lemaitre, B.; Pevet, P.; Challet, E. Increasing the fat-to-carbohydrate ratio in a high-fat diet prevents the development of obesity but not a prediabetic state in rats. *Clin. Sci.* **2007**, *113*, 417–425. [CrossRef] [PubMed]

20. Matveyenko, A.V.; Gurlo, T.; Daval, M.; Butler, A.E.; Butler, P.C. Successful versus failed adaptation to high-fat diet-induced insulin resistance: The role of IAPP-induced beta-cell endoplasmic reticulum stress. *Diabetes* **2009**, *58*, 906–916. [CrossRef] [PubMed]

21. Ouguerram, K.; Nguyen, P. Lipid profile and insulin sensitivity in rats fed with high-fat or high-fructose diets. *Br. J. Nutr.* **2011**, *106*, S206–S210.

22. Tran, L.T.; Yuen, V.G.; McNeill, J.H. The fructose-fed rat: A review on the mechanisms of fructose-induced insulin resistance and hypertension. *Mol. Cell. Biochem.* **2009**, *332*, 145–159. [CrossRef] [PubMed]

23. Miller, A.; Adeli, K. Dietary fructose and the metabolic syndrome. *Curr. Opin. Gastroenterol.* **2008**, *24*, 204–209. [CrossRef] [PubMed]

24. Angelopoulos, T.J.; Lowndes, J.; Zukley, L.; Melanson, K.J.; Nguyen, V.; Huffman, A.; Rippe, J.M. The effect of high-fructose corn syrup consumption on triglycerides and uric acid. *J. Nutr.* **2009**, *139*, 1242S–1245S. [CrossRef] [PubMed]

25. Shulman, G.I. Cellular mechanisms of insulin resistance. *J. Clin. Investig.* **2000**, *106*, 171–176. [CrossRef] [PubMed]

26. Blakely, S.R.; Hallfrisch, J.; Reiser, S.; Prather, E.S. Long-term effects of moderate fructose feeding on glucose tolerance parameters in rats. *J. Nutr.* **1981**, *111*, 307–314. [PubMed]

27. Tappy, L.; Le, K.A. Metabolic effects of fructose and the worldwide increase in obesity. *Physiol. Rev.* **2010**, *90*, 23–46. [CrossRef] [PubMed]

28. Basciano, H.; Federico, L.; Adeli, K. Fructose, insulin resistance, and metabolic dyslipidemia. *Nutr. Metab.* **2005**, *2*, 5–20. [CrossRef] [PubMed]

29. Iida, T.; Yamada, T.; Hayashi, N.; Okuma, K.; Izumori, K.; Ishii, R.; Matsuo, T. Reduction of abdominal fat accumulation in rats by 8-week ingestion of a newly developed sweetener made from high fructose corn syrup. *Food Chem.* **2013**, *138*, 781–785. [CrossRef] [PubMed]

30. Catena, C.; Giacchetti, G.; Novello, M.; Colussi, G.; Cavarape, A.; Sechi, L.A. Cellular mechanisms of insulin resistance in rats with fructose-induced hypertension. *Am. J. Hypertens.* **2003**, *16*, 973–978. [CrossRef]

31. Kho, M.C.; Lee, Y.J.; Ahn, Y.M.; Choi, Y.H.; Kim, A.Y.; Kang, D.G.; Lee, H.S. Effects of ethanol extract of *gastrodia elata blume* on high-fructose induced metabolic syndrome. *FASEB J.* **2013**, *27*, 1108–1113.

32. Dandona, P.; Aljada, A.; Bandyopadhyay, A. Inflammation: The link between insulin resistance, obesity and diabetes. *Trends Immunol.* **2004**, *25*, 4–7. [CrossRef] [PubMed]

33. Fantuzzi, G. Adipose tissue, adipokines, and inflammation. *J. Allergy Clin. Immunol.* **2005**, *115*, 911–999. [CrossRef] [PubMed]

34. Rudin, E.; Barzilai, N. Inflammatory peptides derived from adipose tissue. *Immun. Ageing* **2005**, *2*. [CrossRef] [PubMed]

35. Yudkin, J.S.; Stehouwer, C.D.; Emeis, J.J.; Coppack, S.W. C-reactive protein in healthy subjects: Associations with obesity, insulin resistance, and endothelial dysfunction: A potential role for cytokines originating from adipose tissue? *Arterioscler. Thromb. Vasc. Biol.* **1999**, *19*, 972–978. [CrossRef] [PubMed]

36. Davis, P.H.; Dawson, J.D.; Riley, W.A.; Lauer, R.M. Carotid intimal-medial thickness is related to cardiovascular risk factors measured from childhood through middle age: The Muscatine study. *Circulation* **2001**, *104*, 2815–2819. [CrossRef] [PubMed]

37. Berenson, G.S.; Srinivasan, S.R.; Bao, W.; Newman, W.P.; Tracy, R.E.; Wattigney, W.A. Association between multiple cardiovascular risk factors and atherosclerosis in children and young adults. *N. Engl. J. Med.* **1998**, *338*, 1650–1656. [CrossRef] [PubMed]

38. McGill, H.C., Jr.; McMahan, C.A.; Zieske, A.W.; Malcom, G.T.; Tracy, R.E.; Strong, J.P. Effects of nonlipid risk factors on atherosclerosis in youth with a favorable lipoprotein profile. *Circulation* **2001**, *103*, 1546–1550. [CrossRef] [PubMed]

39. McGill, H.C., Jr.; McMahan, C.A.; Herderick, E.E.; Tracy, R.E.; Malcom, G.T.; Zieske, A.W.; Strong, J.P. Effects of coronary heart disease risk factors on atherosclerosis of selected regions of the aorta and right coronary artery. *Arterioscler. Thromb. Vasc. Biol.* **2000**, *20*, 836–845. [CrossRef] [PubMed]

40. Bonetti, P.O.; Lerman, L.O.; Lerman, A. Endothelial dysfunction: A marker of atherosclerotic risk. *Arterioscler. Thromb. Vasc. Biol.* **2003**, *23*, 168–175. [CrossRef] [PubMed]

41. Pepine, C.J. Clinical implications of endothelial dysfunction. *Clin. Cardiol.* **1998**, *21*, 795–799. [CrossRef] [PubMed]

42. Brunner, H.; Cockcroft, J.R.; Deanfield, J.; Donald, A.; Ferrannini, E.; Halcox, J.; Kiowski, W.; Lüscher, T.F.; Mancia, G.; Natali, A. Endothelial function and dysfunction. Part II: Association with cardiovascular risk factors and diseases. A statement by the working group on endothelins and endothelial factors of the european society of hypertension. *J. Hypertens.* **2005**, *23*, 233–246. [CrossRef] [PubMed]

43. Davignon, J.; Ganz, P. Role of endothelial dysfunction in atherosclerosis. *Circulation* **2004**, *109*, 27–32. [CrossRef] [PubMed]

44. Dawson, V.; Brahmbhatt, H.; Mong, J.; Dawson, T. Expression of inducible nitric oxide synthase causes delayed neurotoxicity in primary mixed neuronal-glial cortical cultures. *Neuropharmacology* **1994**, *33*, 1425–1430. [CrossRef]

45. Rees, D.D.; Palmer, R.M.; Moncada, S. Role of endothelium-derived nitric oxide in the regulation of blood pressure. *Proc. Natl. Acad. Sci. USA* **1989**, *86*, 3375–3378. [CrossRef] [PubMed]

46. Oliver, F.J.; de la Rubia, G.; Feener, E.P.; Lee, M.E.; Loeken, M.R.; Shiba, T.; Quertermous, T.; King, G.L. Stimulation of endothelin-1 gene expression by insulin in endothelial cells. *J. Biol. Chem.* **1991**, *266*, 23251–23256. [PubMed]

47. Verma, S.; Bhanot, S.; McNeill, J.H. Effect of chronic endothelin blockade in hyperinsulinemic hypertensive rats. *Am. J. Physiol.* **1995**, *269*, H2017–H2021. [PubMed]

48. White, J.S. Challenging the fructose hypothesis: New perspectives on fructose consumption and metabolism. *Adv. Nutr.* **2013**, *4*, 246–256. [CrossRef] [PubMed]

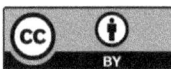

nutrients

MDPI

Article

Fructose in Breast Milk Is Positively Associated with Infant Body Composition at 6 Months of Age

Michael I. Goran [1,*], Ashley A. Martin [1], Tanya L. Alderete [1], Hideji Fujiwara [2] and David A. Fields [3]

[1] Department of Preventive Medicine, University of Southern California, 2250 Alcazar Street, CSC 200, Los Angeles, CA 90033, USA; ashley.ann.martin@gmail.com (A.A.M.); tanya.alderete@usc.edu (T.L.A.)

[2] School of Medicine, Washington University in St. Louis, St. Louis, MO 63110, USA; hideji.fujiwara@gmail.com

[3] Department of Pediatrics, University of Oklahoma Health Sciences Center, Oklahoma City, OK 73104, USA; David-Fields@ouhsc.edu

* Correspondence: goran@usc.edu; Tel.: +323-442-3027; Fax: +323-442-4103

Received: 11 November 2016; Accepted: 8 February 2017; Published: 16 February 2017

Abstract: Dietary sugars have been shown to promote excess adiposity among children and adults; however, no study has examined fructose in human milk and its effects on body composition during infancy. Twenty-five mother–infant dyads attended clinical visits to the Oklahoma Health Sciences Center at 1 and 6 months of infant age. Infants were exclusively breastfed for 6 months and sugars in breast milk (i.e., fructose, glucose, lactose) were measured by Liquid chromatography-mass spectrometry (LC-MS/MS) and glucose oxidase. Infant body composition was assessed using dual-energy X-ray absorptiometry at 1 and 6 months. Multiple linear regression was used to examine associations between breast milk sugars and infant body composition at 6 months of age. Fructose, glucose, and lactose were present in breast milk and stable across visits (means = 6.7 µg/mL, 255.2 µg/mL, and 7.6 g/dL, respectively). Despite its very low concentration, fructose was the only sugar significantly associated with infant body composition. A 1-µg/mL higher breast milk fructose was associated with a 257 g higher body weight ($p = 0.02$), 170 g higher lean mass ($p = 0.01$), 131 g higher fat mass ($p = 0.05$), and 5 g higher bone mineral content ($p = 0.03$). In conclusion, fructose is detectable in human breast milk and is positively associated with all components of body composition at 6 months of age.

Keywords: breastfeeding; breast milk; maternal programming; added sugars; fructose

1. Introduction

Added sugar is an established risk factor for obesity as well as related metabolic diseases including type 2 diabetes, cardiovascular disease and non-alcoholic fatty liver [1–5]. Fructose appears to be at least partially responsible for this detrimental relationship, as fructose metabolism is unregulated [6,7] and fructose has been linked to greater adiposity and metabolic disturbances compared to other sugars that appear to be especially important during critical periods of growth and development [8]. While many studies have examined the impact of fructose and other sugars on body weight in childhood, few studies have examined the impact of early exposures to these sugars during infancy [9,10].

One of the most direct routes by which infants may be exposed to fructose and other sugars is through breastfeeding. During the first six months of life, many infants obtain their nourishment predominately if not exclusively from breast milk, which contains a variety of macronutrients and other relevant factors (e.g., cytokines, appetite hormones) [11–13]. While this exclusive breastfeeding period would appear to preclude any access to fructose exposure in early-life, studies have shown that the composition of breast milk is shaped by the maternal diet [14,15]. Therefore, breast milk may contain varying levels of maternal dietary macronutrients that have the potential to contribute to childhood obesity and future metabolic disease risk [16–19]. For instance, in infants born to mothers diagnosed with gestational diabetes (GDM), consuming greater volumes of 'diabetic' milk in the first week of life has been found to be associated with a 2-fold increased risk of being overweight at age 2 [20]. This effect is attributed, in part, to the higher levels of glucose and insulin observed in the breast milk of mothers with GDM [21,22]. Breast milk concentrations of glucose and insulin have also been found to positively predict adiposity in infants born to non-diabetic mothers [12]. Recent research suggests that even non-nutritive carbohydrates found in breast milk (i.e., human milk oligosaccharides) have the potential to contribute to infant growth and body composition in infancy [23]. Together, these studies highlight the need to better understand the composition of breast milk and whether macronutrient composition affects infant growth and development.

The first aim of this study was to determine whether fructose was detectable in human breast milk. The second aim was to examine if fructose in breast milk was associated with infant weight and body composition at six months of age. We tested this hypothesis within a cohort of 25 mother-infant pairs where infants were exclusively breastfed, analyzing relationships between breast milk sugar composition and infant growth and body composition. To our knowledge, this study is the first to examine the associations between breast milk fructose and infant body composition.

2. Methods

2.1. Study Overview

Thirty-seven mother-infant dyads were enrolled at 1-month ($\pm$5 days) of age for participation in a 6-month longitudinal exclusively breastfeeding growth study. Of the 37 mother-infant pairs initially enrolled in this study, 25 were retained in this analysis. Eleven participants were excluded due to loss of follow-up for milk analyses (either due to dropping out or declining to produce a milk sample) and another participant was excluded because they did not produce enough breast milk for analysis. The overall study design and preliminary results were described in a previous study that examined the relationships between breast milk hormones and inflammatory markers [12]. The data reported here describe relationships between infant body composition and breast milk sugar content that were not explored in the previous work. In brief, participants were instructed to arrive at the University of Oklahoma approximately between 8:00 a.m. and 10:00 a.m. with the mother fasted at least 3 h. Upon arrival, a single breast-milk expression was obtained from the mother with a whole-body dual energy X-ray absorptiometry (DXA) scan conducted on the infant. Measurements were performed when the infant was 1 month of age (used as baseline covariates in this analysis) and were repeated at 6-months of age (all visits were $\pm$ 5 days). All subjects gave their informed consent for inclusion prior to participating in the study. The study was conducted in accordance with the Declaration of Helsinki, and the protocol was approved by the Ethics Committee of the University of Oklahoma Health Sciences Center (IRB #4426 and 5297).

2.2. Participants

The 25 mother-infant dyads were exclusively breast-fed (defined <8 ounces of formula a week though no subject consumed any formula past 7 days of age) with the following inclusion criteria used: (a) maternal age at delivery between 18 and 45 years old; (b) gestation $\geq$37 weeks; (c) singleton birth; and (d) a postpartum hospital stay for mother and infant less than 3 days. Participants were excluded for any of the following: (a) maternal use of tobacco; (b) mothers' alcohol consumption exceeding one drink per week; (c) type 1 or 2 diabetes prior to or during pregnancy; or (d) the infant was born with presumed or known congenital birth defects. All maternal demographic information (age, parity, pre-pregnancy weight and gestational weight gain) was collected by medical chart abstraction when possible.

2.3. Anthropometric and Body Composition Variables

Crown-to-heel length was measured in duplicate using a Seca 416 infantometer (Seca, Hamburg, Germany) with both measures being within 0.1 cm. Nude body weight was measured in duplicate with a Seca 728 scale (Seca, Hamburg, Germany) with both measures being within 10 g. On the rare occasion these measures exceeded the criteria set forth, a third measure was obtained and the two closest values averaged. Weight-for-length z-scores were calculated using World Health Organization data. Total adiposity (% fat), fat mass (g), lean mass (g), bone mineral density (g/cm^2), and bone mineral content (g) were collected using a Lunar iDXA (General Electric, Fairfield, CT, USA) scanner as described previously [12]. During the scan, the infant wore only a diaper and was swaddled in a light blanket. The principal investigator (DAF) positioned all infants and performed subsequent scan analyses.

2.4. Breast-Milk Collection

Mothers came to the University of Oklahoma Health Sciences center for their study visits typically arriving between 8:00 a.m. and 10:00 a.m. The laboratory provided a hospital-grade breast pump for pumping (Symphony® Breast Pump, Medela Inc., McHenry, IL, USA) while the mother was encouraged to completely empty the right breast for the quantification of breast milk sugars. While mothers were encouraged to pump from the right breast for uniformity, each mother was allowed to decide from which breast she pumped.

2.5. Breast-Milk Analyses

Preparation of Fructose Quantification Sample

The protein was removed by precipitating from the breast milk (50 μL) with addition of 200 μL of acetonitrile containing 10 μg of carbon-13 labeled ($^{13}C_6$)-fructose as the internal standard for natural fructose quantification in the breast milk. The supernatant, which contained natural fructose as well as $^{13}C_6$-fructose, was collected after centrifugation of the protein precipitated breast milk for MS analysis. The 5-point calibration samples were prepared for absolute quantification of fructose in the breast milk. QC (quality control) samples were also prepared from pooling some of individual supernatants for monitoring on analytical performance throughout fructose analysis.

Preparation of lactose quantification sample: The original breast milk was initially diluted by 100-fold with water. Then, 5 μL of the diluted breast milk was again diluted by 200-fold with 995 μL of water, containing 5 μg of $^{13}C_{12}$-lactulose as the internal standard. The 4-point calibration samples were prepared for absolute quantification of lactose in the breast milk. QC samples were prepared for lactose analysis.

LC-MS/MS Analyses: The fructose and lactose analyses were performed with a Shimadzu 20AD HPLC system (Shimadzu USA, Columbia, MD, USA) and a Leap PAL (Palparts) autosampler (Leap Technologies, Carrboro, NC, USA) coupled to a triple quadrupole mass spectrometer (API (Atmospheric Pressure Ionization) -4000: Applied Biosystems, Foster City, CA, USA). Initially, 3 μL of fructose and lactose samples were separately injected onto an Imtakt UK-amino HPLC column (3 × 100 mm, 3 μm: Imtakt USA, Portland, OR, USA) with the following mobile phases: (a) 10 m mole ammonium acetate in water; (b) acetonitrile at a flow rate of 1 mL/min. The column was heated at 60 °C throughout the analyses. The positive ion ESI MRM mode was used for detection of fructose (Q1/Q3:198/145) and lactose (Q1/Q3:360/163) as well as $^{13}C_6$ fructose (Q1/Q3:204/151) and $^{13}C_{12}$-lactulose (Q1/Q3:372/169). Data processing was conducted with Analyst 1.5.1 (Applied Biosystems, Foster City, CA, USA). Unlike GC-MS (Gas Chromotrography-Mass Spectrometry) quantification of fructose [24] that can sometimes overestimate concentrations due to incomplete derivatization (see Supplementary Materials Figure S1), our LC-MS/MS method does not require the derivatization of fructose and lactose at all and, thus, is not subject to these concerns.

Glucose and insulin quantification: Milk fat was separated from the aqueous phase by centrifugation with the resulting skimmed milk assayed using commercially available immunoassay kits for insulin described by our group previously [12]. Glucose was measured using the glucose oxidase method (2300 STAT Plus, Yellow Springs Instruments, YSI Incorporated, Yellow Spring, OH, USA).

2.6. Statistical Analysis

Paired *t*-tests were used to assess the change in infant growth and breast milk sugar content from 1 to 6 months. These *t*-tests indicated that sugar and insulin levels in the milk did not significantly vary between 1 and 6 months; thus, all statistical models were conducted using the average of these two values (e.g., average glucose, fructose, lactose, and insulin).

To examine how breast milk levels of fructose, glucose, lactose, and insulin relate to infant growth, separate hierarchical regression models were conducted predicting infant weight, length, weight-for-length z-score, fat mass, lean mass, bone mineral density (BMD), bone mineral content (BMC), and overall percent adiposity at 6 months of age. A priori covariates included mothers' pre-pregnancy body mass index (BMI), 1-month infant weight (g), and infant sex. Pearson correlation coefficients conducted during data exploration indicated that 1-month weight was highly correlated with 1-month length ($r = 0.71$), 1-month fat mass ($r = 0.90$), 1-month fat free mass ($r = 0.95$), and 1-month overall adiposity ($r = 0.68$). Thus, for simplicity and to avoid multicollinearity among predictors, only 1-month weight was retained in the base model. Thus, Step 1 of the hierarchical model consisted of our base model (infant sex, infant 1-month weight, mother prepregnancy BMI) and Step 2 introduced the particular milk component of interest (e.g., average fructose, glucose, lactose, insulin concentration). This approach allowed us to examine the contribution of milk sugar content towards explaining the variance in infant growth after controlling for known predictors of infant weight outcomes. Results are presented as the mean ± standard deviation (M ± SD). Unless otherwise stated, models were conducted with the continuous predictor variables centered on the mean; unstandardized beta coefficients (β) are reported. All assumptions of multiple linear regression were satisfied. Analyses were performed in SPSS version 22 with a priori significance level set at $p < 0.05$ (SPSS, IBM, Armonk, NY, USA).

3. Results

3.1. Variation in Breast Milk Sugar Composition within the First Six Months of Life

The characteristics of the 25 mother–infant pairs enrolled in the study are shown in Table 1. As expected, infants' weight, length, lean mass, fat mass, and overall adiposity significantly increased over the six-month study period ($p < 0.001$). The milk sugar concentration at both one and six months are reported in Table 2. As shown in Figure 1, we were able to accurately measure fructose content in breast milk using LC-MS/MS, displayed as typical chromatographic traces. Milk sugar remained constant over time, as indicated by non-significant *t*-tests comparing one and six months.

Table 1. Participant characteristics.

	1 Month	6 Months	Change [a]
Mother			
Age (years)	29.64 (4.87)		
BMI (kg/m^2)	28.14 (7.32)		
Infant			
Age (days)	39.28 (3.51)		
Sex (F/M)	8/17		
Weight (g)	4766.36 (765.45)	7250.84 (1243.35)	2484.48 (736.89) ‡
Length (cm)	55.82 (2.44)	65.38 (2.92)	9.56 (2.07) ‡
Lean Mass (g) [b]	3753.32 (476.02)	4880.05 (749.21)	1126.72 (494.44) ‡
Fat Mass (g)	1222.84 (309.11)	2485.08 (642.27)	1262.24 (462.29) ‡

Table 1. *Cont.*

	1 Month	6 Months	Change [a]
Infant			
Adiposity (%) [c]	23.96 (3.02)	32.74 (3.75)	8.79 (3.26) ‡
BMC (g)	93.2 (17.85)	134.45 (21.0)	41.28 (19.92) ‡
BMD (g/cm^2)	0.37 (0.04)	0.36 (0.03)	−0.002 (0.03)

Mean (SD) for the 25 mother-infant pairs included in this study. [a] Significance assessed with paired *t*-tests between 1 and 6 months; [b] Lean mass reflects fat-free mass minus BMC (lean tissue only, excluding bone mass); [c] Adiposity calculated as percent of fat mass (g) to total mass (g). SD, standard deviation; BMI, body mass index; F/M, females/male; BMC, bone mineral content; BMD, bone mineral density. * $p < 0.05$, ‡ $p < 0.001$.

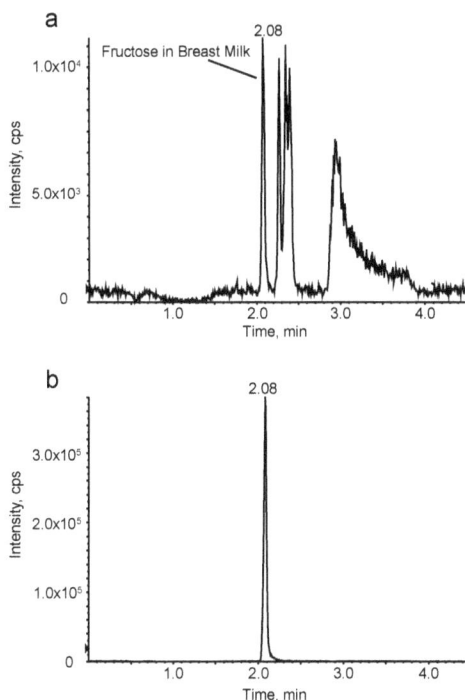

Figure 1. LC-MS/MS (Liquid Chromatography-Mass Spectrometry/Mass Spectrometry) chromatographic traces confirming fructose content in breast milk. (**a**) Natural fructose in breast milk (sample # 108-1); (**b**) Spiked Carbon-13 labeled $^{13}C_6$-fructose as the internal standard (10 μg in 50 μL of breast milk).

Table 2. Changes in milk composition.

	1 Month	6 Month [a]	Average [b]
Insulin (pg/mL) [c]	641.0 (638.0)	640.8 (533.7)	640.9 (469.5)
Fructose (μg/mL)	7.2 (1.72)	6.3 (1.7)	6.7 (1.3)
Glucose (μg/mL)	263.6 (87.5)	246.8 (76.8)	255.2 (75.3)
Lactose (g/dL) [d]	7.8 (0.8)	7.5 (0.7)	7.6 (0.6)

Mean (SD) for 25 mothers included in this study. [a] Change from baseline assessed with paired *t*-test at * $p < 0.05$. All were NS; [b] The average value of each sugar (between 1 and 6 months) was used in all statistical models reported; [c] One participant excluded for extreme hyperinsulinemia; $n = 24$; [d] Data represented in g/dL due to its high concentration in milk.

3.2. Relationships between Breast Milk Sugar Content and Infant Growth

Given that the breast milk concentrations of each sugar did not vary between one and six months, the average concentration of each sugar was calculated and entered into separate hierarchical regression models predicting infant body composition at 6 months of infant age. These results are displayed in Table 3. Even after adjusting for baseline covariates (ome-month infant weight, infant sex, and maternal BMI), breast milk fructose accounted for an additional 8% of the variance in infant weight ($p = 0.02$), an additional 9% of the variance in infant lean mass ($p = 0.01$), an additional 7% of the variance in infant fat mass ($p = 0.05$), and an additional 9% of the variance in infant bone mineral content ($p = 0.03$) at 6 months of age. As shown in Figure 2, each 1-µg/mL increase in fructose was associated with a 257 g increase in body weight ($\beta = 256.9$, $p = 0.02$), 170 g increase in lean mass ($\beta = 170.1$, $p = 0.01$), 131 g increase in fat mass ($\beta = 130.8$, $p = 0.05$), and 5 g increase in bone mineral content ($\beta = 4.7$, $p = 0.03$). A positive relationship was also observed for fructose predicting increased weight-for-length z-scores ($\beta = 0.3$, $p = 0.02$). There was no evidence that infant growth was related to mothers' pre-pregnancy BMI (largest $p = 0.59$; from base model) or to any of the other breast milk components.

Table 3. Relationships between breast milk sugars and infant body composition at 6 months of age [a].

Infant Outcome	Model	β	ΔR^2	ΔR^2 p Value
	Base Model		0.70	0.00
	Fructose	256.9 *	0.08	0.02
Weight (g)	Lactose	26.2	<0.01	0.92
	Glucose	−0.9	<0.01	0.73
	Insulin	0.04	<0.01	0.91
	Base Model		0.56	0.00
	Fructose	0.4	0.03	0.28
Length (cm)	Lactose	−1.1	0.04	0.15
	Glucose	−0.01	0.03	0.23
	Insulin	<0.01	0.03	0.21
	Base Model		0.52	0.00
Weight-for-Length	Fructose	0.3 *	0.12	0.02
z-score	Lactose	0.5	0.05	0.14
	Glucose	<0.01	0.01	0.54
	Insulin	<0.01	0.02	0.39
	Base Model		0.66	0.00
	Fructose	170.1 *	0.09	0.01
Lean Mass (g) [b]	Lactose	224.3	0.03	0.18
	Glucose	−1.8	0.02	0.27
	Insulin	0.30	0.03	0.23
	Base Model		0.59	0.00
	Fructose	130.8 *	0.07	0.05
Fat Mass (g)	Lactose	−31.7	0.00	0.84
	Glucose	−0.2	<0.01	0.88
	Insulin	−0.13	0.01	0.51
	Base Model		0.35	0.03
	Fructose	0.5	0.04	0.29
Adiposity (%) [c]	Lactose	−1.5	0.05	0.20
	Glucose	0.01	0.01	0.56
	Insulin	<0.01	0.09	0.10
	Base Model		0.59	0.00
	Fructose	4.7 *	0.09	0.03
BMC (g)	Lactose	<0.01	0.01	0.57
	Glucose	<0.01	<0.01	0.76
	Insulin	<0.01	<0.01	0.71

Table 3. Relationships between breast milk sugars and infant body composition at 6 months of age [a].

Infant Outcome	Model	β	ΔR^2	ΔR^2 *p* Value
	Base Model		0.47	0.00
	Fructose	<0.01	0.03	0.32
BMD (g/cm^2)	Lactose	<0.01	0.01	0.62
	Glucose	<0.01	0.07	0.09
	Insulin	<0.01	0.01	0.60

Hierarchical linear regression was used to examine the change in R^2 with the addition of each sugar. The base model included infant sex, 1-month infant weight, and maternal BMI. R^2 is reported for the base model and the change in R^2 is reported in response to adding each sugar to the base model. [a] Insulin analyses exclude one participant who was extremely hyperinsulinemic; *n* = 24; [b] Lean mass reflects fat-free mass minus BMC (lean tissue only, excluding bone mass); [c] Adiposity calculated as percent of fat mass (g) to total mass (g). β, unstandardized regression coefficient; BMC, bone mineral content; BMD, bone mineral density.* *p* <0.05.

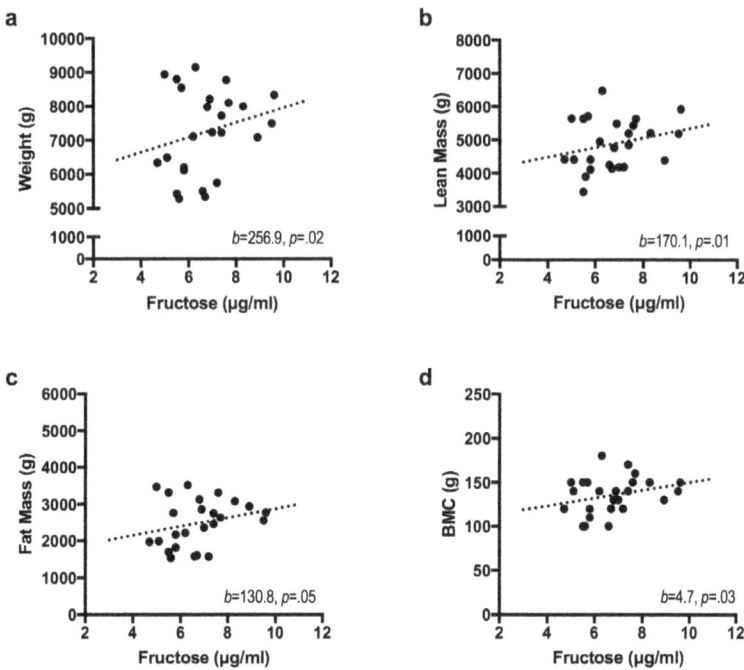

Figure 2. Breast milk fructose is positively associated with infant body composition at 6 months of age. Figures display the unadjusted values for breast milk fructose relative to (**a**) body weight; (**b**) lean mass; (**c**) fat mass; and (**d**) bone mineral content. Hierarchical linear regression was performed to obtain the parameter estimates (*b*) after adjusting for infant sex, one-month infant weight, and maternal body mass index (*n* = 25).

4. Discussion

The detrimental effects of fructose are well documented in children and adults, but no study that we are aware of has examined whether fructose is detectable in human breast milk, and whether this might be associated with growth and body composition, particularly adiposity in infancy. These associations were observed even though the level of fructose in breast milk was extremely low (7 μg/mL), approximately 1/30th the level of glucose. Despite this very low concentration, fructose levels in breastmilk appeared to be biologically relevant. Each 1-μg/mL higher fructose was associated with a 257 g higher body weight, 170 g higher lean mass, 131 g higher fat mass, and 5 g higher bone mineral content at six months of age in our sample. These effects remained significant even after accounting for covariates known to impact infant growth, such as sex, baseline weight, and maternal BMI prior to pregnancy and were not apparent for glucose levels in breastmilk.

In this small proof of concept study, we observed that fructose was significantly associated with higher body weight, and that this effect was distributed across all components of body composition (i.e., fat mass, lean mass, and bone mass). It is important to note that these observed associations do not necessarily imply causation. Further work is needed to examine the possibility that even these very small amounts of fructose can affect musculoskeletal development as well as adipose tissue development in infancy and early life, which is a rapid growth period where significant changes in muscular and skeletal growth are occurring. Indeed, although evidence investigating age-related changes are generally lacking in this area, our results are consistent with a recent paper which found that a high fructose diet led to increased skeletal density and increased length in adolescent rats [25]. Further research is needed examining the effects of fructose in early life, including at low doses, in order to draw more causative conclusions about the specific impact of fructose on infant adiposity and tissue development.

Since human milk does not naturally contain fructose [26], our findings highlight maternal intake of fructose-containing products, such as sugar sweetened beverages, as a targetable intervention for reducing exposure to fructose in early life. While previous studies have shown that fructose can be transmitted in utero through the placenta [27,28], our findings extend this literature by identifying breast milk as a potential route of fructose transmission in the postnatal period. Assuming 800 mL daily intake of breast milk, the concentration we observed in our sample would represent approximately 5 mg/day fructose consumption—an amount roughly equal to 1 mg per kg of body weight for a one-month old infant. We recognize that this amount of fructose is very low and far outside the range where fructose is currently known to have physiological effects. Although very small, this concentration could have meaningful effects in developing infants. For example, fructose may be obesogenic in low concentrations in infants where there can be increased susceptibility to chemicals in the environment, including those delivered indirectly as a result of maternal transmission [29–31]. There is some evidence that fructose may induce obesogenic effects at very low levels of concentration similar to what we have detected in human breastmilk. For example, in a dose-response study, fructose was shown to increase adipogenesis and induce gene expression in cultured pre-adipocytes, with effects seen at levels as low as 55 µM [32]. This concentration is equivalent to 10 µg/mL, which is only slightly above the concentrations in breast milk that we observed. Of particular significance, even the lowest fructose concentration (10 µg/mL) led to a highly significant and four-fold increase in GluT4 expression in pre-adipocytes, a marker of adipogenesis [32]. Collectively, this study supports the idea that even very low levels of fructose could potentially prime pre-adipocytes towards an adipogenic fate.

Unlike glucose, the metabolism of fructose in unregulated by the liver and affects brain development [8]. Studies have shown that increased levels of fructose can contribute to liver fat, resulting in insulin resistance as well as alterations in insulin and glucose metabolism. However, the dose-response of these effects are completely unknown in infants. The first year of life is a critical developmental period, where even small levels of fructose may have detrimental effects on infant metabolism. In addition, it is possible that the very low levels of fructose reported here are indicating "basal" levels, and higher levels of fructose might be delivered via breast milk to the infant when the mother is consuming sugars during the time of feeding. It is also possible that the detected fructose levels are serving as a proxy measure for some other factor affecting infant growth. More studies are needed to examine the pharmacokinetics of fructose transmission through breast milk in response to maternal consumption. Unfortunately, dietary data were not collected as part of this study; thus, it is not possible to formally determine whether mothers' habitual consumption of fructose was positively associated with the level of fructose detected in their breast milk. Future studies examining the relationship between maternal diet and breast milk sugar concentrations will be important for

Nutrients **2017**, *9*, 146

informing guidelines for monitoring sugar and fructose intake during the lactation period, and for determining how the Western diet typically affects breast milk composition and infant growth.

Previous studies have shown that higher breast milk glucose concentrations were associated with greater adiposity in infants [12,20]. In the current study, breast milk glucose levels were not related to infant measures of adiposity. It is possible that this discrepancy may be explained by different study designs, or interactions with maternal factors that were not present in our cohort (i.e., gestational diabetes). Ultimately, more studies are needed to determine whether the effects of breast milk sugars are robust and replicable across a variety of infant cohorts and future studies should consider the potential effects of both fructose and glucose in breast milk.

Limitations of the present study include the small sample size in this proof-of-concept study, limited length of follow-up (six months of age), and a lack of dietary intake data that could help explain the relationship between fructose and breast milk sugar composition. Although women were instructed to exclusively breastfeed, it is possible that food introduction may have occurred in some infants during the study period and contributed to growth and body composition, particularly if infants were given access to fructose-containing food products. Indeed, a recent study which evaluated the sugar content of commercial infant and toddler food products found that between 30% and 50% of snacks, desserts, and juices/drinks targeted at infants contain at least one added sugar, with high fructose corn syrup being present in 2%–4% of these items [33]. Many of these items contain sugars in amounts that differ from nutrition labels and often in excess of recommended daily levels [34]. Together, these findings indicate that it is highly likely that infants are exposed to fructose in the first few months of life (e.g., during breastfeeding and/or weaning when complementary foods are introduced to the diet), highlighting the need for further research into the effects of these sugars on child development. Another potential limitation is that we have limited metabolic variables in the mothers. Although we did exclude mothers with type 1 or 2 diabetes based on standard clinical criteria, we were unable to assess prediabetes in this sample. Therefore, it may be possible that mothers with prediabetes had increased levels of insulin and sugars in breast milk. However, breast milk levels of insulin and glucose were not associated with infant growth and body composition.

5. Conclusions

Overall, this study suggests a novel mechanism by which infants may be inadvertently exposed to fructose through breast milk, before sugar sweetened beverages and other fructose-containing foods are introduced to the infant diet. This work also opens the door for interventions aimed towards decreased consumption of added sugars while lactating. Future work should be performed with larger samples with longer follow-up (>6 months) in order to establish whether the relationships observed between fructose exposure and infant growth meaningfully impact the development of obesity phenotypes in later childhood and to investigative the mechanism of such an effect at very low levels of fructose. In conclusion, we provide preliminary evidence that fructose is present in breast milk and may be transmitted to the infant, impacting growth and body composition by 6 months of age.

Supplementary Materials: The following are available online at http://www.mdpi.com/2072-6643/9/2/146/s1, Figure S1: Fructose Derivatization Scheme with Methoxyamine (NH_2O-Me) and *N*-methyl-*N*-(trimethylsily)-trifluroacetamide (MSTFA) for Gas Chromatography-Mass Spectrometry (GC-MS).

Acknowledgments: Preliminary data in 19 subjects irrespective of maternal BMI from this study were published previously (Fields, D.A.; Demerath, E.W. Relationship of insulin, glucose, leptin, IL-6 and TNF-alpha in human breast milk with infant growth and body composition. *Pediatr Obes.* 2012, *7*, 304–312). We are grateful to the mothers for participating in this study and for Catherine Wolf (study recruitment and testing of subjects) and April Teague (performing breast-milk analyses on glucose and insulin) for their work on the study. Mead Johnson Nutrition provided financial support for the milk collection but provided no financial support for the analysis and the final decision on content was exclusively retained by the authors. A portion of this work was supported by an award from the Harold Hamm Diabetes Center at the University of Oklahoma Health Sciences Center. Support for the Washington University Diabetic Cardiovascular Disease Center came from the NIH (National Institute of Health) (GM103422, DK056341, DK020579). All authors have read and approved the manuscript as submitted.

Author Contributions: D.A.F. and M.I.G. designed the study; T.A.A. conducted the research; A.A.M. analyzed the data and wrote the paper; A.A.M., T.A.A., D.A.F. and M.I.G. had primary responsibility for final content.

Conflicts of Interest: The authors declare no conflict of interest. The founding sponsors had no role in the design of the study; in the collection, analyses, or interpretation of data; in the writing of the manuscript, and in the decision to publish the results.

References

1. Malik, V.S.; Pan, A.; Willett, W.C.; Hu, F.B. Sugar-sweetened beverages and weight gain in children and adults: A systematic review and meta-analysis. *Am. J. Clin. Nutr.* **2013**, *98*, 1084–1102. [CrossRef] [PubMed]
2. Zhang, Z.; Gillespie, C.; Welsh, J.A.; Hu, F.B.; Yang, Q. Usual intake of added sugars and lipid profiles among the U.S. adolescents: National Health and Nutrition Examination Survey, 2005–2010. *J. Adolesc. Health* **2015**, *56*, 352–359. [CrossRef] [PubMed]
3. Welsh, J.A.; Sharma, A.; Cunningham, S.A.; Vos, M.B. Consumption of added sugars and indicators of cardiovascular disease risk among US adolescents. *Circulation* **2011**, *123*, 249–257. [CrossRef] [PubMed]
4. Xi, B.; Huang, Y.; Reilly, K.H.; Li, S.; Zheng, R.; Barrio-Lopez, M.T.; Martinez-Gonzalez, M.A.; Zhou, D. Sugar-sweetened beverages and risk of hypertension and CVD: A dose–response meta-analysis. *Br. J. Nutr.* **2015**, *113*, 709–717. [CrossRef] [PubMed]
5. Ma, J.; Fox, C.S.; Jacques, P.F.; Speliotes, E.K.; Hoffmann, U.; Smith, C.E.; Saltzman, E.; McKeown, N.M. Sugar-sweetened beverage, diet soda, and fatty liver disease in the Framingham Heart Study cohorts. *J. Hepatol.* **2015**, *63*, 462–469. [CrossRef] [PubMed]
6. Bray, G.A.; Popkin, B.M. Calorie-sweetened beverages and fructose: What have we learned 10 years later. *Pediatr. Obes.* **2013**, *8*, 242–248. [CrossRef] [PubMed]
7. Stanhope, K.L.; Schwarz, J.-M.; Havel, P.J. Adverse metabolic effects of dietary fructose: Results from the recent epidemiological, clinical, and mechanistic studies. *Curr. Opin. Lipidol.* **2013**, *24*, 198–206. [CrossRef] [PubMed]
8. Goran, M.I.; Dumke, K.; Bouret, S.G.; Kayser, B.; Walker, R.W.; Blumberg, B. The obesogenic effect of high fructose exposure during early development. *Nat. Rev. Endocrinol.* **2013**, *9*, 494–500. [CrossRef] [PubMed]
9. Pan, L.; Li, R.; Park, S.; Galuska, D.A.; Sherry, B.; Freedman, D.S. A longitudinal analysis of sugar-sweetened beverage intake in infancy and obesity at 6 years. *Pediatrics* **2014**, *134*, S29–S35. [CrossRef] [PubMed]
10. Park, S.; Pan, L.; Sherry, B.; Li, R. The association of sugar-sweetened beverage intake during infancy with sugar-sweetened beverage intake at 6 years of age. *Pediatrics* **2014**, *134*, S56–S62. [CrossRef] [PubMed]
11. Ballard, O.; Morrow, A.L. Human Milk Composition: Nutrients and Bioctive Factors. *Pediatr. Clin. N. Am.* **2013**, *60*, 1–24. [CrossRef] [PubMed]
12. Fields, D.A.; Demerath, E.W. Relationship of insulin, glucose, leptin, IL-6 and TNF-α in human breast milk with infant growth and body composition. *Pediatr. Obes.* **2012**, *7*, 304–312. [CrossRef] [PubMed]
13. Fields, D.A.; Schneider, C.R.; Pavela, G. A narrative review of the associations between six bioactive components in breast milk and infant adiposity. *Obesity* **2016**, *24*, 1213–1221. [CrossRef] [PubMed]
14. Rolls, B.A.; Gurr, M.I.; van Duijvenvoorde, P.M.; Rolls, B.J.; Rowe, E.A. Lactation in lean and obese rats: Effect of cafeteria feeding and of dietary obesity on milk composition. *Physiol. Behav.* **1986**, *38*, 185–190. [CrossRef]
15. Purcell, R.H.; Sun, B.; Pass, L.L.; Power, M.L.; Moran, T.H.; Tamashiro, K.L.K. Maternal stress and high-fat diet effect on maternal behavior, milk composition, and pup ingestive behavior. *Physiol. Behav.* **2011**, *104*, 474–479. [CrossRef] [PubMed]
16. Nicholas, K.R.; Hartmann, P.E. Milk secretion in the rat: Progressive changes in milk composition during lactation and weaning and the effect of diet. *Comp. Biochem. Physiol. A Physiol.* **1991**, *98*, 535–542. [CrossRef]
17. Bayol, S.A.; Farrington, S.J.; Stickland, N.C. A maternal "junk food" diet in pregnancy and lactation promotes an exacerbated taste for "junk food" and a greater propensity for obesity in rat offspring. *Br. J. Nutr.* **2007**, *98*, 843–851. [CrossRef] [PubMed]
18. Gorski, J.N. Postnatal environment overrides genetic and prenatal factors influencing offspring obesity and insulin resistance. *AJP Regul. Integr. Comp. Physiol.* **2006**, *291*, R768–R778. [CrossRef] [PubMed]

19. Plagemann, A.; Harder, T.; Schellong, K.; Schulz, S.; Stupin, J.H. Early postnatal life as a critical time window for determination of long-term metabolic health. *Best Pract. Res. Clin. Endocrinol. Metab.* **2012**, *26*, 641–653. [CrossRef] [PubMed]

20. Plagemann, A.; Harder, T.; Franke, K.; Kohlhoff, R. Long-term impact of neonatal breast-feeding on body weight and glucose tolerance in children of diabetic mothers. *Diabetes Care* **2002**, *25*, 16–22. [CrossRef] [PubMed]

21. Neubauer, S.H. Lactation in insulin-dependent diabetes. *Prog. Food Nutr. Sci.* **1990**, *14*, 333–370. [PubMed]

22. Jovanovic-Peterson, L.; Fuhrmann, K.; Hedden, K.; Walker, L.; Peterson, C.M. Maternal milk and plasma glucose and insulin levels: Studies in normal and diabetic subjects. *J. Am. Coll. Nutr.* **1989**, *8*, 125–131. [CrossRef] [PubMed]

23. Alderete, T.L.; Autran, C.; Brekke, B.E.; Knight, R.; Bode, L.; Goran, M.I.; Fields, D.A. Associations between human milk oligosaccharides and infant body composition in the first 6 mo of life. *Am. J. Clin. Nutr.* **2015**, *102*, 1381–1388. [CrossRef] [PubMed]

24. Scano, P.; Murgia, A.; Demuru, M.; Consonni, R.; Caboni, P. Metabolite profiles of formula milk compared to breast milk. *Food Res. Int.* **2016**, *87*, 76–82. [CrossRef]

25. Bass, E.F.; Baile, C.A.; Lewis, R.D.; Giraudo, S.Q. Bone quality and strength are greater in growing male rats fed fructose compared with glucose. *Nutr. Res.* **2013**, *33*, 1063–1071. [CrossRef] [PubMed]

26. Jenness, R. The composition of human milk. *Semin. Perinatol.* **1979**, *3*, 225–239. [PubMed]

27. Hagerman, D.D.; Villee, C.A. The transport of fructose by human placenta. *J. Clin. Investig.* **1952**, *31*, 911–913. [CrossRef] [PubMed]

28. Holmberg, N.G.; Kaplan, B.; Karvonen, M.J.; Lind, J.; Malm, M. Permeability of human placenta to glucose, fructose, and xylose. *Acta Physiol. Scand.* **1956**, *36*, 291–299. [CrossRef] [PubMed]

29. Bailey, K.A.; Smith, A.H.; Tokar, E.J.; Graziano, J.H.; Kim, K. Mechanisms Underlying Latent Disease Risk Associated with Early-Life Arsenic Exposure: Current Research Trends and Scientific Gaps. *Environ. Health Perspect.* **2016**, *124*, 170–176. [CrossRef] [PubMed]

30. Rauh, V.A.; Perera, F.P.; Horton, M.K.; Whyatt, R.M.; Bansal, R.; Hao, X.; Liu, J.; Barr, D.B.; Slotkin, T.A.; Peterson, B.S. Brain anomalies in children exposed prenatally to a common organophosphate pesticide. *Proc. Natl. Acad. Sci. USA* **2012**, *109*, 7871–7876. [CrossRef] [PubMed]

31. Whyatt, R.M.; Rauh, V.; Barr, D.B.; Camann, D.E.; Andrews, H.F.; Garfinkel, R.; Hoepner, L.A.; Diaz, D.; Dietrich, J.; Reyes, A.; et al. Prenatal insecticide exposures and birth weight and length among an urban minority cohort. *Environ. Health Perspect.* **2004**, *112*, 1125–1132. [CrossRef] [PubMed]

32. Du, L.; Heaney, A.P. Regulation of Adipose Differentiation by Fructose and GluT5. *Mol. Endocrinol.* **2012**, *26*, 1773–1782. [CrossRef] [PubMed]

33. Cogswell, M.E.; Gunn, J.P.; Yuan, K.; Park, S.; Merritt, R. Sodium and sugar in complementary infant and toddler foods sold in the United States. *Pediatrics* **2015**, *135*, 416–423. [CrossRef] [PubMed]

34. Walker, R.; Goran, M. Laboratory determined sugar content and composition of commercial infant formulas, baby foods and common grocery items targeted to children. *Nutrients* **2015**, *7*, 5850–5867. [CrossRef] [PubMed]

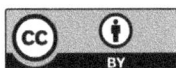

nutrients

MDPI

Article

Lifetime Exposure to a Constant Environment Amplifies the Impact of a Fructose-Rich Diet on Glucose Homeostasis during Pregnancy

Aleida Song [1,†], Stuart Astbury [1,2,†], Abha Hoedl [1], Brent Nielsen [1], Michael E. Symonds [2,*] and Rhonda C. Bell [1,3,*]

1   Division of Human Nutrition, Department of Agricultural, Food and Nutritional Sciences, University of Alberta, Edmonton, AB T6G 2E1, Canada; aleida@ualberta.ca (A.S.); stuart.astbury@nottingham.ac.uk (S.A.); abha@ualberta.ca (A.H.); banielse@ualberta.ca (B.N.)
2   Early Life Research Group, Academic Division of Child Health, Obstetrics & Gynaecology, and NIHR Nottingham Digestive Diseases Biomedical Research Unit, School of Medicine, University of Nottingham and Nottingham University Hospitals NHS Trust, Nottingham NG7 2UH, UK
3   Women and Children's Health Research Institute, University of Alberta, Edmonton, AB T6G 2E1, Canada
*   Correspondences: michael.symonds@nottingham.ac.uk (M.E.S.); rhonda.bell@ualberta.ca (R.C.B.); Tel.: +44-(0)-115-823-0625 (M.E.S.); +1-780-492-7742 (R.C.B.)
†   These authors contributed equally to this work.

Received: 27 February 2017; Accepted: 21 March 2017; Published: 25 March 2017

Abstract: The need to refine rodent models of human-related disease is now being recognized, in particular the rearing environment that can profoundly modulate metabolic regulation. Most studies on pregnancy and fetal development purchase and transport young females into the research facility, which after a short period of acclimation are investigated (Gen0). We demonstrate that female offspring (Gen1) show an exaggerated hyperinsulinemic response to pregnancy when fed a standard diet and with high fructose intake, which continues throughout pregnancy. Markers of maternal hepatic metabolism were differentially influenced, as the gene expression of acetyl-CoA-carboxylase was raised in Gen1 given fructose and controls, whereas glucose transporter 5 and fatty acid synthase expression were only raised with fructose. Gen1 rats weighed more than Gen0 throughout the study, although fructose feeding raised the percent body fat but not body weight. We show that long-term habituation to the living environment has a profound impact on the animal's metabolic responses to nutritional intervention and pregnancy. This has important implications for interpreting many studies investigating the influence of maternal consumption of fructose on pregnancy outcomes and offspring to date.

Keywords: fructose; development; pregnancy; metabolism; type II diabetes

1. Introduction

Diabetes and metabolic syndrome are normally considered to result from exposure to an obesogenic environment together with an individual's genotype [1]. It is also recognized that in populations that migrate to more affluent countries, it is the next generation that is at greater risk of becoming diabetic, in part due to early life exposures [2,3]. These factors are seldom considered in animal models of diabetes, especially those examining the impact of exposure to an adverse maternal nutritional environment on the offspring. Although there is increasing awareness of the role of high intakes of fructose in metabolic syndrome–associated diseases, such as non-alcoholic fatty liver disease [4], coronary artery disease [5] and type II diabetes [6], and a growing body of literature covering high intakes of fructose during pregnancy [7–10], there is still a lack of longer-term rodent studies following the offspring into adulthood and pregnancy. Rodent studies have demonstrated that fructose in pregnancy can significantly reduce the weight of the placenta [11], and increase the expression of genes related to lipogenesis in the offspring liver [12].

Rodent models of nutritional programming usually use young females that are shipped into a research facility and, after a brief period of acclimation, are exposed to a dietary intervention. This experimental approach seldom accounts for the fact that the mothers experienced a significant change in environment while offspring were not moved from their home environment. Failure to account for these differences could mask important adverse consequences that are expressed only in subsequent generations that are fully habituated to their living environment. This could account for how diet-induced maternal obesity can result in glucose intolerance in the offspring in some [13,14] but not all studies [15,16]. We therefore examined whether offspring born and reared in a single research facility (Gen1) exhibit a more pronounced diabetes-related phenotype than their mothers (Gen0). Half of the animals were given fructose (F) in drinking water as a 10% solution (vs. distilled water) prior to and during pregnancy to establish whether fructose would amplify these effects. Fructose was chosen since it produces a gestational diabetes mellitus (GDM)-type phenotype of metabolic dysfunction in the adult offspring [8,11,17]. A 10% solution was chosen to more closely mimic fructose consumption in humans (i.e., as an added sweetener), and previous work has shown this concentration has significant metabolic effects in rodents [18]. The extent to which metabolic outcomes differ between generations has not been previously examined.

2. Materials and Methods

2.1. Animals and Diets

Seven-week-old female Wistar rats (Charles River Canada, Montreal, Quebec, Canada) were pair-housed in shoebox cages in a temperature-controlled room (21–23 °C; 40%–70% humidity) with a 12 h light:dark cycle. All rats were allowed access to food ad libitum (Purina 5001; Purina Mills, St. Louis, MO, USA) throughout the study and distilled water was available to all rats during the standard one week acclimation period. At eight weeks of age, rats were randomly assigned to receive either a 10% fructose solution (w/v in distilled water, Amresco, Solon, OH, USA; Gen0-F, $n = 15$) or distilled water (Gen0-C, $n = 15$). At 11 weeks of age, they were co-housed with males which had been maintained on distilled water. Pregnancy was confirmed by vaginal lavage and a positive sperm test was considered gestational day (GD) 0. Animals remained on this intervention for three weeks prior to mating and during mating and pregnancy. Ten Gen0-C and 10 Gen0-F were euthanized at GD 21 (details described below). The remaining pregnant dams were left to litter out and all litters were culled to 10–12 pups/litter at birth. Dams continued their assigned diet during lactation (until 21 days after delivery), at which point two female pups were randomly selected to remain in the study as offspring. Eight-week-old female offspring were placed on the same diet as their dams (either 10% fructose solution (Gen1-F, $n = 10$) or distilled water (Gen1-C, $n = 10$). These diets continued through mating and pregnancy. Pregnant offspring were euthanized at GD 21. The study was approved by the Research Ethics Office of the University of Alberta.

2.2. Regular Monitoring of Body Weight and Plasma Metabolites

Body weights were recorded weekly during the study, beginning at eight weeks of age and in early (GD4-7), mid (GD14-17) and late pregnancy (GD19-20). Morning blood samples were also collected, mixed with anti-coagulant (K_2 EDTA, BD, Franklin Lakes, NJ, USA) and remained on ice until centrifugation (Eppendorf Centrifuge 5415C, Germany, $16,000 \times g$, 5 min). Plasma was stored at -20 °C until being analyzed for glucose (Trinder assay kit, Genzyme Diagnostics, Charlottetown, PEI, Canada), insulin (Rat Ultrasensitive ELISA Immunoassay kit, ALPCO Diagnostics, Salem, NH, USA), and triglycerides (Triglyceride-SL assay kit, Genzyme Diagnostics, Cambridge, MA, USA).

2.3. Oral Glucose Tolerance Tests (OGTT)

OGTT were carried out on GD19 after a 4 h fast, this was chosen both to avoid inducing a starvation state overnight [19,20] and to avoid the stress fasting places on pregnant rodents due to their increased glucose utilization [21]. Following collection of a baseline blood sample a 3 g·kg^{-1} glucose solution was administered by gavage. Blood samples were collected at 15, 30, 45, 60 and 90 min after glucose administration. Plasma was separated and stored as above before assaying for glucose and insulin. The incremental area under the curve (IAUC) for glucose and insulin from 0 to 90 min was calculated.

2.4. Determination of Body Composition and Tissue Collection

On GD 21 the proportions of fat and lean tissue of each animal were measured using quantitative magnetic resonance imaging (EchoMRI LLC 4-in-1 whole-body composition analyzer; Echo Medical Systems, Houston, TX, USA). Following euthanasia, the liver was excised from each rat, snap-frozen in liquid nitrogen and stored at −80 °C until analysis. Placentae and fetuses were dissected from the uterus, counted, individually weighed, and the placental:fetal weight ratio calculated.

2.5. RNA Extraction and Determination of Hepatic Gene Expression

Total RNA was extracted from frozen liver that had been homogenized in TRI Reagent (Ambion Diagnostics, Austin, TX, USA), using the RNeasy Mini Kit (Qiagen N.V., Hilden, Germany). RNA concentration and purity were confirmed using a Nanodrop spectrophotometer (Thermo Scientific, Waltham, MA, USA), and reverse transcription PCR was carried out using the High Capacity cDNA reverse transcription kit (Applied Biosystems, Waltham, MA, USA). Quantitative polymerase chain reaction (qPCR) was carried out using SYBR Green dye and the StepOne Plus PCR machine (Applied Biosystems). Primers were designed using Primer3 [22] to the rat genome; primer sequences and GenBank references are included in Supplementary Table S1. Primers were designed to be intron-spanning to avoid amplification of genomic DNA. Product sizes and primer specificity were confirmed using classical PCR and gel electrophoresis before qPCR and melt-curves following qPCR. All qPCR results were adjusted to two reference genes (RPLP0 and GAPDH) using GeNorm for Microsoft Excel [23] and are presented as fold change in arbitrary units relative to the Gen0-C group, according to the $2^{-\Delta\Delta CT}$ method [24].

2.6. Statistical Analysis

Following a Shapiro Wilk test for normality all data were compared using unpaired *t*-tests, with a Bonferroni correction applied where necessary for multiple comparisons. Analyses were carried out using SPSS (version 23, IMB Corp., Armonk, NY, USA).

3. Results and Discussion

Fructose feeding caused hyperinsulinemia to a greater extent in Gen1 than in Gen0 (Figure 1A). Hyperinsulinemia began prior to pregnancy, was exacerbated during pregnancy, and was also observed during the OGTT at the end of pregnancy (Figure 1B). This suggests increased insulin resistance in Gen1 that is exacerbated by a high intake of fructose and was corroborated by the fact that the insulin IAUC was greater in Gen1 than in Gen0 and exaggerated in Gen1-F. Consistent with evidence in humans and rats [25,26], circulating triglycerides were higher in Gen0-F and Gen1-F prior to and during pregnancy, and more so in Gen1.

Body weight was raised in Gen1, but composition did not differ between generations. Fructose enhanced the proportion of fat in Gen0 and Gen1 (Table 1). Litter size was not different between generations or diet groups but fetal weight was reduced in Gen0-F and Gen1-F, and placentae were smaller in Gen1-F (Table 1). Reductions in placental but not fetal weight following fructose intake have been previously demonstrated [11]. Further investigation into the generational effects of fructose on placental blood flow and nutrient transport would be worthwhile.

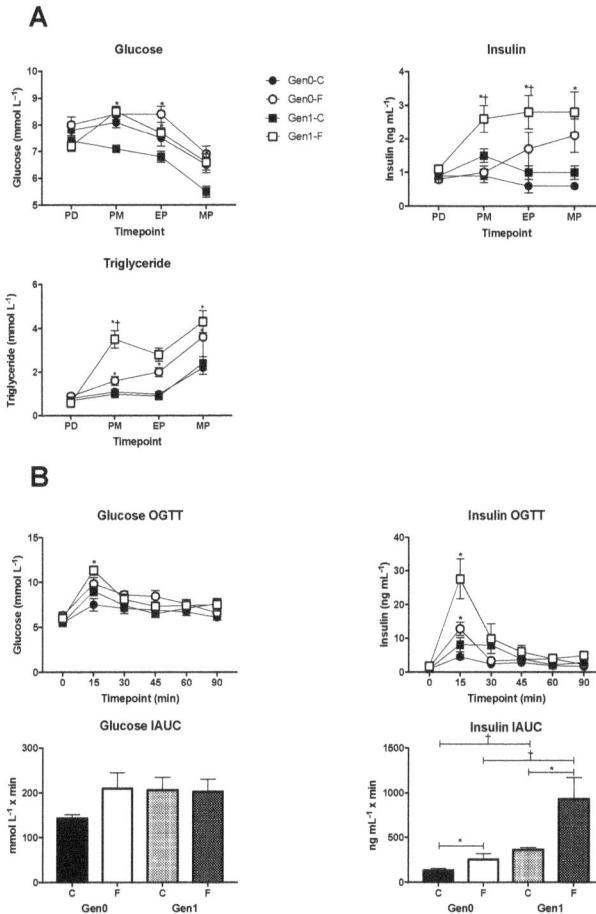

Figure 1. (**A**) Plasma glucose, insulin and triglyceride concentrations measured regularly throughout the study. Gen0-C n = 15, Gen0-F n = 15, Gen1-C n = 10, Gen1-F n = 10. Time points were as follows: PD/pre-diet treatment = eight weeks of age, PM/pre-mating = 11 weeks, EP/early pregnancy = 12 weeks/gestational day (GD) 4–7, MP/mid pregnancy = 13 weeks/GD14–17. Whole blood was collected from non-fasted rats and plasma was separated and stored at −20 °C before analysis. (**B**) Oral glucose tolerance tests (OGTT) were conducted on GD19. Rats were fasted for 4 h. Following collection of a baseline blood sample 3 g·kg^{-1} body weight of glucose was administered by gavage. Blood samples were collected at 15, 30, 45, 60 and 90 min post glucose bolus. * $p < 0.05$, Gen0-C vs. Gen0-F, or Gen1-C vs. Gen1-F (effect of diet) and † $p < 0.05$, Gen0-C vs. Gen1-C and Gen0-F vs. Gen1-F (effect of generation), unpaired t-test with a Bonferroni correction applied for multiple comparisons.

Given the importance of the liver in responding to high fructose intake [27], we examined the mRNA abundance of genes involved in liver glucose and fructose transport [28,29]. Though *GLUT2* expression was raised by fructose in Gen0 and *GLUT5* was raised in Gen0 and Gen1, neither was affected by generation (Figure 2). Generational effects were observed in *FAS* and *ACC1* expression, and *FAS* expression also displayed a fructose effect. This suggests an upregulation in lipid metabolism in Gen1 that is more pronounced with fructose intake.

Table 1. Body weights (g) before and throughout pregnancy, and body composition and feto-placental unit near to term.

Age/Pregnancy Stage	Gen0-C	Gen0-F	Gen1-C	Gen1-F
Body Weight (g)				
Week 8/Pre-diet	200.6 ± 3.3	204.1 ± 3.1	225.1 ± 6.3 [†]	226.4 ± 5.7 [†]
Week 9	227.0 ± 2.0	238.3 ± 2.9	254.5 ± 6.6 [†]	252.3 ± 6.5 [†]
Week 10	247.3 ± 2.3	257.2 ± 3.1	280.7 ± 6.8 [†]	285.9 ± 7.7 [†]
Week 11/Pre-mating	261.5 ± 3.0	277.7 ± 4.7	305.5 ± 7.4 [†]	316.3 ± 9.3 [†]
Week 12/ Early pregnancy	290.5 ± 2.3	304.9 ± 5.3	332.2 ± 6.8 [†]	352.3 ± 12.9 [†]
Week 13/ Mid pregnancy	329.4 ± 5.1	337.6 ± 5.9	383.8 ± 7.6 [†]	393.3 ± 14.3 [†]
Week 14/ Late pregnancy	386.5 ± 5.4	403.1 ± 6.7	428.7 ± 12.3 [†]	444.4 ± 15.6 [†]
Body Composition (%)				
Fat mass at GD21	11.2 ± 0.7	15.2 ± 1.0 *	11.4 ± 0.5	16.7 ± 1.3 *
Feto-placental unit				
Number of pups	15.5 ± 1.7	16.0 ± 3.2	16.3 ± 2.3	17.0 ± 3.3
Placental weight (g)	0.53 ± 0.02	0.48 ± 0.02	0.57 ± 0.02	0.47 ± 0.01 *
Fetal weight (g)	3.88 ± 0.19	3.36 ± 0.14 *	4.07 ± 0.05	3.57 ± 0.09 *
The ratio of placental:fetal weight	0.14 ± 0.01	0.15 ± 0.01	0.14 ± 0.00	0.13 ± 0.01

All values are means $\pm$ SEM. Gen0-C $n = 10$, Gen0-F $n = 10$, Gen1-C $n = 10$, Gen1-F $n = 10$. * $p < 0.05$, Gen0-C vs. Gen0-F, or Gen1-C vs. Gen1-F (effect of diet) and † $p < 0.05$, Gen0-C vs. Gen1-C and Gen0-F vs. Gen1-F (effect of generation), unpaired *t*-test with a Bonferroni correction applied for multiple comparisons.

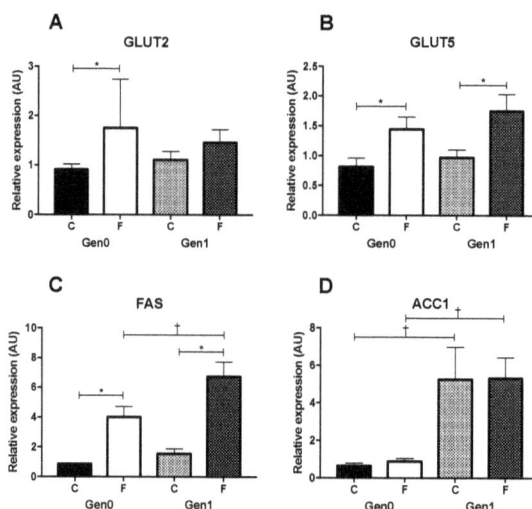

Figure 2. Hepatic gene expression. Gen0-C $n = 10$, Gen0-F $n = 10$, Gen1-C $n = 10$, Gen1-F $n = 10$. Livers were excised on gestational day 21 and snap frozen before RNA extraction and cDNA production by reverse transcription PCR. Expression of glucose transporter 2 (*GLUT2*) (**A**), fructose transporter *GLUT5* (**B**), fatty acid synthase (*FAS*) (**C**) and acetyl-CoA-carboxylase (*ACC1*) (**D**) were measured by real-time PCR, relative to the reference genes glyceraldehyde-3-phosphate dehydrogenase (*GAPDH*) and 60 s acidic ribosomal protein P0 (*RPLP0*) using GeNorm [15] and the $2^{-\Delta\Delta CT}$ method [16]. * $p < 0.05$, Gen0-C vs. Gen0-F, or Gen1-C vs. Gen1-F (effect of diet) and † $p < 0.05$, Gen0-C vs. Gen1-C and Gen0-F vs. Gen1-F (effect of generation), unpaired *t*-test with a Bonferroni correction applied for multiple comparisons.

The substantial difference in insulin resistance and hypertriglyceridemia through pregnancy between Gen0 dams that were recently transported to the facility and Gen1 dams that were born and maintained in the same environment for their life has not been previously demonstrated. Moreover, the nutritional intervention negatively impacted insulin resistance and triglyceride concentrations before and through pregnancy, and these responses were enhanced in Gen1. This is consistent with previous work, which suggests that intake of fructose inversely correlates with insulin receptor expression in a number of organs [30]. To our knowledge, no previous studies have compared the insulin response to fructose in pregnancy between dams and their offspring. The fact that insulin responses were higher in both groups of offspring, who were heavier and fatter than their mothers, suggests that body weight and adiposity could play a role. Previous reports on fructose consumption leading to hyperleptinemia support this [27,31]. The amplified insulin response to glucose in Gen1 has clear implications for the interpretation of studies previously conducted examining the impact of maternal diet on long-term outcomes in offspring. It also highlights the importance of thoroughly characterizing both the mother and her offspring so that true programming effects can be identified. It is likely that in studies in which young rodents were shipped to a research facility and studied a few weeks later, animals were still adapting to this transition. Based on our findings, we suggest that the negative impact of nutritional programming on offspring glucose and lipid homeostasis mediated by fructose feeding [11,12,32] has been significantly underestimated.

A primary factor in enabling us to identify the profound effect on insulin and lipid profiles was our focus on pregnancy as a major physiological challenge. As expected, plasma insulin became raised during pregnancy, but this adaptation was greatly amplified by fructose exposure. At the start of the study (i.e., when the animals were eight weeks old), age-matched offspring were heavier than their dams, and interestingly, the increased Gen1 body weight was not accompanied with greater adiposity, although it was raised in both groups by fructose (Table 1). The impact of adding purified fructose to the diet in human beings remains controversial due in part to the inconsistency in metabolic outcomes [33]. Studying animals which have recently been subjected to the combined stress of transportation and a new living environment may mask many of the metabolic consequences of fructose.

4. Conclusions

In conclusion, substantial adaptations in metabolic profiles through pregnancy are seen between generations that are greatly amplified when offspring are maintained in the research environment as opposed to being transported into the facility and then studied. The magnitude of this adaptation is most apparent in the regulation of plasma insulin and lipids and is exacerbated when the animals are allowed ad libitum access to a fructose solution. It is therefore likely that many studies examining the impact of dietary modulation through pregnancy underestimate the magnitude of the effect on both the mother and her offspring.

Supplementary Materials: The following are available online at www.mdpi.com/1999-4907/9/04/327/s1, Table S1: Primer sequences.

Acknowledgments: Funding sources: University of Alberta Faculty of Medicine and Dentistry Emerging Team Grant (with the Women and Children's Health Research Institute); Natural Science and Engineering Research Council Canada, the Alberta Diabetes Institute and The Faculty of Medicine and Health Sciences, University of Nottingham. The authors are grateful to Nicole Coursen for her assistance with all aspects of animal care.

Author Contributions: All authors contributed to the research and reviewed the manuscript. A.S., S.A. and R.C.B. designed the study; A.S., S.A., B.N., and A.H. carried out all animal husbandry, sample collection and laboratory work; A.S., B.N. and S.A. prepared the table, figures and supplementary material. A.S., S.A., B.N., M.E.S. and R.C.B. led the biological interpretation of results. A.S., S.A., M.E.S. and R.C.B. drafted the manuscript. All authors extensively discussed the analysis, results, interpretation and presentation of results.

Conflicts of Interest: The authors declare no conflict of interest.

References

1. Roche, H.M.; Phillips, C.; Gibney, M.J. The metabolic syndrome: The crossroads of diet and genetics. *Proc. Nutr. Soc.* **2005**, *64*, 371–377. [CrossRef] [PubMed]
2. Misra, A.; Ganda, O.P. Migration and its impact on adiposity and type 2 diabetes. *Nutrition* **2007**, *23*, 696–708. [CrossRef] [PubMed]
3. Symonds, M.E.; Sebert, S.P.; Hyatt, M.A.; Budge, H. Nutritional programming of the metabolic syndrome. *Nat. Rev. Endocrinol.* **2009**, *5*, 604–610. [CrossRef] [PubMed]
4. Vos, M.B.; Lavine, J.E. Dietary fructose in nonalcoholic fatty liver disease. *Hepatology* **2013**, *57*, 2525–2531. [CrossRef] [PubMed]
5. Hollenbeck, C.B. Dietary fructose effects on lipoprotein metabolism and risk for coronary artery disease. *Am. J. Clin. Nutr.* **1993**, *58*, 800S–809S. [PubMed]
6. Imamura, F.; O'Connor, L.; Ye, Z.; Mursu, J.; Hayashino, Y.; Bhupathiraju, S.N.; Forouhi, N.G. Consumption of sugar sweetened beverages, artificially sweetened beverages, and fruit juice and incidence of type 2 diabetes: Systematic review, meta-analysis, and estimation of population attributable fraction. *BMJ* **2015**, *351*, h3576. [CrossRef] [PubMed]
7. Sloboda, D.M.; Li, M.; Patel, R.; Clayton, Z.E.; Yap, C.; Vickers, M.H. Early Life Exposure to Fructose and Offspring Phenotype: Implications for Long Term Metabolic Homeostasis. *J. Obes.* **2014**, *2014*, 1–10. [CrossRef] [PubMed]
8. Lineker, C.; Kerr, P.M.; Nguyen, P.; Bloor, I.; Astbury, S.; Patel, N.; Budge, H.; Hemmings, D.G.; Plane, F.; Symonds, M.E.; et al. High fructose consumption in pregnancy alters the perinatal environment without increasing metabolic disease in the offspring. *Reprod. Fertil. Dev.* **2016**, *28*, 2007–2015. [CrossRef] [PubMed]
9. Alzamendi, A.; Del Zotto, H.; Castrogiovanni, D.; Romero, J.; Giovambattista, A.; Spinedi, E. Oral Metformin Treatment Prevents Enhanced Insulin Demand and Placental Dysfunction in the Pregnant Rat Fed a Fructose-Rich Diet. *Int. Sch. Res. Not.* **2012**, *2012*, e757913. [CrossRef] [PubMed]
10. Rodríguez, L.; Panadero, M.I.; Rodrigo, S.; Roglans, N.; Otero, P.; Álvarez-Millán, J.J.; Laguna, J.C.; Bocos, C. Liquid fructose in pregnancy exacerbates fructose-induced dyslipidemia in adult female offspring. *J. Nutr. Biochem.* **2016**, *32*, 115–122. [CrossRef] [PubMed]
11. Vickers, M.H.; Clayton, Z.E.; Yap, C.; Sloboda, D.M. Maternal fructose intake during pregnancy and lactation alters placental growth and leads to sex-specific changes in fetal and neonatal endocrine function. *Endocrinology* **2011**, *152*, 1378–1387. [CrossRef] [PubMed]
12. Mukai, Y.; Kumazawa, M.; Sato, S. Fructose intake during pregnancy up-regulates the expression of maternal and fetal hepatic sterol regulatory element-binding protein-1c in rats. *Endocrine* **2012**, *44*, 79–86. [CrossRef] [PubMed]
13. Bayol, S.A.; Simbi, B.H.; Stickland, N.C. A maternal cafeteria diet during gestation and lactation promotes adiposity and impairs skeletal muscle development and metabolism in rat offspring at weaning. *J. Physiol.* **2005**, *567*, 951–961. [CrossRef] [PubMed]
14. Nivoit, P.; Morens, C.; Assche, F.A.V.; Jansen, E.; Poston, L.; Remacle, C.; Reusens, B. Established diet-induced obesity in female rats leads to offspring hyperphagia, adiposity and insulin resistance. *Diabetologia* **2009**, *52*, 1133–1142. [CrossRef] [PubMed]
15. McCurdy, C.E.; Bishop, J.M.; Williams, S.M.; Grayson, B.E.; Smith, M.S.; Friedman, J.E.; Grove, K.L. Maternal high-fat diet triggers lipotoxicity in the fetal livers of nonhuman primates. *J. Clin. Investig.* **2009**, *119*, 323–335. [CrossRef] [PubMed]
16. Pereira, T.J.; Moyce, B.L.; Kereliuk, S.M.; Dolinsky, V.W. Influence of maternal overnutrition and gestational diabetes on the programming of metabolic health outcomes in the offspring: Experimental evidence. *Biochem. Cell Biol.* **2014**, *93*, 438–451. [CrossRef] [PubMed]
17. Battaglia, F.C.; Meschia, G. Principal substrates of fetal metabolism. *Physiol. Rev.* **1978**, *58*, 499–527. [PubMed]
18. Rawana, S.; Clark, K.; Zhong, S.; Buison, A.; Chackunkal, S.; Jen, K.L. Low dose fructose ingestion during gestation and lactation affects carbohydrate metabolism in rat dams and their offspring. *J. Nutr.* **1993**, *123*, 2158–2165. [PubMed]
19. Bowe, J.E.; Franklin, Z.J.; Hauge-Evans, A.C.; King, A.J.; Persaud, S.J.; Jones, P.M. Metabolic phenotyping guidelines: Assessing glucose homeostasis in rodent models. *J. Endocrinol.* **2014**, *222*, G13–G25. [CrossRef] [PubMed]

20. Andrikopoulos, S.; Blair, A.R.; Deluca, N.; Fam, B.C.; Proietto, J. Evaluating the glucose tolerance test in mice. *Am. J. Physiol. Endocrinol. Metab.* **2008**, *295*, E1323–E1332. [CrossRef] [PubMed]

21. Nolan, C.J.; Proietto, J. The feto-placental glucose steal phenomenon is a major cause of maternal metabolic adaptation during late pregnancy in the rat. *Diabetologia* **1994**, *37*, 976–984. [CrossRef] [PubMed]

22. Untergasser, A.; Cutcutache, I.; Koressaar, T.; Ye, J.; Faircloth, B.C.; Remm, M.; Rozen, S.G. Primer3—New capabilities and interfaces. *Nucleic Acids Res.* **2012**, *40*, e115–e115. [CrossRef] [PubMed]

23. Vandesompele, J.; De Preter, K.; Pattyn, F.; Poppe, B.; Van Roy, N.; De Paepe, A.; Speleman, F. Accurate normalization of real-time quantitative RT-PCR data by geometric averaging of multiple internal control genes. *Genome Biol.* **2002**. [CrossRef] [PubMed]

24. Livak, K.J.; Schmittgen, T.D. Analysis of relative gene expression data using real-time quantitative PCR and the $2^{-\Delta\Delta CT}$ method. *Methods* **2001**, *25*, 402–408. [CrossRef] [PubMed]

25. Bocarsly, M.E.; Powell, E.S.; Avena, N.M.; Hoebel, B.G. High-fructose corn syrup causes characteristics of obesity in rats: Increased body weight, body fat and triglyceride levels. *Pharmacol. Biochem. Behav.* **2010**, *97*, 101–106. [CrossRef] [PubMed]

26. Teff, K.L.; Elliott, S.S.; Tschöp, M.; Kieffer, T.J.; Rader, D.; Heiman, M.; Townsend, R.R.; Keim, N.L.; D'Alessio, D.; Havel, P.J. Dietary Fructose Reduces Circulating Insulin and Leptin, Attenuates Postprandial Suppression of Ghrelin, and Increases Triglycerides in Women. *J. Clin. Endocrinol. Metab.* **2004**, *89*, 2963–2972. [CrossRef] [PubMed]

27. Dekker, M.J.; Su, Q.; Baker, C.; Rutledge, A.C.; Adeli, K. Fructose: A highly lipogenic nutrient implicated in insulin resistance, hepatic steatosis, and the metabolic syndrome. *Am. J. Physiol. Endocrinol. Metab.* **2010**, *299*, E685–E694. [CrossRef] [PubMed]

28. Wood, I.S.; Trayhurn, P. Glucose transporters (GLUT and SGLT): Expanded families of sugar transport proteins. *Br. J. Nutr.* **2003**, *89*, 3–9. [CrossRef] [PubMed]

29. Lim, J.S.; Mietus-Snyder, M.; Valente, A.; Schwarz, J.-M.; Lustig, R.H. The role of fructose in the pathogenesis of NAFLD and the metabolic syndrome. *Nat. Rev. Gastroenterol. Hepatol.* **2010**, *7*, 251–264. [CrossRef] [PubMed]

30. Catena, C.; Giacchetti, G.; Novello, M.; Colussi, G.; Cavarape, A.; Sechi, L.A. Cellular mechanisms of insulin resistance in rats with fructose-induced hypertension. *Am. J. Hypertens.* **2003**, *16*, 973–978. [CrossRef]

31. Mooradian, A.D.; Chehade, J.; Hurd, R.; Haas, M.J. Monosaccharide-enriched diets cause hyperleptinemia without hypophagia. *Nutrition* **2000**, *16*, 439–441. [CrossRef]

32. Gray, C.; Long, S.; Green, C.; Gardiner, S.M.; Craigon, J.; Gardner, D.S. Maternal Fructose and/or Salt Intake and Reproductive Outcome in the Rat: Effects on Growth, Fertility, Sex Ratio, and Birth Order. *Biol. Reprod.* **2013**, *89*, 51. [CrossRef] [PubMed]

33. Tappy, L.; Lê, K.-A. Metabolic Effects of Fructose and the Worldwide Increase in Obesity. *Physiol. Rev.* **2010**, *90*, 23–46. [CrossRef] [PubMed]

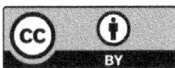

nutrients

MDPI

Article

Fructose and Sucrose Intake Increase Exogenous Carbohydrate Oxidation during Exercise

Jorn Trommelen [1], Cas J. Fuchs [1], Milou Beelen [1], Kaatje Lenaerts [1], Asker E. Jeukendrup [2], Naomi M. Cermak [1] and Luc J. C. van Loon [1,*]

[1]   NUTRIM School of Nutrition and Translational Research in Metabolism, Maastricht University Medical Centre, P.O. Box 616, 6200 MD Maastricht, The Netherlands; jorn.trommelen@maastrichtuniversity.com (J.T.); cas.fuchs@maastrichtuniversity.nl (C.J.F.); milou.beelen@maastrichtuniversity.nl (M.B.); kaatje.lenaerts@maastrichtuniversity.nl (K.L.); naomi.cermak1234@gmail.com (N.M.C.)
[2]   School of Sport, Exercise and Health Sciences, Loughborough University, Loughborough LE11 3TU, UK; asker@mysportscience.com
*   Correspondence: l.vanloon@maastrichtuniversity.com; Tel.: +31-43-388-1397

Received: 6 January 2017; Accepted: 16 February 2017; Published: 20 February 2017

Abstract: Peak exogenous carbohydrate oxidation rates typically reach ~1 g·min^{-1} during exercise when ample glucose or glucose polymers are ingested. Fructose co-ingestion has been shown to further increase exogenous carbohydrate oxidation rates. The purpose of this study was to assess the impact of fructose co-ingestion provided either as a monosaccharide or as part of the disaccharide sucrose on exogenous carbohydrate oxidation rates during prolonged exercise in trained cyclists. Ten trained male cyclists (VO$_2$peak: 65 ± 2 mL·kg^{-1}·min^{-1}) cycled on four different occasions for 180 min at 50% W$_{max}$ during which they consumed a carbohydrate solution providing 1.8 g·min^{-1} of glucose (GLU), 1.2 g·min^{-1} glucose + 0.6 g·min^{-1} fructose (GLU + FRU), 0.6 g·min^{-1} glucose + 1.2 g·min^{-1} sucrose (GLU + SUC), or water (WAT). Peak exogenous carbohydrate oxidation rates did not differ between GLU + FRU and GLU + SUC (1.40 ± 0.06 vs. 1.29 ± 0.07 g·min^{-1}, respectively, $p = 0.999$), but were 46% ± 8% higher when compared to GLU (0.96 ± 0.06 g·min^{-1}: $p < 0.05$). In line, exogenous carbohydrate oxidation rates during the latter 120 min of exercise were 46% ± 8% higher in GLU + FRU or GLU + SUC compared with GLU (1.19 ± 0.12, 1.13 ± 0.21, and 0.82 ± 0.16 g·min^{-1}, respectively, $p < 0.05$). We conclude that fructose co-ingestion (0.6 g·min^{-1}) with glucose (1.2 g·min^{-1}) provided either as a monosaccharide or as sucrose strongly increases exogenous carbohydrate oxidation rates during prolonged exercise in trained cyclists.

Keywords: substrate utilization; stable isotopes; metabolism; sugar

1. Introduction

It has been well established that carbohydrate ingestion during prolonged moderate-to high-intensity endurance-type exercise increases exercise capacity and performance [1–3]. The observed improvements in performance with carbohydrate ingestion have been attributed to maintenance of plasma glucose concentrations and high rates of carbohydrate oxidation during the latter stages of exercise [1,4].

Glucose ingestion during exercise results in a maximal exogenous carbohydrate oxidation rate of ~1 g·min^{-1} [5,6]. The rate of exogenous glucose oxidation appears limited by intestinal glucose absorption [5,7]. The intestinal sodium-dependent glucose transporter 1 (SGLT1) may become saturated when large amounts of glucose or glucose polymers are ingested [7,8]. Interestingly, the intestine contains a distinct class of carbohydrate transporters, glucose transporter 5 (GLUT5), that absorbs fructose and most likely fructose released during the hydrolysis from the disaccharide sucrose [9–11]. More recently, other intestinal carbohydrate transporters have been implicated in glucose (GLUT2) and fructose (GLUT2, GLUT8, GLUT 12) absorption [12–14]. Because of the distinct transport routes for glucose and fructose, higher total intestinal carbohydrate absorption rates can be expected when glucose and fructose are co-ingested. In agreement, combined glucose and fructose ingestion has been shown to enhance intestinal carbohydrate absorption rates and results in higher exogenous carbohydrate oxidation rates during exercise compared with an equivalent amount of glucose [8,15,16].

Sucrose combines glucose and fructose monomers, and its hydrolysis is typically not rate-limiting for intestinal absorption [15,17]. In addition, recent work suggests that intact sucrose can also be transported as a disaccharide across the intestinal membrane [18]. Therefore, sucrose may represent an (even more) effective dietary source of fructose co-ingestion. In agreement, sucrose co-ingestion has been shown to further increase exogenous carbohydrate oxidation rates during exercise compared to glucose only [19,20]. However, sucrose co-ingestion during exercise does not seem to elevate exogenous carbohydrate oxidation rates beyond 1.2–1.3 $g \cdot min^{-1}$ [19,20], which is typically lower than 1.3–1.8 $g \cdot min^{-1}$ when fructose is co-ingested with glucose during exercise [8,16,21,22]. Exogenous carbohydrate oxidation rates do not appear to level off when increasing amounts of fructose are co-ingested [21]. In contrast, exogenous carbohydrate oxidation rates have been shown to plateau when moderate amounts of sucrose are co-ingested [19]. This may suggest that sucrose digestion and/or absorption becomes a limiting factor when large amounts of sucrose are co-ingested. Therefore, it remains unclear whether sucrose co-ingestion can be as effective as fructose co-ingestion to further augment exogenous carbohydrate oxidation rates when glucose ingestion is increased above 1.0–1.1 $g \cdot min^{-1}$.

We have recently shown that endurance-type exercise induces splanchnic hypoperfusion, resulting in a rapid increase in plasma I-FABP, a novel biomarker of intestinal damage [23]. Hypoperfusion-induced intestinal compromise may hamper athletic performance and can jeopardize early post-exercise recovery [24]. Meal ingestion and intestinal nutrient supply have the ability to increase the superior mesenteric artery blood flow and, hence, splanchnic perfusion [25,26]. Therefore, carbohydrate ingestion during endurance-type exercise may represent an effective nutritional strategy to attenuate splanchnic hypoperfusion and, as such, prevent exercise-induced gastrointestinal injury.

The present study assesses the impact of the combined ingestion of fructose or sucrose with glucose on exogenous carbohydrate oxidation rates. We hypothesized that both fructose and sucrose co-ingestion augment exogenous carbohydrate oxidation rates during exercise when compared to an isoenergetic amount of glucose. Furthermore, we hypothesized that fructose provided as part of the disaccharide sucrose is less effective as the same amount of fructose provided as a monosaccharide to further augment exogenous carbohydrate oxidation rates during exercise. We tested our hypothesis by subjecting 10 male cyclists to a 180 min exercise bout on four occasions, during which they ingested GLU (1.8 $g \cdot min^{-1}$ glucose), GLU + FRU (1.2 $g \cdot min^{-1}$ glucose + 0.6 $g \cdot min^{-1}$ fructose), GLU + SUC (0.6 $g \cdot min^{-1}$ glucose + 1.2 $g \cdot min^{-1}$ sucrose), or WAT (water placebo).

2. Materials and Methods

2.1. Subjects

Ten trained male cyclists or triathletes participated in this study (age: 26 ± 1 years, body weight: 74.8 ± 2.1 kg, body mass index: 21.5 ± 0.5 $kg \cdot m^{-2}$, maximal workload capacity (W_{max}): 5.5 ± 0.1 $W \cdot kg^{-1}$, peak oxygen consumption (VO_2peak): 65 ± 2 $mL \cdot kg^{-1} \cdot min^{-1}$). Subjects cycled at least 100 $km \cdot wk^{-1}$ and had a training history of >3 years. Subjects were fully informed on the nature and possible risks of the experimental procedures before their written informed consent was obtained. The study was approved by the Medical Ethical Committee of the Maastricht University Medical Centre, The Netherlands and conformed to standards for the use of human subjects in research outlined in the most recent version of the Helsinki Declaration. This trial was registered at clinicaltrials.gov as NCT0109617.

2.2. Pretesting

Baseline characteristics were determined during screening. Subject's maximal workload capacity (W_{max}) and peak oxygen consumption (VO_2peak) were determined while performing a stepwise exercise test to exhaustion on an electronically braked cycle (Lode Excalibur, Groningen, The Netherlands), using an online gas-collection system (Omnical, Maastricht University, Maastricht, The Netherlands). After a 5 min warm up at 100 W, workload was set at 150 W and increased 50 W every 2.5 min until exhaustion. VO_2peak was defined as the median of the highest consecutive values over 30 s. Maximal workload capacity was calculated as the workload in the last completed stage + workload relative to the time spent in the last incomplete stage: (time in seconds)/150 × 50 (W).

2.3. Diet and Activity before Testing

Subjects recorded their food intake and activity pattern 2 days before the first experimental exercise trial and followed the same diet and exercise activities prior to the other three trials. In addition, 5–7 days before each experimental testing day, subjects performed an intense exercise training session to deplete (^{13}C-enriched) glycogen stores. Subjects were further instructed not to consume any food products with a high natural ^{13}C abundance (carbohydrates derived from C_4 plants: maize, sugar cane) at least 1 week before and during the entire experimental period to minimize any shift in background $^{13}CO_2$ enrichment.

2.4. Experimental Design

Each subject performed four exercise trials which consisted of 180 min of cycling at 50% W_{max} while ingesting a glucose drink (GLU), an isoenergetic glucose + fructose drink (GLU + FRU), an isoenergetic glucose + sucrose drink (GLU + SUC), or plain water (WAT). To quantify exogenous carbohydrate oxidation rates, corn-derived glucose monohydrate (Cargill, Sas van Gent, The Netherlands), crystalline fructose and sugar cane-derived sucrose (Rafti Sugar Solutions BV, Wijchen, The Netherlands) were used, all of which have a high natural ^{13}C abundance (−11.2, −11.4 and −11.2 δ‰ vs. Pee Dee Bellemnitella (PDB), respectively). The ^{13}C enrichment of the ingested glucose, fructose, and sucrose were determined by gas chromatography-combustion-isotope ratio mass spectrometry (GC/C/IRMS; Agilent 7890A/GC5975C; MSD, Wilmington, DE, USA). To all drinks 20 mmol·L^{-1} of sodium chloride was added. The order of the experimental drinks was randomly assigned in a cross-over double-blinded design. Experimental trials were separated by 7–28 days.

2.5. Protocol

Subjects reported to the laboratory in the morning at 08:00 a.m. after an overnight fast (10 h) and having refrained from any strenuous activity or drinking any alcohol in the previous 24 h. On arrival in the laboratory, a Teflon catheter was inserted in an antecubital vein of an arm to allow repeated blood sampling during exercise. The subjects then mounted a cycle ergometer and a resting breath sample was collected in 10 mL Exetainer tubes (Labco Limited, Lampeter, UK), which were filled directly from a mixing chamber in duplicate to determine the $^{13}C/^{12}C$ ratio in the expired CO_2. Next a resting blood sample (10 mL) was taken. Subjects then started a 180-min exercise bout at a work rate equivalent to 50% W_{max}. Blood samples were collected at 30-min intervals throughout the 180 min exercise period. Expired breath samples were collected every 15 min until cessation of exercise. Measurements of oxygen consumption (VO_2), carbon dioxide production (VCO_2) and respiratory exchange ratio (RER) were obtained every 15 min for periods of 4 min through the use of a respiratory facemask, connected to an online gas-collection system [27].

During the first 3 min of exercise, subjects drank an initial bolus (600 mL) of one of the four experimental drinks: GLU, GLU + FRU, GLU + SUC, or WAT. Thereafter, every 15 min a beverage volume of a 150 mL was provided. The total fluid provided during the 180 min-exercise bout was 2.25 L. The GLU, GLU + FRU, and GLU + SUC drinks provided 1.8 g carbohydrate·min^{-1}. The GLU drink provided 1.8 g·min^{-1} glucose, the GLU + FRU drink provided 1.2 g·min^{-1} glucose + 0.6 g·min^{-1} fructose, and the GLU + SUC drink provided 0.6 g·min^{-1} glucose + 1.14 g·min^{-1} sucrose. The amount of sucrose (1.14 vs. 1.2 g·min^{-1}) was selected to allow exactly the same equimolar amounts of glucose and fructose provided in the GLU + SUC, GLU and GLU + FRU drinks.

Subjects were asked to rate their perceived exertion (RPE) every 30 min on a scale from 6 to 20 using the Borg category scale [28]. In addition, subjects were asked every 30 min to fill in questionnaire to rate possible gastrointestinal (GI) problems using a ten-point scale (1 = no complaints at all, 10 = very severe complaints). The questions consisted of six questions related to upper GI symptons (nausea, general stomach problems, belching, urge to vomit, heartburn, and stomach cramps), four questions related to lower GI complaints (flatulence, urge to defecate, intestinal cramps, and diarrhea), and four questions related to central or other symptoms (dizziness, headache, urge to urinate, and bloated feeling). All exercise tests were performed under normal and standard environmental conditions (18–22 °C dry bulb temperature and 55%–65% relative humidity). During the exercise trials, subjects were cooled with standing floor fans.

2.6. Analyses

Blood samples (10 mL) were collected in EDTA-containing tubes and centrifuged at 1000× *g* and 4 °C for 10 min. Aliquots of plasma were frozen in liquid nitrogen and stored at −80 °C until analysis. Plasma glucose and lactate were analyzed with a COBAS FARA semiautomatic analyzer (Roche). Plasma insulin concentrations were analyzed using commercially available kits (Elecsys Insulin assay, Roche, Ref: 12017547122; Mannheim, Germany). Plasma I-FABP levels were measured using an in-house developed enzyme-linked immunosorbent assay. The detection window of the I-FABP assay is 12.5–800 pg·mL^{-1}, with an intra-assay and inter-assay coefficient of variation of 4.1% and 6.2%, respectively [23,29]. Breath samples were analyzed for $^{13}C/^{12}C$ ratio by gas chromatography continuous flow isotope ratio mass spectrometry (GC/C/IRMS; Finnigan, Bremen, Germany). From indirect calorimetry (VO_2 and VCO_2) and stable isotope measurements (breath $^{13}CO_2/^{12}CO_2$ ratio), oxidation rates of total fat, total carbohydrate and exogenous carbohydrate were calculated.

2.7. Calculations

From VCO_2 and VO_2 (L·min^{-1}), total carbohydrate and fat oxidation rates (g·min^{-1}) were calculated using the stoichiometric equations of Frayn [30] with the assumption that protein oxidation during exercise was negligible:

$$\text{Carbohydrate oxidation} = 4.55 \, VCO_2 - 3.21 \, VO_2 \tag{1}$$

$$\text{Fat oxidation} = 1.67 \, VO_2 - 1.67 \, VCO_2 \tag{2}$$

The isotopic enrichment was expressed as δ per mil difference between the $^{13}C/^{12}C$ ratio of the sample and a known laboratory reference standard according to the formula of Craig [31]:

$$\delta^{13}C = \left(\left(\frac{^{13}C/^{12}C \text{ sample}}{^{13}C/^{12}C \text{ standard}} \right) - 1 \right) \cdot 10^3 \tag{3}$$

The $\delta^{13}C$ was then related to an international standard (PDB-1). In the GLU, GLU + FRU, and GLU + SUC treatments, the rate of exogenous carbohydrate oxidation was calculated using the following [32]:

$$\text{Exogenous glucose oxidation} = VCO_2 \cdot \left(\frac{\delta \, Exp - \delta \, Exp_{bkg}}{\delta \, Ing - \delta \, Exp_{bkg}} \right) \left(\frac{1}{k} \right) \tag{4}$$

in which δ Exp is the ^{13}C enrichment of expired air during exercise at different time points, δ Ing is the ^{13}C enrichment of the ingested carbohydrate solution, δ Exp$_{bkg}$ is the ^{13}C enrichment of expired air in the WAT treatment (background) at different time points and k is the amount of CO_2 (in L) produced by the oxidation of 1 g of glucose ($k = 0.7467$ L of $CO_2 \cdot g^{-1}$ of glucose).

A methodological consideration when using $^{13}CO_2$ in expired air to calculate exogenous substrate oxidation is the trapping of $^{13}CO_2$ in the bicarbonate pool, in which an amount of CO_2 arising from decarboxylation of energy substrates is temporarily trapped [33]. However, during exercise the CO_2 production increases several-fold so that a physiological steady state condition will occur relatively rapidly, and $^{13}CO_2$ in the expired air will be equilibrated with the $^{13}CO_2/H^{13}CO_3^-$ pool, respectively. Recovery of the $^{13}CO_2$ from oxidation will approach 100% after 60 min of exercise when dilution in the bicarbonate pool becomes negligible [33,34]. As a consequence of this, calculations on substrate oxidation were performed over the last 120 min of exercise (60–180 min).

2.8. Statistical Analyses

Plasma and substrate utilization parameters are expressed as means $\pm$ SEM, RPE and GI distress scores are expressed as median and interquartile range. A sample size of 10 was calculated with a power of 80% and an alpha level of 0.05 to detect a ~20% difference in exogenous carbohydrate oxidation between treatments [20]. For all data, the normality of the distribution was confirmed after visual inspection and the use of Shapiro-Wilk tests. A one-way repeated measures ANOVA with treatment as factor was used to compare differences in substrate utilization parameters between treatments. In case of significant F-ratios, Bonferroni post-hoc tests were applied to locate the differences. A two-way repeated measures ANOVA with time and treatment as factors was used to compare differences in plasma parameters between treatments and over time. In case of significant F-ratios, paired t-tests were used to locate the differences. A Friedman test was performed to compare RPE and GI distress scores between treatments. In case of significant χ^2, post hoc analysis with Wilcoxon signed-rank test was conducted. Data evaluation was performed using SPSS (version 21.0, IBM Corp., Armonk, NY, USA). Statistical significance was set at $p < 0.05$.

3. Results

3.1. Indirect Calorimetry

Data for VO_2, RER, and total carbohydrate and fat oxidation rates over the 60 to 180 min exercise period are presented in Table S1. VO_2 did not differ between the four experimental treatments ($p = 0.301$). RER in WAT was lower compared with GLU + FRU and GLU + SUC ($p < 0.05$). Total carbohydrate oxidation rates were lower in WAT compared with GLU + FRU and GLU + SUC treatments ($p < 0.05$). No significant differences in total carbohydrate oxidation rates were observed between GLU, GLU + FRU and GLU + SUC (pairwise comparisons: all $p \geq 0.172$). Total fat oxidation rates were higher in WAT compared to GLU + SUC ($p = 0.010$). No significant differences in total fat oxidation rates were observed between GLU, GLU + FRU and GLU + SUC (pairwise comparisons: all $p \geq 0.443$).

3.2. Stable-Isotope Measurements

Changes in isotopic composition of expired CO_2 in response to exercise with ingestion of GLU, GLU + FRU, GLU + SUC or WAT are presented in Figure 1A. Resting breath $^{13}CO_2$ enrichments did not differ between treatments, and averaged -26.55 ± 0.13, -26.86 ± 0.16, -26.69 ± 0.14, -26.83 ± 0.18 δ‰ versus PDB for WAT, GLU, GLU + FRU, and GLU + SUC, respectively. No significant increases in expired breath $^{13}CO_2$ enrichments were observed in the water only treatment (WAT; $p = 0.096$). In contrast, expired breath $^{13}CO_2$ enrichments strongly increased to up to -22.36 ± 0.33, -20.70 ± 0.18, and -20.97 ± 0.34 δ‰ versus PDB in the GLU, GLU + FRU, and GLU + SUC treatments, respectively (time x treatment, $p < 0.001$). The slight shift in expired breath $^{13}CO_2$ enrichments in the

WAT treatment was used as a background correction for the calculation of exogenous carbohydrate oxidation rates in the GLU, GLU + FRU and GLU + SUC treatments.

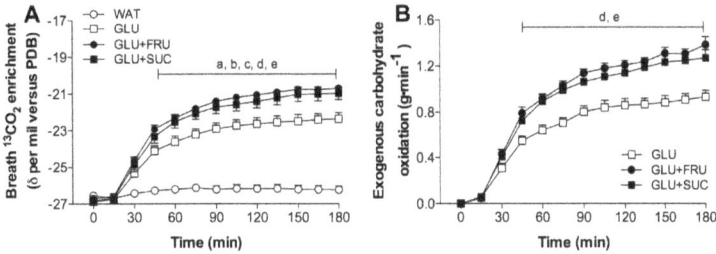

Figure 1. Breath $^{13}CO_2$ enrichments (**A**) and exogenous carbohydrate oxidation rates (**B**) during exercise without ingestion of carbohydrate (WAT), with the ingestion of glucose (GLU), with the ingestion of glucose and fructose (GLU + FRU), or with the ingestion of glucose and sucrose (GLU + SUC). Data were analsysed with a two-way repeated measures ANOVA (time-treatment). Data are presented as means ± SEM. $N = 10$. a, denotes GLU significantly different from WAT; b, denotes GLU + FRU significantly different from WAT; c, denotes GLU + SUC significantly different from WAT; d, denotes GLU + FRU significantly different from GLU; e, denotes GLU + SUC significantly different from GLU ($p < 0.05$).

3.3. Exogenous and Endogenous Carbohydrate Oxidation Rates

In the GLU, GLU + FRU, and GLU + SUC treatments, the calculated exogenous carbohydrate oxidation rates increased significantly over time (Figure 1B, $p < 0.001$). Peak exogenous carbohydrate oxidation rates were 51% ± 9% and 40% ± 12% higher in GLU + FRU and GLU + SUC when compared to GLU (1.40 ± 0.06 and 1.29 ± 0.07 vs. 0.96 ± 0.06 g·min^{-1}, respectively: $p < 0.05$). Peak exogenous carbohydrate oxidation rates did not differ between GLU + FRU and GLU + SUC ($p = 0.999$). Assessed over the last 120 min of exercise, average exogenous carbohydrate oxidation rates were higher in the GLU + FRU and GLU + SUC treatments compared to the GLU treatments (1.19 ± 0.12, 1.13 ± 0.21, and 0.82 ± 0.16 g·min^{-1}, respectively: $p < 0.05$). No differences were observed in exogenous carbohydrate oxidation rates between GLU + FRU and GLU + SUC ($p = 0.999$). No significant differences in endogenous carbohydrate oxidation rates were observed between treatments ($p = 0.112$). The relative contribution of substrates to total energy expenditure during exercise is presented in Figure 2.

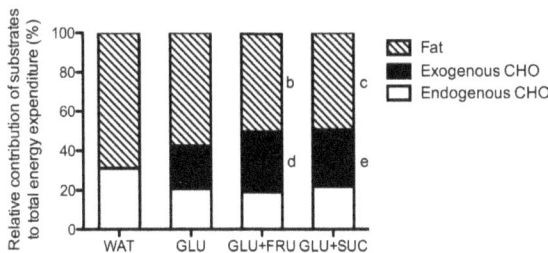

Figure 2. Relative contribution of substrates to total energy expenditure calculated for the 60- to 180 min period of exercise without the ingestion of carbohydrate (WAT), with the ingestion of glucose (GLU), with the ingestion of glucose and fructose (GLU + FRU), or with the ingestion of glucose and sucrose (GLU + SUC). Data were analsysed with a repeated measures ANOVA (treatment). Data are presented as means ± SEM. $N = 10$; b, denotes GLU + FRU significantly different from WAT; c, denotes GLU + SUC significantly different from WAT; d, denotes GLU + FRU significantly different from GLU; e, denotes GLU + SUC significantly different from GLU ($p < 0.05$).

3.4. Plasma Metabolites

Plasma glucose, insulin, and lactate concentrations are shown in Figure 3. Plasma glucose concentrations showed a transient increase at $t = 30$ min in the GLU, GLU + FRU and GLU + SUC treatments, but plasma glucose concentrations at $t = 30$ min were only significantly higher in GLU + SUC compared to WAT ($p = 0.028$). Plasma glucose concentrations decreased in the WAT treatment compared to the GLU, GLU + FRU and GLU + SUC treatments (time x treatment interaction: $p < 0.001$). Plasma glucose concentrations were significantly lower in the WAT treatment compared to the GLU, GLU + FRU and GLU + SUC treatments from $t = 90$ min onwards ($p < 0.05$). Plasma insulin concentrations increased in the GLU, GLU + FRU and GLU + SUC treatments, peaking at $t = 30$ after glucose ingestion (8.2 ± 1.2, 8.3 ± 1.1, and 10.6 ± 2.2 mU·L^{-1}, respectively), and then declined throughout exercise. In contrast, plasma insulin concentrations declined throughout the entire exercise bout in the WAT treatment (time x treatment interaction: $p < 0.001$).

Plasma lactate concentrations increased in all treatments, but this increase was much greater in the GLU + FRU and GLU + SUC treatments when compared with the WAT and GLU treatments (time x treatment interaction: $p < 0.001$). Plasma I-FABP levels, depicted as a percentage change from individual baseline values, did not change significantly over time ($p = 0.764$; Figure 4A). Area under the curve (AUC) calculations of the percentage change from individual I-FABP baseline values did not differ between treatments ($p = 0.101$; Figure 4B).

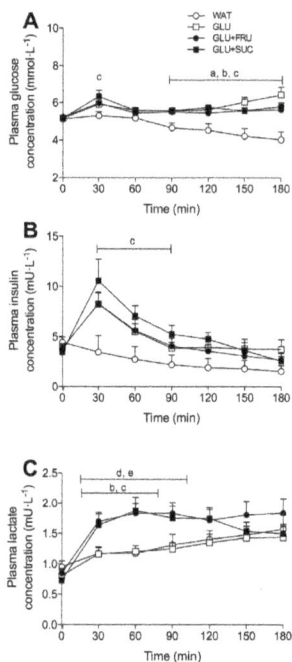

Figure 3. Plasma glucose (**A**), insulin (**B**), and lactate (**C**) concentrations during exercise without ingestion of carbohydrate (WAT), with the ingestion of glucose (GLU), with the ingestion of glucose and fructose (GLU + FRU), or with the ingestion of glucose and sucrose (GLU + SUC). Data were analsysed with a two-way repeated measures ANOVA (time-treatment). Data are presented as means ± SEM. $N = 10$; a, denotes GLU significantly different from WAT; b, denotes GLU + FRU significantly different from WAT; c, denotes GLU + SUC significantly different from WAT; d, denotes GLU + FRU significantly different from GLU; e, denotes GLU + SUC significantly different from GLU ($p < 0.05$).

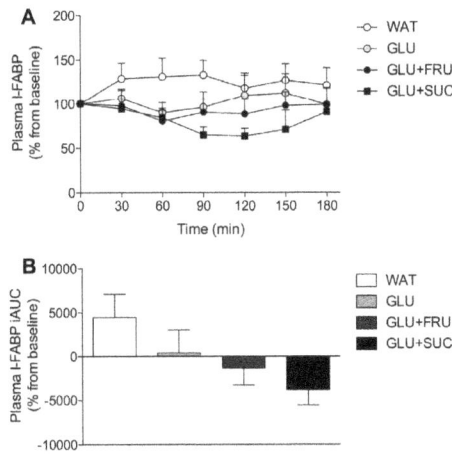

Figure 4. Plasma I-FABP concentrations during exercise (**A**) and (area under the curve (AUC) of percentage I-FABP change during exercise (**B**) without ingestion of carbohydrate (WAT), with the ingestion of glucose (GLU), with the ingestion of glucose and fructose (GLU + FRU), or with the ingestion of glucose and sucrose (GLU + SUC). Plasma I-FABP (**A**) was analsysed with a two-way repeated measures ANOVA (time-treatment). Plasma I-FABP iAUC was analysed with a repeated measures ANOVA (treatment). Data are presented as means ± SEM. $N = 10$. Differences between treatments did not reach statistical significance ($p > 0.05$).

3.5. Gastrointestinal Distress and Rating of Percieved Exertion

Total upper GI distress scores were 62 (53–83), 109 (67–147), 69 (57–96) and 74 (53–79), in the WAT, GLU, GLU + FRU, GLU + SUC treatments, respectively, and were significantly higher in the GLU compared to the WAT, GLU + FRU, and GLU + SUC treatments ($p < 0.05$). Low GI distress scores were observed for other symptons, with the exception of urge to urinate which did not differ between treatments ($p = 0.455$). Ratings of perceived exertion did not differ between treatments and averaged 13 (11–14), 14 (13–14), 13 (12–13), and 13 (12–14) for WAT, GLU, GLU + FRU, and GLU + SUC, respectively ($p = 0.056$).

4. Discussion

The present study shows that the combined ingestion of glucose and fructose (1.2 g·min^{-1} glucose plus 0.6 g·kg^{-1} fructose or 0.6 g·min^{-1} glucose plus 1.2 g·min^{-1} sucrose) further increases exogenous carbohydrate oxidation rates compared to the ingestion of an isocaloric amount of glucose only. Furthermore, combined ingestion of glucose plus fructose or sucrose resulted in less GI complaints when compared with the ingestion of glucose only.

Previous work suggests that exogenous glucose oxidation rates are limited by intestinal glucose absorption [5,7]. Because fructose is absorbed through a different intestinal transport route, higher total intestinal carbohydrate absorption rates can be expected when glucose and fructose are co-ingested. Therefore, we hypothesized that fructose co-ingestion with glucose would increase total carbohydrate oxidation rates during prolonged exercise. Furthermore, we hypothesized that fructose provided as part of the disaccharide sucrose is less effective as the same amount of fructose provided as a monosaccharide to further augment exogenous glucose oxidation rates during exercise.

In the present study, we observed that the ingestion of an ample amount of glucose only results in peak exogenous carbohydrate oxidation rates of 0.96 ± 0.06 g·min^{-1} (Figure 1). These rates are in line with previous work and confirm that exogenous glucose oxidation rates will not rise above 1.0–1.1 g·min^{-1} when only glucose is ingested during exercise [7,16,22,35,36]. Combined ingestion of glucose plus fructose or glucose plus sucrose in the present study resulted in peak exogenous carbohydrate oxidation rates of 1.40 ± 0.06 and 1.29 ± 0.07 g·min^{-1}, respectively (Figure 1). These data confirm previous observations showing 35%–55% higher exogenous carbohydrate oxidation rates following fructose co-ingestion when compared to the ingestion of glucose only during exercise [8,16]. While sucrose co-ingestion has also been shown to increase exogenous carbohydrate oxidation rates [19,20], maximal exogenous carbohydrate oxidation rates appear lower when sucrose [19,20] as opposed to fructose [8,16,21,22] is co-ingested during exercise (1.2–1.3 vs. 1.3–1.8 g·min^{-1}, respectively). In the present study, we compared the impact of equimolar amounts of fructose co-ingestion provided as its monosaccharide or provided as sucrose on exogenous carbohydrate oxidation rates during exercise in the same cohort of athletes. We extend on previous work by showing no significant differences in peak exogenous carbohydrate oxidation rates between the GLU + FRU and GLU + SUC treatments ($p = 0.999$). These results suggest that sucrose intestinal digestion and/or absorption are not rate-limiting for subsequent oxidation. Consequently, we demonstrate that fructose co-ingestion provided as part of the disaccharide sucrose does not differ from an equivalent amount of fructose provided as a monosaccharide to augment exogenous carbohydrate oxidation rates during endurance type exercise.

The ingestion of glucose only resulted in substantially higher GI distress when compared to the WAT, GLU + FRU and GLU + SUC treatments ($p < 0.05$). The lower total GI distress with fructose or sucrose co-ingestion seems to suggest that these treatments result in less carbohydrate accumulation in the GI tract, possibly caused by more rapid intestinal carbohydrate absorption when compared with the ingestion of glucose only [37]. To further evaluate potential underlying mechanisms of the GI discomfort, we also measured plasma I-FABP as a marker of intestinal damage. Previous work has shown that exercise resulted in a rapid appearance of this marker in blood, which correlated with splanchnic hypoperfusion [23]. Though not significant, we observed lower I-FABP release in the GLU, GLU + FRU, and GLU + SUC groups compared with the WAT treatment ($p = 0.101$, Figure 4). The observed increase in plasma I-FABP in the WAT treatment was lower when compared to our previous work [29]. This may be explained by differences in the exercise protocols. In our previous work, subjects cycled for 60 min at 70% W$_{max}$ vs. 180 min at 50% W$_{max}$ in the current study. This suggests that exercise intensity may be a more important modulator of peak plasma I-FABP levels than exercise duration. It remains to be established whether carbohydrate ingestion may reduce exercise-induced GI compromise during higher intensity exercise.

After ingestion and intestinal absorption, fructose is metabolized in the liver and subsequently released in the systemic circulation as lactate or converted to glucose via gluconeogenesis, which is mainly released or used for liver glycogen synthesis depending on the need to maintain plasma glucose levels [38]. We observed no significant differences in plasma glucose concentrations between the GLU, GLU + FRU, and the GLU + SUC treatments (Figure 3). We have recently shown that sucrose ingestion does not preserve liver glycogen concentrations more than glucose ingestion during exercise [39]. Therefore, it seems unlikely that hepatic glycogenesis was a major fate of the ingested fructose during exercise. We did observe elevated plasma lactate concentrations in the GLU + FRU and GLU + SUC treatments when compared to the GLU treatment. Fructose co-ingestion has been shown to increase plasma lactate production and oxidation, with a minimal amount of fructose being directly oxidized [40]. Therefore, fructose or sucrose co-ingested with glucose appears to be effectively absorbed in the intestine and transported to the liver where it is metabolized to lactate, released in the circulation and subsequently oxidized.

Exogenous glucose oxidation rates have been shown to correlate with exercise performance during prolonged, moderate- to high-intensity exercise [2]. Fructose co-ingestion further improves exogenous carbohydrate oxidation rates and has shown to improve exercise performance compared to an isocaloric amount of glucose [8,14,16,22,41–43]. The latter has been attributed to a combination of higher exogenous carbohydrate oxidation rates and decreased GI distress [41,43]. Although we did not assess exercise performance, we observed increased exogenous carbohydrate rates and lower GI distress following fructose co-ingestion. Furthermore, exogenous carbohydrate oxidation rates and GI distress levels did not differ between the GLU + FRU and GLU + SUC treatments. Therefore, our data suggest that both fructose and sucrose represents proper ingredients for sports drinks to further increase exogenous carbohydrate oxidation rates during exercise.

This study presents several limitations. First, we assessed whole-body exogenous carbohydrate oxidation rates following fructose co-ingestion, which does not provide insight in the specific site of oxidation. The increased exogenous carbohydrate oxidation rates following fructose co-ingestion is likely largely attributed to increased lactate oxidation in muscle [40,44]. However, hepatic fructose conversion into glucose and/or lactate costs energy [45], thereby decreasing energy efficiency and possibly increasing hepatic carbohydrate oxidation rates. Therefore, the observed 46% ± 8% higher exogenous carbohydrate oxidation rates following fructose co-ingestion may slightly overestimate increased energy availability and exogenous carbohydrate oxidation rates in muscle. Secondly, we cannot exclude the possibility that sucrose co-ingestion is less effective at increasing exogenous carbohydrate oxidation when compared to fructose monosaccharide co-ingestion when total carbohydrate ingestion rates are higher than provided in the current study. It has been suggested that sucrose digestion and/or absorption becomes a limiting factor to further increase exogenous carbohydrate oxidation rates when total carbohydrate intakes levels exceed 1.8 g·min^{-1} [19]. However, such carbohydrate ingestion rates may be impractically high and result in GI distress that may be detrimental to exercise performance [43]. Therefore, we provided total carbohydrate ingestion rates that are more practical and have shown to increase performance [42].

5. Conclusions

We conclude that fructose co-ingestion provided either as a monosaccharide or as sucrose strongly increases exogenous carbohydrate oxidation rates during prolonged exercise in trained cyclists. When ingesting large amounts of carbohydrates during exercise, co-ingestion of fructose or sucrose will lower GI distress and increase the capacity for exogenous carbohydrate oxidation.

Supplementary Materials: The following are available online at http://www.mdpi.com/2072-6643/9/2/167/s1, Table S1: Oxygen uptake (VO$_2$), respiratory exchange ratio (RER), total carbohydrate (CHO) oxidation (CHOtot), total fat oxidation (FATtot), endogenous carbohydrate (Endogenous CHO), exogenous carbohydrate (Exogenous CHO) oxidation and peak exogenous carbohydrate oxidation (peak exogenous CHO) rates during cycling exercise with ingestion of GLU, GLU + FRU, and GLU + SUC, and WAT.

Acknowledgments: We gratefully acknowledge the assistance of Janneau van Kranenburg and the enthusiastic support of the volunteers who participated in these experiments. This project was partly funded by a research grant from Kenniscentrum Suiker & Voeding, Utrecht, The Netherlands and Sugar Nutrition UK, London, UK.

Author Contributions: A.E.J., N.M.C. and L.J.C.v.L. conceived and designed the experiments; J.T. and C.J.F. performed the experiments; J.T. and K.L. analyzed the data; K.L. contributed reagents/materials/analysis tools; J.T., M.B. and L.J.C.v.L wrote the paper.

Conflicts of Interest: The authors declare no conflict of interest. The founding sponsors had no role in the design of the study; in the collection, analyses, or interpretation of data; in the writing of the manuscript, and in the decision to publish the results.

References

1. Coyle, E.F.; Coggan, A.R.; Hemmert, M.K.; Ivy, J.L. Muscle glycogen utilization during prolonged strenuous exercise when fed carbohydrate. *J. Appl. Physiol. (1985)* **1986**, *61*, 165–172.
2. Smith, J.W.; Zachwieja, J.J.; Peronnet, F.; Passe, D.H.; Massicotte, D.; Lavoie, C.; Pascoe, D.D. Fuel selection and cycling endurance performance with ingestion of [13C]glucose: Evidence for a carbohydrate dose response. *J. Appl. Physiol. (1985)* **2010**, *108*, 1520–1529. [CrossRef] [PubMed]
3. Stellingwerff, T.; Cox, G.R. Systematic review: Carbohydrate supplementation on exercise performance or capacity of varying durations. *Appl. Physiol. Nutr. Metab.* **2014**, *39*, 998–1011. [CrossRef] [PubMed]
4. Coggan, A.R.; Coyle, E.F. Reversal of fatigue during prolonged exercise by carbohydrate infusion or ingestion. *J. Appl. Physiol. (1985)* **1987**, *63*, 2388–2395.

5. Jeukendrup, A.E.; Wagenmakers, A.J.; Stegen, J.H.; Gijsen, A.P.; Brouns, F.; Saris, W.H. Carbohydrate ingestion can completely suppress endogenous glucose production during exercise. *Am. J. Physiol.* **1999**, *276*, E672–E683. [PubMed]

6. Jeukendrup, A.E.; Jentjens, R. Oxidation of carbohydrate feedings during prolonged exercise: Current thoughts, guidelines and directions for future research. *Sports Med.* **2000**, *29*, 407–424. [CrossRef] [PubMed]

7. Jeukendrup, A.E. Carbohydrate and exercise performance: The role of multiple transportable carbohydrates. *Curr. Opin. Clin. Nutr. Metab. Care* **2010**, *13*, 452–457. [CrossRef] [PubMed]

8. Jentjens, R.L.P.G.; Moseley, L.; Waring, R.H.; Harding, L.K.; Jeukendrup, A.E. Oxidation of combined ingestion of glucose and fructose during exercise. *J. Appl. Physiol. (1985)* **2004**, *96*, 1277–1284. [CrossRef] [PubMed]

9. Davidson, R.E.; Leese, H.J. Sucrose absorption by the rat small intestine in vivo and in vitro. *J. Physiol.* **1977**, *267*, 237–248. [CrossRef] [PubMed]

10. Ferraris, R.P.; Diamond, J. Regulation of intestinal sugar transport. *Physiol. Rev.* **1997**, *77*, 257–302. [PubMed]

11. Sandle, G.I.; Lobley, R.W.; Warwick, R.; Holmes, R. Monosaccharide absorption and water secretion during disaccharide perfusion of the human jejunum. *Digestion* **1983**, *26*, 53–60. [CrossRef] [PubMed]

12. DeBosch, B.J.; Chi, M.; Moley, K.H. Glucose transporter 8 (GLUT8) regulates enterocyte fructose transport and global mammalian fructose utilization. *Endocrinology* **2012**, *153*, 4181–4191. [CrossRef] [PubMed]

13. Leturque, A.; Brot-Laroche, E.; Le Gall, M.; Stolarczyk, E.; Tobin, V. The role of GLUT2 in dietary sugar handling. *J. Physiol. Biochem.* **2005**, *61*, 529–537. [CrossRef] [PubMed]

14. Rowlands, D.S.; Houltham, S.; Musa-Veloso, K.; Brown, F.; Paulionis, L.; Bailey, D. Fructose-Glucose Composite Carbohydrates and Endurance Performance: Critical Review and Future Perspectives. *Sports Med.* **2015**, *45*, 1561–1576. [CrossRef] [PubMed]

15. Shi, X.; Summers, R.W.; Schedl, H.P.; Flanagan, S.W.; Chang, R.; Gisolfi, C.V. Effects of carbohydrate type and concentration and solution osmolality on water absorption. *Med. Sci. Sports Exerc.* **1995**, *27*, 1607–1615. [CrossRef] [PubMed]

16. Wallis, G.A.; Rowlands, D.S.; Shaw, C.; Jentjens, R.L.; Jeukendrup, A.E. Oxidation of Combined Ingestion of Maltodextrins and Fructose during Exercise. *Med. Sci. Sports Exerc.* **2005**, *37*, 426–432. [CrossRef] [PubMed]

17. Wallis, G.A.; Wittekind, A. Is there a specific role for sucrose in sports and exercise performance? *Int. J. Sport Nutr. Exerc. Metab.* **2013**, *23*, 571–583. [CrossRef] [PubMed]

18. Likely, R.; Johnson, E.; Ahearn, G.A. Functional characterization of a putative disaccharide membrane transporter in crustacean intestine. *J. Comp. Physiol. B* **2015**, *185*, 173–183. [CrossRef] [PubMed]

19. Jentjens, R.L.; Shaw, C.; Birtles, T.; Waring, R.H.; Harding, L.K.; Jeukendrup, A.E. Oxidation of combined ingestion of glucose and sucrose during exercise. *Metabolism* **2005**, *54*, 610–618. [CrossRef] [PubMed]

20. Jentjens, R.L.; Venables, M.C.; Jeukendrup, A.E. Oxidation of exogenous glucose, sucrose, and maltose during prolonged cycling exercise. *J. Appl. Physiol. (1985)* **2004**, *96*, 1285–1291. [CrossRef] [PubMed]

21. Jentjens, R.L.; Jeukendrup, A.E. High rates of exogenous carbohydrate oxidation from a mixture of glucose and fructose ingested during prolonged cycling exercise. *Br. J. Nutr.* **2005**, *93*, 485–492. [CrossRef] [PubMed]

22. Roberts, J.D.; Tarpey, M.D.; Kass, L.S.; Tarpey, R.J.; Roberts, M.G. Assessing a commercially available sports drink on exogenous carbohydrate oxidation, fluid delivery and sustained exercise performance. *J. Int. Soc. Sports Nutr.* **2014**, *11*, 8. [CrossRef] [PubMed]

23. Van Wijck, K.; Lenaerts, K.; van Loon, L.J.C.; Peters, W.H.M.; Buurman, W.A.; Dejong, C.H.C. Exercise-induced splanchnic hypoperfusion results in gut dysfunction in healthy men. *PLoS ONE* **2011**, *6*, e22366. [CrossRef] [PubMed]

24. Van Wijck, K.; Lenaerts, K.; Grootjans, J.; Wijnands, K.A.P.; Poeze, M.; van Loon, L.J.C.; Dejong, C.H.C.; Buurman, W.A. Physiology and pathophysiology of splanchnic hypoperfusion and intestinal injury during exercise: Strategies for evaluation and prevention. *Am. J. Physiol. Gastrointest. Liver Physiol.* **2012**, *303*, G155–G168. [CrossRef] [PubMed]

25. Chou, C.C.; Coatney, R.W. Nutrient-induced changes in intestinal blood flow in the dog. *Br. Vet. J.* **1994**, *150*, 423–437. [CrossRef]

26. Gentilcore, D.; Nair, N.S.; Vanis, L.; Rayner, C.K.; Meyer, J.H.; Hausken, T.; Horowitz, M.; Jones, K.L. Comparative effects of oral and intraduodenal glucose on blood pressure, heart rate, and splanchnic blood flow in healthy older subjects. *Am. J. Physiol. Regul. Integr. Comp. Physiol.* **2009**, *297*, R716–R722. [CrossRef] [PubMed]

27. Cermak, N.M.; Gibala, M.J.; van Loon, L.J.C. Nitrate supplementation's improvement of 10-km time-trial performance in trained cyclists. *Int. J. Sport Nutr. Exerc. Metab.* **2012**, *22*, 64–71. [CrossRef] [PubMed]

28. Borg, G. Ratings of perceived exertion and heart rates during short-term cycle exercise and their use in a new cycling strength test. *Int. J. Sports Med.* **1982**, *3*, 153–158. [CrossRef] [PubMed]

29. Van Wijck, K.; Wijnands, K.A.P.; Meesters, D.M.; Boonen, B.; van Loon, L.J.C.; Buurman, W.A.; Dejong, C.H.C.; Lenaerts, K.; Poeze, M. L-Citrulline Improves Splanchnic Perfusion and Reduces Gut Injury during Exercise. *Med. Sci. Sports Exerc.* **2014**, *46*, 2039–2046. [CrossRef] [PubMed]

30. Frayn, K.N. Calculation of substrate oxidation rates in vivo from gaseous exchange. *J. Appl. Physiol. (1985)* **1983**, *55*, 628–634.

31. Craig, H. Isotopic standards for carbon and oxygen and correction factors for mass-spectrometric analysis of carbon dioxide. *Geochim. Cosmoch. Acta* **1957**, *12*, 133–149. [CrossRef]

32. Pirnay, F.; Lacroix, M.; Mosora, F.; Luyckx, A.; Lefebvre, P. Glucose oxidation during prolonged exercise evaluated with naturally labeled [13C]glucose. *J. Appl. Physiol.* **1977**, *43*, 258–261.

33. Robert, J.J.; Koziet, J.; Chauvet, D.; Darmaun, D.; Desjeux, J.F.; Young, V.R. Use of 13C-labeled glucose for estimating glucose oxidation: Some design considerations. *J. Appl. Physiol. (1985)* **1987**, *63*, 1725–1732.

34. Pallikarakis, N.; Sphiris, N.; Lefebvre, P. Influence of the bicarbonate pool and on the occurrence of $13CO_2$ in exhaled air. *Eur. J. Appl. Physiol. Occup. Physiol.* **1991**, *63*, 179–183. [CrossRef] [PubMed]

35. Wagenmakers, A.J.; Brouns, F.; Saris, W.H.; Halliday, D. Oxidation rates of orally ingested carbohydrates during prolonged exercise in men. *J. Appl. Physiol. (1985)* **1993**, *75*, 2774–2780.

36. Rowlands, D.S.; Wallis, G.A.; Shaw, C.; Jentjens, R.L.P.G.; Jeukendrup, A.E. Glucose polymer molecular weight does not affect exogenous carbohydrate oxidation. *Med. Sci. Sports Exerc.* **2005**, *37*, 1510–1516. [CrossRef] [PubMed]

37. Jentjens, R.L.; Achten, J.; Jeukendrup, A.E. High oxidation rates from combined carbohydrates ingested during exercise. *Med. Sci. Sports Exerc.* **2004**, *36*, 1551–1558. [CrossRef] [PubMed]

38. Laughlin, M.R. Normal roles for dietary fructose in carbohydrate metabolism. *Nutrients* **2014**, *6*, 3117–3129. [CrossRef] [PubMed]

39. Gonzalez, J.T.; Fuchs, C.J.; Smith, F.E.; Thelwall, P.E.; Taylor, R.; Stevenson, E.J.; Trenell, M.I.; Cermak, N.M.; van Loon, L.J.C. Ingestion of glucose or sucrose prevents liver but not muscle glycogen depletion during prolonged endurance-type exercise in trained cyclists. *Am. J. Physiol. Endocrinol. Metab.* **2015**, *309*, E1032–E1039. [CrossRef] [PubMed]

40. Lecoultre, V.; Benoit, R.; Carrel, G.; Schutz, Y.; Millet, G.P.; Tappy, L.; Schneiter, P. Fructose and glucose co-ingestion during prolonged exercise increases lactate and glucose fluxes and oxidation compared with an equimolar intake of glucose. *Am. J. Clin. Nutr.* **2010**, *92*, 1071–1079. [CrossRef] [PubMed]

41. Baur, D.A.; Schroer, A.B.; Luden, N.D.; Womack, C.J.; Smyth, S.A.; Saunders, M.J. Glucose-fructose enhances performance versus isocaloric, but not moderate, glucose. *Med. Sci. Sports Exerc.* **2014**, *46*, 1778–1786. [CrossRef] [PubMed]

42. Currell, K.; Jeukendrup, A.E. Superior endurance performance with ingestion of multiple transportable carbohydrates. *Med. Sci. Sports Exerc.* **2008**, *40*, 275–281. [CrossRef] [PubMed]

43. Rowlands, D.S.; Swift, M.; Ros, M.; Green, J.G. Composite versus single transportable carbohydrate solution enhances race and laboratory cycling performance. *Appl. Physiol. Nutr. Metab.* **2012**, *37*, 425–436. [CrossRef] [PubMed]

44. Brooks, G.A.; Dubouchaud, H.; Brown, M.; Sicurello, J.P.; Butz, C.E. Role of mitochondrial lactate dehydrogenase and lactate oxidation in the intracellular lactate shuttle. *Proc. Natl. Acad. Sci. USA* **1999**, *96*, 1129–1134. [CrossRef] [PubMed]

45. Tappy, L.; Egli, L.; Lecoultre, V.; Schneider, P. Effects of fructose-containing caloric sweeteners on resting energy expenditure and energy efficiency: A review of human trials. *Nutr. Metab.* **2013**, *10*, 54. [CrossRef] [PubMed]

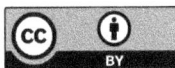

nutrients

MDPI

Article

Metabolic Effects of Glucose-Fructose Co-Ingestion Compared to Glucose Alone during Exercise in Type 1 Diabetes

Lia Bally [1], Patrick Kempf [1], Thomas Zueger [1], Christian Speck [1], Nicola Pasi [1], Carlos Ciller [2,3], Katrin Feller [1], Hannah Loher [1], Robin Rosset [4], Matthias Wilhelm [5], Chris Boesch [6], Tania Buehler [6], Ayse S. Dokumaci [6], Luc Tappy [4] and Christoph Stettler [1,*]

[1]   Department of Diabetes, Endocrinology, Clinical Nutrition and Metabolism, Inselspital,
      Bern University Hospital, University of Bern, 3010 Bern, Switzerland; lia.bally@insel.ch (L.B.);
      patrick.kempf@insel.ch (P.K.); t.zueger@bluewin.ch (T.Z.); christian.speck@outlook.com (C.S.);
      nicola.pasi@students.unibe.ch (N.P.); katrin.feller2@insel.ch (K.F.); hannah.loher@bluewin.ch (H.L.)
[2]   Department of Radiology, University Hospital Centre and University of Lausanne,
      1011 Lausanne, Switzerland; ciller@gmail.com
[3]   Centre for Biomedical Imaging (CIBM), Signal Processing Core, 1015 Lausanne, Switzerland
[4]   Department of Physiology, Faculty of Biology and Medicine, University of Lausanne,
      1005 Lausanne, Switzerland; robin.Rosset@unil.ch (R.R.); luc.tappy@unil.ch (L.T.)
[5]   Department of Cardiology, Interdisciplinary Center for Sports Medicine, Inselspital,
      Bern University Hospital, University of Bern, 3010 Bern, Switzerland; matthias.wilhelm@insel.ch
[6]   Department of Clinical Research and Department of Radiology, University of Bern, 3010 Bern, Switzerland;
      chris.boesch@insel.ch (C.B.); buehler_tania@gmx.net (T.B.); ayse.dokumaci@insel.ch (A.S.D.)
*   Correspondence: christoph.stettler@insel.ch; Tel.: +41-31-632-40-70; Fax: +41-31-632-84-14

Received: 19 January 2017; Accepted: 15 February 2017; Published: 21 February 2017

Abstract: This paper aims to compare the metabolic effects of glucose-fructose co-ingestion (GLUFRU) with glucose alone (GLU) in exercising individuals with type 1 diabetes mellitus. Fifteen male individuals with type 1 diabetes (HbA1c 7.0% $\pm$ 0.6% (53 $\pm$ 7 mmol/mol)) underwent a 90 min iso-energetic continuous cycling session at 50% VO_{2max} while ingesting combined glucose-fructose (GLUFRU) or glucose alone (GLU) to maintain stable glycaemia without insulin adjustment. GLUFRU and GLU were labelled with ^{13}C-fructose and ^{13}C-glucose, respectively. Metabolic assessments included measurements of hormones and metabolites, substrate oxidation, and stable isotopes. Exogenous carbohydrate requirements to maintain stable glycaemia were comparable between GLUFRU and GLU ($p = 0.46$). Fat oxidation was significantly higher (5.2 $\pm$ 0.2 vs. 2.6 $\pm$ 1.2 mg·kg^{-1}·min^{-1}, $p < 0.001$) and carbohydrate oxidation lower (18.1 $\pm$ 0.8 vs. 24.5 $\pm$ 0.8 mg·kg^{-1}·min^{-1} $p < 0.001$) in GLUFRU compared to GLU, with decreased muscle glycogen oxidation in GLUFRU (10.2 $\pm$ 0.9 vs. 17.5 $\pm$ 1.0 mg·kg^{-1}·min^{-1}, $p < 0.001$). Lactate levels were higher (2.2 $\pm$ 0.2 vs. 1.8 $\pm$ 0.1 mmol/L, $p = 0.012$) in GLUFRU, with comparable counter-regulatory hormones between GLUFRU and GLU ($p > 0.05$ for all). Glucose and insulin levels, and total glucose appearance and disappearance were comparable between interventions. Glucose-fructose co-ingestion may have a beneficial impact on fuel metabolism in exercising individuals with type 1 diabetes without insulin adjustment, by increasing fat oxidation whilst sparing glycogen.

Keywords: carbohydrates; glucose; fructose; type 1 diabetes; exercise; glycaemia; substrate oxidation

---

1. Introduction

The beneficial effects of exercise on cardiovascular health and general well-being in patients with type 1 diabetes are well documented [1,2], however, maintaining glycaemic control during exercise remains complex and demanding. The use of exogenous insulin which leads to supraphysiological peripheral insulin levels, in addition to the exercise-induced increase in muscle glucose uptake, predisposes to hypoglycaemia (e.g., dangerous fall in blood glucose levels, below the normal physiological range). Consequently, fear of exercise-related hypoglycaemia is an important factor deterring patients with type 1 diabetes from exercising, despite the fact that many of these individuals are physically fit and wish to be active [3].

Current exercise management guidelines provide pragmatic recommendations, such as adjusting insulin doses and/or increasing the amount of carbohydrates (CHO) ingested before, during, or after exercise [4]. However, simple reduction of insulin dosages require pre-planning and may not always achieve desired results [5]. Several studies have evaluated the dosing and administration schedules of CHO to mitigate against hypoglycaemia [6,7]. The metabolic effects of differing types of CHO in the context of physical activity, however, remain under-studied, particularly in individuals with type 1 diabetes. Although the glycaemic effects of different types of CHO under conditions of insulin dose adjustment have been studied [8–11], the metabolic responses under usual insulin dose conditions remain unclear.

Fructose is a monosaccharide with a considerably different metabolism from that of glucose. Orally-ingested fructose is absorbed via specific intestinal transporter (GLUT5) [12] and is then almost completely extracted by the liver and metabolized by a specific set of enzymes [13]. Fructose, as a subsidiary energy source, is converted to primary energy substrates such as lactate, glucose, and lipids which can either be released into circulation and used by other organs (e.g., the exercising muscle) or stored in the liver [13]. Fructose may therefore act as an alternative to glucose in meeting energy requirements, without the need for insulin, thereby being of particular interest to patients with type 1 diabetes. While the co-ingestion of glucose and fructose under exercise conditions has been previously investigated in healthy non-diabetic individuals [14–16], there is no systematic analysis to date in patients with type 1 diabetes. Therefore, we aimed to investigate the effects of glucose-fructose co-ingestion (GLUFRU) compared to glucose alone (GLU) in exercising type 1 diabetes individuals, on glycaemic stability and exercise-associated metabolism.

2. Material and Methods

2.1. Inclusion Criteria

Fifteen recreationally active male adults with well-controlled type 1 diabetes were recruited for this study. Eleven participants were insulin pump users and four were multiple daily injection users. Volunteers were eligible if they had undetectable C-peptide (<100 pmol/L with concomitant blood glucose $\geq$4 mmol/L), had no known diabetes-related complications, were on stable insulin regime for at least three months prior to the study, and were not on any medications other than insulin. All participants signed informed consent prior to the start of study-related procedures. The study was approved by the Ethics Committee Bern (KEK 001/14).

2.2. Experimental Design and Protocol

This was a prospective non-randomised cross-over design study. Baseline study visits included indirect calorimetry to determine basal metabolic rate (BMR), bioimpedance analysis for lean body mass calculation (BIA 101, Akern, Pontassieve FI, Italy), and a stepwise incremental exercise test on a bicycle ergometer with breath-to-breath spiroergometry (Cardiovit AT-104 PC; Schiller, Baar, Switzerland), as previously described [17].

A 1:1 glucose-fructose mixture (GLUFRU) or glucose alone (GLU) was given orally to maintain stable glycaemia over a 90 min cycling session at 50% VO_{2max}. GLUFRU and GLU consisted of 20% (1:1 glucose-fructose) and 10% CHO solution (Glucosum monohydricum, Hänseler AG, Herisau, Switzerland, D-Fructose, Fluka Analytic, Sigma Aldrich, Buchs, Switzerland), respectively. The concentration of GLUFRU solution was higher compared to GLU to ensure that both solutions provided comparable immediate glycaemic effects at the same volume. GLUFRU or GLU were provided based on personalised CHO-intake regimens which were pre-determined during the familiarisation period (90 min cycling session) in order to account for variable individual responses. The primary outcome of the study was the CHO requirements to maintain stable glycaemia during the final 30 min of the exercise period. Secondary endpoints included assessment of whole body substrate oxidation, glucose turnover, as well as measurements of metabolites and hormones. Ten participants underwent GLU first, followed by GLUFRU. Conversely, five participants underwent GLUFRU first, followed by GLU.

2.3. Pre-Study Standardization Procedures

Participants consumed a standardized diet with a pre-defined daily CHO quantity corresponding to 50% of their calculated energy expenditure 48 h before the main study intervention day. The diet was replicated prior to the second intervention. Foods naturally-enriched in ^{13}C-CHO were avoided to limit baseline shifts in expired $^{13}CO_2$ [18]. Participants were additionally requested to avoid strenuous exercise (pedometer record <5000 steps per day), alcohol, and caffeine. Patients adhered to their usual insulin regime, and daily glycaemia levels were assessed using a continuous glucose monitor (CGM) and capillary glucose measurements. On the main study day, participants were given a standardized breakfast containing one-sixth of each individual's estimated daily CHO amount at 0700, for which participants bolused according to their carbohydrate-to-insulin ratio. Participants were admitted to the research facility at 0930. Basal insulin delivery was not adjusted prior to exercise, and kept identical during both study interventions.

2.4. Sampling Procedures for Metabolites and Hormones

An 18 G cannula was inserted into the antecubital vein of each forearm upon arrival to the research facility. Blood glucose was measured every 10 min (YSI 2300; Yellow Springs Instruments, Yellow Springs, OH, USA). Blood sampling for insulin, counter-regulatory hormones (catecholamines, growth hormone (GH), glucagon, cortisol) and metabolites (lactate, non-esterified fatty acids (NEFAs)) was performed 50 min prior to exercise, at 10, 30, 60, and 80 min of exercise, as well as in the recovery phase (120 min after exercise completion). Insulin, GH, and cortisol were measured using commercially available immunoassay kits (insulin: Architect, Abbott, Baar, Switzerland; GH: Immulite, Siemens, Zurich, Switzerland; cortisol: Modular, Roche, Rotkreuz, Switzerland). Glucagon was measured using a double radioimmunoassay (Siemens, Zurich, Switzerland) in ethylenediaminetetraacetic acid (EDTA) plasma mixed with aprotinin, immediately cooled and frozen after separation. NEFA levels were assessed using a kit from Wako Chemicals (Dietikon, Switzerland). Lactate and pH were determined electrochemically using the ABL 835/837 FLEX (Radiometer, Thalwil, Switzerland) analyser. Plasma catecholamines were quantified using ultraperformance liquid chromatography-tandem mass spectrometry (Waters Acquity UPLC/TQD, Manchester, UK) [19].

2.5. Respiratory Gas Exchange, Cardiopulmonary Monitoring, and Substrate Oxidation

VCO_2 and VO_2 were measured immediately before, during, and 120 min after exercise completion. The 90 min exercise session involved six spirometric recording phases, each performed over 5 min periods at 15, 35, 55, 65, 75, and 85 min of exercise. Net substrate oxidation and energy expenditure were calculated from standard indirect calorimetry equations [20].

Heart rate was recorded continuously by a portable three channel electrocardiogram (ECG) (Lifecard CF, Del Mar Reynolds Medical Inc., Irvine, CA, USA). Rate of perceived exertion (RPE) was assessed by the Borg scale every 10 min.

2.6. Stable Isotopes

Orally supplied CHO solutions were labelled with 0.5% U-$^{13}C_6$-fructose for GLUFRU and 0.5% U-$^{13}C_6$-glucose for GLU. 6,6-$^2H_2$-glucose (Cambridge Isotope Laboratories, Tewksbury, MA, USA) was infused for both interventions. Double background enrichment measurements (blood and breath samples) were taken immediately after intravenous cannulation. Twenty minutes before exercise, a primed (0.6 mg·kg^{-1}(mmol/L)$^{-1}$) constant infusion of 30 μg 6,6-^{2}H$_2$-glucose kg^{-1}·min^{-1} was initiated. At the onset of exercise, the 6,6-^{2}H$_2$-glucose infusion rate was quadrupled to minimize changes in enrichment [21]. Blood and breath samples were obtained during exercise at 59, 69, 79, and 89 min. Plasma 6,6-^{2}H$_2$-glucose and ^{13}C-glucose isotopic enrichment (IE) were measured using gas-chromatography mass-spectrometry (GC-MS) (Hewlett-Packard Instruments, Palo Alto, CA, USA) in chemical ionization mode, as previously described [22]. ^{13}CO$_2$-IE was measured by isotope-ratio mass spectrometry (SerCon, Crewe, UK). Plasma fructose concentrations were measured using a previously published protocol from Petersen and colleagues [23].

2.7. Calculations of Glucose and Fructose Turnover

Glucose and fructose turnover were computed during the last 30 min of exercise, to ensure plateau enrichment was achieved. The rate of glucose appearance (R$_a$) and disappearance (R$_d$) were calculated from 6,6-deuterated glucose dilution using Steele's equation for non-steady state conditions, assuming an effective fraction of 0.65 and a distribution volume of 0.22 L/kg [24]. Glucose metabolic clearance rate (MCR) was calculated as R$_d$/glucose concentration. Muscle glycogen oxidation was estimated as the difference between net CHO oxidation and glucose R$_d$, assuming that 100% of plasma glucose uptake was oxidized during exercise [25]. Gluconeogenesis from fructose was assessed by the product of R$_a$ and isotope enrichment ratio of plasma glucose (M + 3) and ingested fructose (M + 6). The ratio of ^{13}C-abundance in the expired air and ingested glucose and fructose, using a recovery factor of 1.0, provided an estimate of the oxidised amount of fructose (GLUFRU) and glucose (GLU) [26]. A bicarbonate correction factor, assuming a bicarbonate pool of 14.2 mmol/kg, was applied to estimate ^{13}C-fructose/glucose oxidation [27].

2.8. Statistical Analysis

We estimated that twelve participants would provide 95% power to detect a mean difference of 8.2 g of glucose given during the last 30 min, at a level of 5% significance [15]. Assuming a SD of 7 g (based on previous metabolic studies in participants with type 1 diabetes with inherent glycaemic variability [28]), we estimated a sample size of 12, which was increased to 15 to account for drop outs (related to the complexity of study procedures and visits). Data were analysed using Stata 13.0 (Stata Corporation, College Station, TX, USA), Matlab R2015a (The MathWorks, Inc., Natick, MA, USA), and GraphPad Prism software 5.0 (GraphPad Software Inc., San Diego, CA, USA). Differences in hormones, metabolites, and substrate oxidation were evaluated using paired comparisons of area under the curve. Glucose turnover was compared using values obtained during the last 30 min of exercise. Continuous variables were analysed for normality using the Shapiro-Wilk test and qq-plots. Student's paired t tests were used to identify differences for normally distributed variables, and Wilcoxon's signed rank tests were used for non-normally distributed variables. A *p*-value <0.05 was considered statistically significant. Values are expressed as mean ± standard error of the mean (SEM), unless otherwise specified.

3. Results

3.1. Baseline Characteristics and Pre-Study Conditions

Baseline characteristics are shown in Table 1. Total daily CHO intake and insulin dosage were similar for GLUFRU and GLU during the 48 h prior to the main study intervention (CHO: 353 ± 13 vs. 351 ± 11 g/day, *p* = 0.83; insulin dose: 71 ± 4 vs. 70 ± 3 U/day, *p* = 0.49).

Table 1. Baseline characteristics. Data presented as mean (SD).

	$n = 15$
Age (years)	26.1 ± 4.8
Weight (kg)	80.4 ± 10.7
Height (m)	1.81 ± 0.08
BMI (kg/m^2)	24.5 ± 3.2
Fat-free mass (%)	78.8 ± 7.1
BMR (MJ/day)	8.3 ± 0.9
VO_{2max} $(mL \cdot (kg \cdot body \cdot weight)^{-1} \cdot min^{-1})$	47 ± 9
Diabetes duration (years)	13.3 ± 6.7
Haemoglobin A1c (%)	7.0 ± 0.6
Haemoglobin A1c (mmol/mol)	53 ± 7
Total average daily insulin $(U \cdot kg^{-1} \cdot day^{-1})$	0.7 ± 0.1

BMI = body mass index. BMR = basal metabolic rate. VO_{2max} = maximal oxygen uptake.

3.2. CHO Requirements

The primary endpoint (CHO requirements within the last 30 min of exercise) did not differ significantly between interventions: 7.7 ± 2.9 vs. 14.1 ± 3.2 g ($p = 0.14$) in GLUFRU and GLU, respectively. Total CHO requirements to maintain stable glycaemia over the whole exercise period were similar (34.0 ± 2.9 g in GLUFRU and 37.8 ± 5.3 g in GLU, $p = 0.46$). Notably, half of the supplied CHO in GLUFRU consisted of fructose (17 g) (Figure 1).

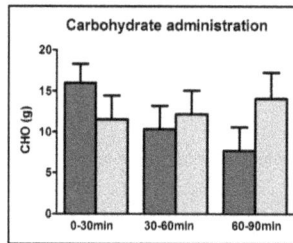

Figure 1. Carbohydrate administration during first, second, and third 30 min-intervals of exercise. GLUFRU (glucose-fructose co-ingestion) = dark grey bar and GLU (glucose alone ingestion) = light grey bar. Results are expressed as mean $\pm$ SEM.

3.3. Energy Expenditure

Total energy expenditure during exercise was 3.3 ± 0.2 and 3.2 ± 0.1 MJ ($p = 0.34$), in GLUFRU and GLU, respectively. Average heart rate did not differ between GLUFRU and GLU (138.6 ± 3.1 vs. 133.4 ± 3.1 beats per minutewhich corresponded to $73\% \pm 2\%$ and $71\% \pm 2\%$ of maximal heart rate, respectively ($p = 0.12$). The measured oxygen consumption was similar during both GLUFRU (24 ± 1 $mg \cdot kg^{-1} \cdot min^{-1}$) and GLU ($23 \pm 1$ $mg \cdot kg^{-1} \cdot min^{-1}$), which corresponded to $53\% \pm 2\%$ VO_{2max} and $51\% \pm 3\%$ VO_{2max}, respectively ($p = 0.20$).

3.4. Glycaemia and Insulin Levels

During exercise, glucose (8.1 ± 0.3 vs. 7.7 ± 0.2 mmol/L, $p = 0.67$) and insulin (138.3 ± 0.8 vs. 141.8 ± 0.9 pmol/L, $p = 0.23$) levels were not significantly different between GLUFRU and GLU (Figure 2). Insulin levels 120 min after exercise were 106.7 ± 32.6 pmol/L in GLUFRU and 103.2 ± 18.7 pmol/L in GLU ($p = 0.89$). Corresponding glucose levels were 8.7 ± 0.7 and 8.9 ± 0.6 mmol/L for GLUFRU and GLU, respectively ($p = 0.72$) (Figure 2).

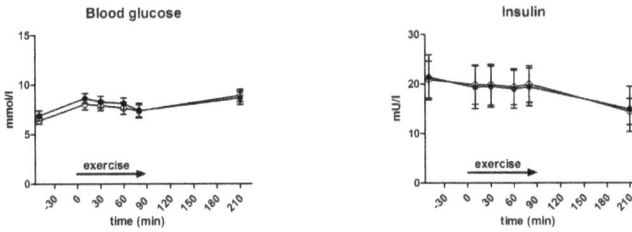

Figure 2. Measured blood glucose and insulin during GLUFRU (black circle) and GLU (white circle). Left to right: blood glucose, $p = 0.67$; insulin, $p = 0.89$. Results are expressed as mean $\pm$ SEM.

3.5. Metabolites and Counter-Regulatory Hormones

Measured metabolites and hormones are shown in Figure 3. During exercise, lactate levels were significantly higher (2.2 ± 0.2 vs. 1.8 ± 0.1 mmol/L, $p = 0.012$), but not at 120 min after exercise completion ($p = 0.58$), in GLUFRU compared to GLU. No differences in pH levels were observed between GLUFRU and GLU (7.39 ± 0.01 vs. 7.38 ± 0.00, $p = 0.33$). NEFA levels during exercise were 0.5 ± 0.04 mmol/L in GLUFRU and 0.4 ± 0.03 mmol/L in GLU ($p = 0.43$). During exercise, mean glucagon levels were 10.7 ± 0.6 and 11.6 ± 0.6 pmol/L ($p = 0.16$) in GLUFRU and GLU, respectively. Mean GH levels (9.7 ± 1.1 vs. 10.8 ± 1.1 ng/mL, $p = 0.50$), noradrenaline (5.9 ± 0.3 vs. 5.5 ± 0.3 nmol/L, $p = 0.45$), adrenaline (0.6 ± 0.1 nmol/L vs. 0.6 ± 0.1 nmol/L, $p = 0.39$), and cortisol (417.6 ± 28.2 and 436.8 ± 23.1 nmol, $p = 0.54$) were comparable between GLUFRU and GLU. Dopamine levels were significantly higher in GLUFRU compared to GLU (0.13 ± 0.02 vs. 0.08 ± 0.02 nmol/L, $p = 0.037$).

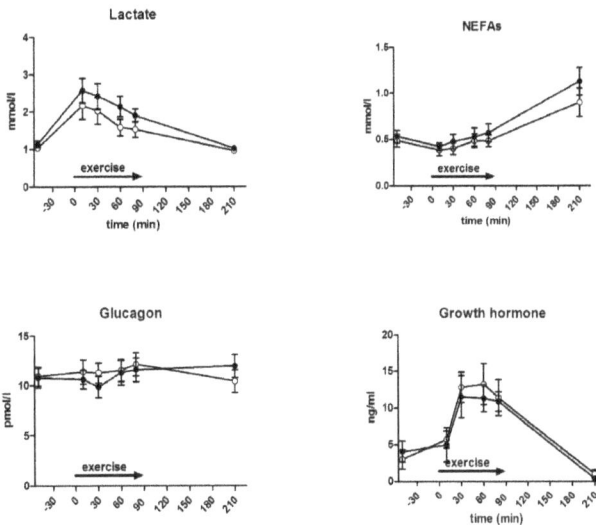

Figure 3. *Cont.*

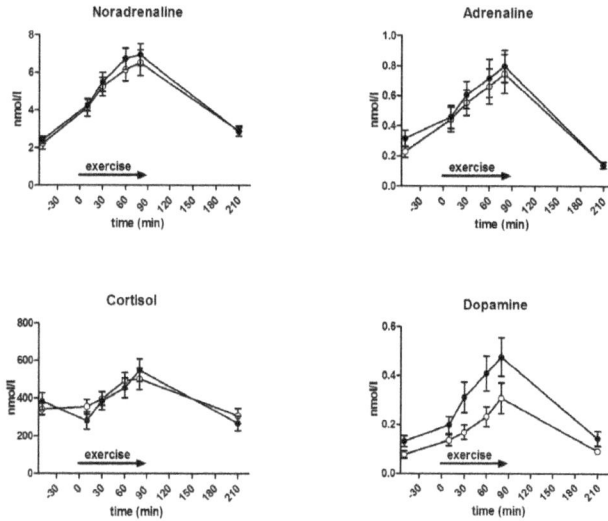

Figure 3. Measured hormones and metabolites during GLUFRU (black circle) and GLU (white circle). Clockwise from top left: lactate, $p = 0.012$; non-esterified fatty acids (NEFAs), $p = 0.43$; growth hormone, $p = 0.50$; adrenaline, $p = 0.39$; dopamine, $p = 0.037$; cortisol, $p = 0.54$; noradrenaline, $p = 0.45$; glucagon, $p = 0.16$. Results are expressed as mean $\pm$ SEM.

3.6. Substrate Oxidation and Turnover

Substrate oxidation is outlined in Figure 4 and Table 2. Fat (1.5 ± 0.1 and 1.6 ± 0.2 mg·kg^{-1}·min^{-1}, $p = 0.69$) and CHO (1.7 ± 0.5 and 2.5 ± 0.3 mg·kg^{-1}·min^{-1}, $p = 0.10$) oxidation at baseline were comparable between GLUFRU and GLU. During the 90 min exercise period, fat oxidation was significantly higher and CHO oxidation lower in GLUFRU compared to GLU (5.2 ± 0.2 vs. 2.6 ± 1.2 mg·kg^{-1}·min^{-1} and 18.1 ± 0.8 mg·kg^{-1}·min^{-1} vs. 24.5 ± 0.8 mg·kg^{-1}·min^{-1}, $p < 0.001$ for both). Respiratory exchange ratio was lower during GLUFRU compared to GLU (0.86 ± 0.01 vs. 0.93 ± 0.00, $p < 0.001$). Fat oxidation contributed to $45.8\% \pm 1.8\%$ of overall energy production in GLUFRU, and $25.5\% \pm 1.4\%$ in GLU ($p < 0.001$). Energy yield contribution from CHO oxidation was $54.2\% \pm 1.8\%$ in GLUFRU and $74.8\% \pm 1.4\%$ in GLU ($p = 0.02$). Fat (1.9 ± 0.21 vs. 1.7 ± 0.2 mg·kg^{-1}·min^{-1}, $p = 0.41$) and CHO (0.5 ± 0.3 vs. 1.2 ± 0.4 mg·kg^{-1}·min^{-1}, $p = 0.09$) oxidation were comparable 120 min after exercise completion between GLUFRU and GLU.

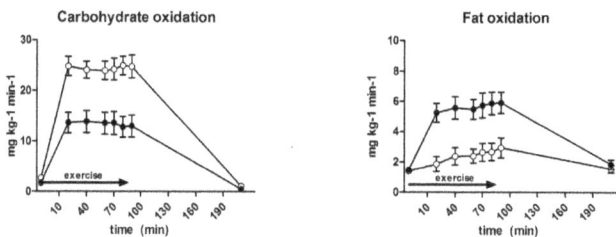

Figure 4. Carbohydrate (CHO) and fat oxidation during GLUFRU (black circle) and GLU (white circle). Results are expressed as mean $\pm$ SEM. Left to right: CHO oxidation, $p < 0.001$; fat oxidation, $p < 0.001$.

Table 2. Metabolic measures during last 30 min of exercise in GLUFRU and GLU. Values are mean (SEM). GLUFRU = glucose-fructose co-ingestion, GLU = glucose alone ingestion.

	GLUFRU (*n* = 15)	GLU (*n* = 15)	*p* Value
Carbohydrate requirements (g)	34.0 ± 2.9	37.8 ± 5.3	0.46
Carbohydrate oxidation (mg·kg^{-1}·min^{-1})	18.1 ± 0.8	24.5 ± 0.8	<0.001
Fat oxidation (mg·kg^{-1}·min^{-1})	5.2 ± 0.2	2.6 ± 1.2	<0.001
Glucose appearance, R_a (mg·kg^{-1}·min^{-1})	7.0 ± 0.4	7.3 ± 0.4	0.53
Glucose disappearance, R_d (mg·kg^{-1}·min^{-1})	7.8 ± 0.3	7.6 ± 0.5	0.57
Metabolic clearance rate, MCR (mg·kg^{-1}·min^{-1})	6.0 ± 0.3	5.9 ± 0.4	0.80

There was no significant difference in glucose turnover between GLUFRU and GLU during the last 30 min of exercise (Table 2). R_a was 7.0 ± 0.4 vs. 7.3 ± 0.4 mg·kg^{-1}·min^{-1} (p = 0.53) in GLUFRU and GLU, respectively. R_d and MCR were comparable between GLUFRU and GLU (7.8 ± 0.3 vs. 7.6 ± 0.5 mL·kg^{-1}·min^{-1} and 6.0 ± 0.3 vs. 5.9 ± 0.4 mL·kg^{-1}·min^{-1}; p = 0.57 and p = 0.80, respectively). Estimated muscle glycogen oxidation was significantly lower in GLUFRU compared to GLU (10.2 ± 0.9 vs. 17.5 ± 1.0 mg·kg^{-1}·min^{-1}, p < 0.001).

Gluconeogenesis from fructose in GLUFRU was 0.9 ± 0.1 mg·kg^{-1}·min^{-1}, contributing to 12.1% ± 1.1% of total Ra. Plasma fructose concentration in the last 30 min of exercise in GLUFRU was 154.7 ± 8.4 μmol/L.

^{13}C-isotopic enrichment in breath samples showed exogenous fructose and glucose oxidation rates of 1.5 ± 0.1 mg·kg^{-1}·min^{-1} in GLUFRU and 3.0 ± 0.3 mg·kg^{-1}·min^{-1} in GLU, in concordance with the 50% lower administered amount of ^{13}C-labeled CHO in GLUFRU when compared to GLU (0.09 vs. 0.19 g).

4. Discussion

The metabolic and hormonal effects of two different CHO supplementation approaches during exercise in patients with type 1 diabetes under identical insulin levels were compared in this study: glucose-fructose co-ingestion (GLUFRU) and glucose alone (GLU). Although the total amount of exogenous CHO needed to maintain stable glycaemia during the whole exercise period did not differ significantly, there was a tendency towards lower CHO requirements during GLUFRU (approximately 50% lower amounts compared to GLU) within the last 30 min of exercise (primary outcome). In daily clinical settings, this may have practical implications as the frequency of CHO supplementation could be reduced when using GLUFRU, thereby potentially providing convenience and safety to the exercising individual with type 1 diabetes.

GLUFRU resulted in significantly higher fat oxidation and lower CHO oxidation, and this was related to lower muscle glycogen oxidation in GLUFRU. Although identical exercise protocols were followed, GLUFRU increased lactate levels, suggesting that ingested fructose was partially converted into lactate. Thus, the benefits of GLUFRU supplementation in exercising individuals with type 1 diabetes may be its more sustainable glycaemic effect, in conjunction with increased fat utilization and sparing of muscle glycogen.

To our knowledge, this is the first study in type 1 diabetes to investigate the metabolic effects of fructose when used in combination with glucose as a CHO supplementation to maintain stable glycaemia during exercise. The observed higher fat oxidation in GLUFRU compared to GLU is in line with a previous study in type 1 diabetes comparing a single oral load of 75 g glucose with an equivalent amount of isomaltulose (a disaccharide of glucose and fructose linked by an alpha-1,6-glycosidic bond), covered with identical insulin boluses 2 h pre-exercise. The authors observed lower CHO oxidation and greater lipid oxidation when 45 min of treadmill running was performed at 80% VO$_{2max}$ [10]. Most studies assessing the effects of glucose-fructose ingestion compared to glucose alone, however, were performed in healthy non-diabetic individuals [15,29]. These studies adopted notably higher CHO feeding rates than those used in the present study (up to 2.4 g/min vs. 0.45 g/min), to maximize CHO absorption, which is the limiting factor for glucose-only supplementation regimes [30]. The authors were able to confirm their hypothesis that glucose-fructose co-ingestion increased total CHO absorption, and consequently metabolic substrate availability, which translated to greater exogenous CHO oxidation and improved endurance performance. Findings related to net substrate oxidation have been inconsistent, however, with some showing either similar [14] or higher [15,31] CHO oxidation with glucose-fructose co-ingestion, whereas others showed tendency to lower CHO oxidation [16]. Direct comparison between type 1 diabetes and healthy non-diabetic individuals is challenging, as CHO intake elicits endogenous insulin secretion in the latter, which is the main determinant in fuel selection [32]. Therefore, studies in individuals with type 1 diabetes, if performed under standardized conditions with identical insulinemia, may offer a unique opportunity to investigate isolated metabolic effects of fructose in an exercise context.

Our finding of increased lactate levels for GLUFRU is in line with other studies reporting partial conversion of ingested fructose into lactate following first pass hepatic metabolism [33–36]. It has been well reported that lactate is readily oxidized by the working muscle [37], therefore fructose-derived lactate may provide an efficient fuel during exercise. This statement is supported by a study comparing glucose-fructose co-ingestion with glucose alone in exercising healthy non-diabetic individuals, which showed that fructose-derived lactate oxidation and fructose-derived glucose oxidation each accounted for approximately 50% of net fructose oxidation [15]. Notably, the present study observed a net ^{13}C-fructose oxidation of 1.5 mg·kg^{-1}·min^{-1} in conjunction with a gluconeogenesis from fructose of 0.9 mg·kg^{-1}·min^{-1}, suggesting that the difference (approximately 0.6 mg·kg^{-1}·min^{-1}) may be accounted for by fructose-derived lactate oxidation.

The findings of higher fat oxidation and lower CHO oxidation under GLUFRU in the present study were unexpected, given the comparable levels of insulin, blood glucose, and gluco-regulatory hormones. The CHO concentration (20% vs. 10% solutions) and administration regime (tendency towards lower CHO supply in GLUFRU within last 30 min of exercise) were the only accountable differences between GLUFRU and GLU. The resulting differences in CHO intake-related glucose appearance is further compounded by the two-step metabolisation of fructose, which requires initial conversion into primary energy substrates such as glucose and lactate, for it to be used as fuel in the working muscle.

Could one therefore hypothesise that the observed increased fat oxidation may be related to an increased utilization of fructose-derived lactate? Continuous low rate of fructose-derived lactate oxidation through lactate dehydrogenase reaction increases the NADH/NAD+ ratio, which then may lower pyruvate dehydrogenase (PDH) activity, thereby favouring acetyl-CoA production by β-oxidation [38]. At a certain level of β-oxidation, associated energy provision becomes self-sustaining as the generated acetyl-CoA and NADH further diminish PDH activity [39]. Testing this hypothesis, however, is beyond the scope of the present work and would need further investigation. Despite differences in fat oxidation, NEFA levels were comparable between GLUFRU and GLU. Such a constellation (higher fat oxidation despite comparable NEFA levels) has also been reported by others [10,40] and may suggest that differences in fat utilization may be attributable to intramyocellular lipid (IMCL), rather than peripheral adipose tissue lipolysis. This is further supported by the well-known fact that in comparison to peripheral lipolysis, intramyocellular hormone-sensitive lipase is not suppressed by the relatively high and constant exogenous insulin levels in our study population [41]. However, we acknowledge that the lack of IMCL assessment in the present study precludes statements regarding intramyocellular lipid utilization.

Interestingly, dopamine levels were significantly higher in GLUFRU compared to GLU in the present study. Due to the standardized setting dietary effects are unlikely to have contributed to this this finding. Although it is known that renal tubular cells can metabolize fructose [42], there is no data suggesting that this could alter the clearance of dopamine leading to higher circulating levels. We acknowledge that the observed difference in dopamine may entirely be due to chance. Although there is limited evidence suggesting dopamine to increase fat oxidation, further studies are needed to validate this hypothesis [43,44].

Post-exercise glycogen repletion has been shown to be related to a decline in blood glucose levels and, consequently, an increased risk for hypoglycaemia in exercising individuals with type 1 diabetes [45]. Therefore, the higher fat oxidation and glycogen-sparing effect observed in GLUFRU may be particularly beneficial for these individuals, pointing towards a potential role of fructose as a supplementary CHO for exercising individuals with type 1 diabetes. Of note, concerns have emerged related to adverse metabolic effects of fructose, albeit in sedentary individuals with relatively high intake of fructose-enriched diet [46–48]. These adverse metabolic effects have been shown to be potentially reversed by physical activity [49,50]. This is in line with the present findings that oxidation is the predominant metabolic fate of ingested fructose which thereby serves as an efficient fuel under exercising conditions.

The strengths of the present study are its standardized design, which comprehensively combines independent techniques to investigate exercise-related fuel metabolism in a commonly encountered clinical situation (e.g., performing exercise without adjustment of insulin doses). The adoption of the study intervention in daily practice is feasible, and potentially provides metabolic benefits to exercising individuals with type 1 diabetes.

Due to the complexity of the chosen technical approach, this study has several limitations, and therefore our results will need to be interpreted with caution. The non-significant difference of the primary endpoint may have been related to the relatively small sample size, and the variability in carbohydrate absorption. In addition, the study had a non-randomised design, and the exclusive recruitment of well-controlled male participants may have limited the generalizability of our findings. The latter was to mitigate against metabolic differences related to sex hormones [51,52]. Larger randomised studies will be needed to validate findings from the present study. The tracer calculations used were based on a one compartment model [53], which may not be fully appropriate for non-steady state conditions. Muscle glycogen oxidation may have been underestimated if less than 100% of glucose R_d was oxidised. However, the probability that a major amount of glucose may have been oxidised in non-muscle tissue under exercise conditions is low. Of note, the metabolic fate of co-ingested glucose could not be determined during GLUFRU, as only fructose was labelled. Additionally, for logistical reasons the amount of fructose disposed though systemic lactate was not measured by our tracer methods, as this would have required duplication of tests for each participant to separately monitor glucose and lactate kinetics.

5. Conclusions

In conclusion, the present study shows that GLUFRU is equally effective as GLU in stabilizing glycaemia in type 1 diabetes during exercise, and induces a shift towards higher fat oxidation with concomitant glycogen-sparing effect in the working muscle. These findings corroborate the flexibility of exercise-related fuel metabolism in type 1 diabetes, indicating that glucose-fructose co-ingestion may be a promising strategy to optimise fuel metabolism during exercise in type 1 diabetes. Further studies are needed to explore the related mechanisms in more detail, such as evaluating different fructose intake doses and schedules under reduced insulin doses, as per clinical guidelines [4].

Acknowledgments: The authors would like to thank all the volunteers for their participation and enthusiasm. Special thanks go to M. Fiedler and A. Leichtle from the Centre of Laboratory Medicine at the University Hospital Bern for great support in diagnostic aspects, to the study nurses involved in the study, and to E. Grouzmann from the University of Lausanne for support in the analysis of catecholamines. Clinical Trial Registration Number: www.clinicaltrials.gov NCT02068638. This study was supported by unrestricted grants from the Swiss National Science Foundation (grant number 320030_149321/1 to C. Stettler).

Author Contributions: The following authors contributed to conception and design of the study: Lia Bally, Luc Tappy, Matthias Wilhelm, and Christoph Stettler; acquisition of data: Lia Bally, Patrick Kempf, Thomas Zueger, Nicola Pasi, Christian Speck, Katrin Feller, Hannah Loher, Robin Rosset, Matthias Wilhelm, and Luc Tappy; analysis: Lia Bally, Patrick Kempf, Christian Speck, Thomas Zueger, Nicola Pasi, Carlos Ciller, Robin Rosset,

Luc Tappy, Chris Boesch, and Christoph Stettler; and interpretation of data: Lia Bally, Robin Rosset, Luc Tappy, and Christoph Stettler. All authors were involved in drafting the article (Lia Bally, Luc Tappy, and Christoph Stettler), or revising it critically for important intellectual content (Lia Bally, Patrick Kempf, Thomas Zueger, Nicola Pasi, Christian Speck, Carlos Ciller, Katrin Feller, Hannah Loher, Robin Rosset, Matthias Wilhelm, Ayse S. Dokumaci, Tania Buehler, Chris Boesch, Luc Tappy, and Christoph Stettler). Christoph Stettler is responsible for the integrity of the work as a whole.

Conflicts of Interest: The authors declare no conflict of interest.

References

1. LaPorte, R.E.; Dorman, J.S.; Tajima, N.; Cruickshanks, K.J.; Orchard, T.J.; Cavender, D.E.; Becker, D.J.; Drash, A.L. Pittsburgh Insulin-Dependent Diabetes Mellitus Morbidity and Mortality Study: Physical activity and diabetic complications. *Pediatrics* **1986**, *78*, 1027–1033.

2. Zoppini, G.; Carlini, M.; Muggeo, M. Self-reported exercise and quality of life in young type 1 diabetic subjects. *Diabetes Nutr. Metab.* **2003**, *16*, 77–80. [PubMed]

3. Brazeau, A.S.; Rabasa-Lhoret, R.; Strychar, I.; Mircescu, H. Barriers to physical activity among patients with type 1 diabetes. *Diabetes Care* **2008**, *31*, 2108–2109. [CrossRef] [PubMed]

4. Riddell, M.C.; Gallen, I.W.; Smart, C.E.; Taplin, C.E.; Adolfsson, P.; Lumb, A.N.; Kowalski, A.; Rabasa-Lhoret, R.; McCrimmon, R.J.; Hume, C.; et al. Exercise management in type 1 diabetes: A consensus statement. *Lancet Diabetes Endocrinol.* **2017**. [CrossRef]

5. McAuley, S.A.; Horsburgh, J.C.; Ward, G.M.; La Gerche, A.; Gooley, J.L.; Jenkins, A.J.; MacIsaac, R.J.; O'Neal, D.N. Insulin pump basal adjustment for exercise in type 1 diabetes: A randomised crossover study. *Diabetologia* **2016**, *59*, 1636–1644. [CrossRef] [PubMed]

6. Grimm, J.J.; Ybarra, J.; Berné, C.; Muchnick, S.; Golay, A. A new table for prevention of hypoglycaemia during physical activity in type 1 diabetic patients. *Diabetes Metab.* **2004**, *30*, 465–470. [CrossRef]

7. Francescato, M.P.; Stel, G.; Stenner, E.; Geat, M. Prolonged exercise in type 1 diabetes: Performance of a customizable algorithm to estimate the carbohydrate supplements to minimize glycemic imbalances. *PLoS ONE* **2015**, *10*, E0125220. [CrossRef]

8. Gray, B.J.; Page, R.; Turner, D.; West, D.J.; Campbell, M.D.; Kilduff, L.P.; Stephens, J.W.; Bain, S.C.; Bracken, R.M. Improved end-stage high-intensity performance but similar glycemic responses after waxy barley starch ingestion compared to dextrose in type 1 diabetes. *J. Sports Med. Phys. Fit.* **2016**, *56*, 1392–1400.

9. Bracken, R.M.; Page, R.; Gray, B.; Kilduff, L.P.; West, D.J.; Stephens, J.W.; Bain, S.C. Isomaltulose improves glycemia and maintains run performance in type 1 diabetes. *Med. Sci. Sports Exerc.* **2012**, *44*, 800–808. [CrossRef] [PubMed]

10. West, D.J.; Morton, R.D.; Stephens, J.W.; Bain, S.C.; Kilduff, L.P.; Luzio, S.; Still, R.; Bracken, R.M. Isomaltulose Improves Postexercise Glycemia by Reducing CHO Oxidation in T1DM. *Med. Sci. Sports Exerc.* **2011**, *43*, 204–210. [CrossRef] [PubMed]

11. West, D.J.; Stephens, J.W.; Bain, S.C.; Kilduff, L.P.; Luzio, S.; Still, R.; Bracken, R.M. A combined insulin reduction and carbohydrate feeding strategy 30 min before running best preserves blood glucose concentration after exercise through improved fuel oxidation in type 1 diabetes mellitus. *J. Sports Sci.* **2011**, *29*, 279–289. [CrossRef] [PubMed]

12. Wood, I.S.; Trayhurn, P. Glucose transporters (GLUT and SGLT): Expanded families of sugar transport proteins. *Br. J. Nutr.* **2003**, *89*, 3–9. [CrossRef] [PubMed]

13. Mayes, P.A. Intermediary metabolism of fructose. *Am. J. Clin. Nutr.* **1993**, *58*, 754S–765S. [PubMed]

14. Jeukendrup, A.E.; Moseley, L. Multiple transportable carbohydrates enhance gastric emptying and fluid delivery. *Scand. J. Med. Sci. Sports* **2010**, *20*, 112–121. [CrossRef] [PubMed]

15. Lecoultre, V.; Benoit, R.; Carrel, G.; Schutz, Y.; Millet, G.P.; Tappy, L.; Schneiter, P. Fructose and glucose co-ingestion during prolonged exercise increases lactate and glucose fluxes and oxidation compared with an equimolar intake of glucose. *Am. J. Clin. Nutr.* **2010**, *92*, 1071–1079. [CrossRef]

16. Wilson, P.B.; Ingraham, S.J. Glucose-fructose likely improves gastrointestinal comfort and endurance running performance relative to glucose-only. *Scand. J. Med. Sci. Sports* **2015**, *25*, E613–E620. [CrossRef] [PubMed]

17. Jenni, S.; Oetliker, C.; Allemann, S.; Ith, M.; Tappy, L.; Wuerth, S.; Egger, A.; Boesch, C.; Schneiter, P.; Diem, P.; et al. Fuel metabolism during exercise in euglycaemia and hyperglycaemia in patients with type 1 diabetes mellitus—A prospective single-blinded randomised crossover trial. *Diabetologia* **2008**, *51*, 1457–1465. [CrossRef] [PubMed]
18. Lefebvre, P.J. From plant physiology to human metabolic investigations. *Diabetologia* **1985**, *28*, 255–263. [CrossRef] [PubMed]
19. Dunand, M.; Gubian, D.; Stauffer, M.; Abid, K.; Grouzmann, E. High-throughput and sensitive quantitation of plasma catecholamines by ultraperformance liquid chromatography-tandem mass spectrometry using a solid phase microwell extraction plate. *Anal. Chem.* **2013**, *85*, 3539–3544. [CrossRef] [PubMed]
20. Peronnet, F.; Massicotte, D. Table of nonprotein respiratory quotient: An update. *Can. J. Sport Sci.* **1991**, *16*, 23–29. [PubMed]
21. Wolfe, R.R.; Chinkes, D.L. *Isotope Tracers in Metabolic Research: Principles and Practice of Kinetic Analysis*; Wiley: Hoboken, NJ, USA, 2005.
22. Tounian, P.; Schneiter, P.; Henry, S.; Delarue, J.; Tappy, L. Effects of dexamethasone on hepatic glucose production and fructose metabolism in healthy humans. *Am. J. Physiol.* **1997**, *273*, E315–E320. [PubMed]
23. Petersen, K.F.; Laurent, D.; Yu, C.; Cline, G.W.; Shulman, G.I. Stimulating effects of low-dose fructose on insulin-stimulated hepatic glycogen synthesis in humans. *Diabetes* **2001**, *50*, 1263–1268. [CrossRef] [PubMed]
24. Steele, R.; Wall, J.S.; De Bodo, R.C.; Altszuler, N. Measurement of size and turnover rate of body glucose pool by the isotope dilution method. *Am. J. Physiol.* **1956**, *187*, 15–24. [PubMed]
25. Romijn, J.A.; Coyle, E.F.; Sidossis, L.S.; Gastaldelli, A.; Horowitz, J.F.; Endert, E.; Wolfe, R.R. Regulation of endogenous fat and carbohydrate metabolism in relation to exercise intensity and duration. *Am. J. Physiol.* **1993**, *265*, E380–E391. [PubMed]
26. Robert, J.J.; Koziet, J.; Chauvet, D.; Darmaun, D.; Desjeux, J.F.; Young, V.R. Use of 13C-labeled glucose for estimating glucose oxidation: Some design considerations. *J. Appl. Physiol. (1985)* **1987**, *63*, 1725–1732.
27. Schneiter, P.; Pasche, O.; Di Vetta, V.; Jequier, E.; Tappy, L. Noninvasive assessment of in vivo glycogen kinetics in humans: Effect of increased physical activity on glycogen breakdown and synthesis. *Eur. J. Appl. Physiol. Occup. Physiol.* **1994**, *69*, 557–563. [CrossRef] [PubMed]
28. Dube, M.C.; Lavoie, C.; Weisnagel, S.J. Glucose or intermittent high-intensity exercise in glargine/glulisine users with T1DM. *Med. Sci. Sports Exerc.* **2013**, *45*, 3–7. [CrossRef]
29. Rowlands, D.S.; Houltham, S.; Musa-Veloso, K.; Brown, F.; Paulionis, L.; Bailey, D. Fructose-Glucose Composite Carbohydrates and Endurance Performance: Critical Review and Future Perspectives. *Sports Med.* **2015**, *45*, 1561–1576. [CrossRef] [PubMed]
30. Shi, X.; Summers, R.W.; Schedl, H.P.; Flanagan, S.W.; Chang, R.; Gisolfi, C.V. Effects of carbohydrate type and concentration and solution osmolality on water absorption. *Med. Sci. Sports Exerc.* **1995**, *27*, 1607–1615. [CrossRef] [PubMed]
31. Roberts, J.D.; Tarpey, M.D.; Kass, L.S.; Tarpey, R.J.; Roberts, M.G. Assessing a commercially available sports drink on exogenous carbohydrate oxidation, fluid delivery and sustained exercise performance. *J. Int. Soc. Sports Nutr.* **2014**, *11*, 8. [CrossRef] [PubMed]
32. Dimitriadis, G.; Mitrou, P.; Lambadiari, V.; Maratou, E.; Raptis, S.A. Insulin effects in muscle and adipose tissue. *Diabetes Res. Clin. Pract.* **2011**, *93* (Suppl. 1), S52–S59. [CrossRef]
33. Macdonald, I.; Keyser, A.; Pacy, D. Some effects, in man, of varying the load of glucose, sucrose, fructose, or sorbitol on various metabolites in blood. *Am. J. Clin. Nutr.* **1978**, *31*, 1305–1311. [PubMed]
34. Sahebjami, H.; Scalettar, R. Effects of fructose infusion on lactate and uric acid metabolism. *Lancet* **1971**, *1*, 366–369. [CrossRef]
35. Chandramouli, V.; Kumaran, K.; Ekberg, K.; Wahren, J.; Landau, B.R. Quantitation of the pathways followed in the conversion of fructose to glucose in liver. *Metabolism* **1993**, *42*, 1420–1423. [CrossRef]
36. Coss-Bu, J.A.; Sunehag, A.L.; Haymond, M.W. Contribution of galactose and fructose to glucose homeostasis. *Metabolism* **2009**, *58*, 1050–1058. [CrossRef] [PubMed]
37. Brooks, G.A.; Dubouchaud, H.; Brown, M.; Sicurello, J.P.; Butz, C.E. Role of mitochondrial lactate dehydrogenase and lactate oxidation in the intracellular lactate shuttle. *Proc. Natl. Acad. Sci. USA* **1999**, *96*, 1129–1134. [CrossRef] [PubMed]
38. Randle, P.J.; Garland, P.B.; Hales, C.N.; Newsholme, E.A. The glucose fatty-acid cycle. Its role in insulin sensitivity and the metabolic disturbances of diabetes mellitus. *Lancet* **1963**, *1*, 785–789. [CrossRef]

39. Sugden, M.C.; Holness, M.J. Recent advances in mechanisms regulating glucose oxidation at the level of the pyruvate dehydrogenase complex by PDKs. *Am. J. Physiol. Endocrinol. Metab.* **2003**, *284*, E855–E862. [CrossRef] [PubMed]

40. Massicotte, D.; Péronnet, F.; Allah, C.; Hillaire-Marcel, C.; Ledoux, M.; Brisson, G. Metabolic response to [13C]glucose and [13C]fructose ingestion during exercise. *J. Appl. Physiol. (1985)* **1986**, *61*, 1180–1184.

41. Moberg, E.; Sjöberg, S.; Hagström-Toft, E.; Bolinder, J. No apparent suppression by insulin of in vivo skeletal muscle lipolysis in nonobese women. *Am. J. Physiol. Endocrinol. Metab.* **2002**, *283*, E295–E301. [CrossRef] [PubMed]

42. Björkman, O.; Felig, P. Role of the kidney in the metabolism of fructose in 60-hour fasted humans. *Diabetes* **1982**, *31*, 516–520. [CrossRef] [PubMed]

43. Thompson, G.E. Dopamine and lipolysis in adipose tissue of the sheep. *Q. J. Exp. Physiol.* **1984**, *69*, 155–159. [CrossRef] [PubMed]

44. Ruttimann, Y.; Schutz, Y.; Jéquier, E.; Lemarchand, T.; Chioléro, R. Thermogenic and metabolic effects of dopamine in healthy men. *Crit. Care Med.* **1991**, *19*, 1030–1036. [CrossRef]

45. Bogardus, C.; Thuillez, P.; Ravussin, E.; Vasquez, B.; Narimiga, M.; Azhar, S. Effect of muscle glycogen depletion on in vivo insulin action in man. *J. Clin. Investig.* **1983**, *72*, 1605–1610. [CrossRef] [PubMed]

46. Wei, Y.; Pagliassotti, M.J. Hepatospecific effects of fructose on c-jun NH2-terminal kinase: Implications for hepatic insulin resistance. *Am. J. Physiol. Endocrinol. Metab.* **2004**, *287*, E926–E933. [CrossRef] [PubMed]

47. Lecoultre, V.; Egli, L.; Carrel, G.; Theytaz, F.; Kreis, R.; Schneiter, P.; Boss, A.; Zwygart, K.; Lê, K.A.; Bortolotti, M.; et al. Effects of fructose and glucose overfeeding on hepatic insulin sensitivity and intrahepatic lipids in healthy humans. *Obesity (Silver Spring)* **2013**, *21*, 782–785. [CrossRef] [PubMed]

48. Faeh, D.; Minehira, K.; Schwarz, J.M.; Periasamy, R.; Park, S.; Tappy, L. Effect of fructose overfeeding and fish oil administration on hepatic de novo lipogenesis and insulin sensitivity in healthy men. *Diabetes* **2005**, *54*, 1907–1913. [CrossRef] [PubMed]

49. Egli, L.; Lecoultre, V.; Theytaz, F.; Campos, V.; Hodson, L.; Schneiter, P.; Mittendorfer, B.; Patterson, B.W.; Fielding, B.A.; Gerber, P.A.; et al. Exercise prevents fructose-induced hypertriglyceridemia in healthy young subjects. *Diabetes* **2013**, *62*, 2259–2265. [CrossRef] [PubMed]

50. Bidwell, A.J.; Fairchild, T.J.; Redmond, J.; Wang, L.; Keslacy, S.; Kanaley, J.A. Physical activity offsets the negative effects of a high-fructose diet. *Med. Sci. Sports Exerc.* **2014**, *46*, 2091–2098. [CrossRef] [PubMed]

51. Galassetti, P.; Tate, D.; Neill, R.A.; Morrey, S.; Wasserman, D.H.; Davis, S.N. Effect of sex on counterregulatory responses to exercise after antecedent hypoglycemia in type 1 diabetes. *Am. J. Physiol. Endocrinol. Metab.* **2004**, *287*, E16–E24. [CrossRef] [PubMed]

52. Devries, M.C.; Hamadeh, M.J.; Phillips, S.M.; Tarnopolsky, M.A. Menstrual cycle phase and sex influence muscle glycogen utilization and glucose turnover during moderate-intensity endurance exercise. *Am. J. Physiol. Regul. Integr. Comp. Physiol.* **2006**, *291*, R1120–R1128. [CrossRef] [PubMed]

53. Hovorka, R.; Jayatillake, H.; Rogatsky, E.; Tomuta, V.; Hovorka, T.; Stein, D.T. Calculating glucose fluxes during meal tolerance test: A new computational approach. *Am. J. Physiol. Endocrinol. Metab.* **2007**, *293*, E610–E619. [CrossRef] [PubMed]

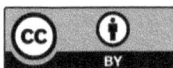

nutrients

MDPI

Review

Glucose Plus Fructose Ingestion for Post-Exercise Recovery—Greater than the Sum of Its Parts?

Javier T. Gonzalez [1,*], Cas J. Fuchs [2], James A. Betts [1] and Luc J. C. van Loon [2]

[1] Department for Health, University of Bath, Bath BA2 7AY, UK; j.betts@bath.ac.uk
[2] Department of Human Biology and Movement Sciences, NUTRIM School of Nutrition and Translational Research in Metabolism, Maastricht University Medical Centre+ (MUMC+), P.O. Box 616, 6200 MD Maastricht, The Netherlands; cas.fuchs@maastrichtuniversity.nl (C.J.F.); l.vanloon@maastrichtuniversity.nl (L.J.C.v.L.)
*   Correspondence: J.T.Gonzalez@bath.ac.uk

Received: 27 February 2017; Accepted: 27 March 2017; Published: 30 March 2017

Abstract: Carbohydrate availability in the form of muscle and liver glycogen is an important determinant of performance during prolonged bouts of moderate- to high-intensity exercise. Therefore, when effective endurance performance is an objective on multiple occasions within a 24-h period, the restoration of endogenous glycogen stores is the principal factor determining recovery. This review considers the role of glucose–fructose co-ingestion on liver and muscle glycogen repletion following prolonged exercise. Glucose and fructose are primarily absorbed by different intestinal transport proteins; by combining the ingestion of glucose with fructose, both transport pathways are utilised, which increases the total capacity for carbohydrate absorption. Moreover, the addition of glucose to fructose ingestion facilitates intestinal fructose absorption via a currently unidentified mechanism. The co-ingestion of glucose and fructose therefore provides faster rates of carbohydrate absorption than the sum of glucose and fructose absorption rates alone. Similar metabolic effects can be achieved via the ingestion of sucrose (a disaccharide of glucose and fructose) because intestinal absorption is unlikely to be limited by sucrose hydrolysis. Carbohydrate ingestion at a rate of $\geq$1.2 g carbohydrate per kg body mass per hour appears to maximise post-exercise muscle glycogen repletion rates. Providing these carbohydrates in the form of glucose–fructose (sucrose) mixtures does not further enhance muscle glycogen repletion rates over glucose (polymer) ingestion alone. In contrast, liver glycogen repletion rates are approximately doubled with ingestion of glucose–fructose (sucrose) mixtures over isocaloric ingestion of glucose (polymers) alone. Furthermore, glucose plus fructose (sucrose) ingestion alleviates gastrointestinal distress when the ingestion rate approaches or exceeds the capacity for intestinal glucose absorption (~1.2 g/min). Accordingly, when rapid recovery of endogenous glycogen stores is a priority, ingesting glucose–fructose mixtures (or sucrose) at a rate of $\geq$1.2 g·kg body mass^{-1}·h^{-1} can enhance glycogen repletion rates whilst also minimising gastrointestinal distress.

Keywords: carbohydrates; glycogen; liver; metabolism; muscle; resynthesis; sports nutrition; sucrose

1. Introduction

Carbohydrates are a major substrate for oxidation during almost all exercise intensities [1]. The main determinants of carbohydrate utilisation during exercise are the intensity and duration of exercise [1,2], followed by training and nutritional status [3,4]. In the fasted state, the main forms of carbohydrate utilised during exercise are skeletal muscle glycogen and plasma glucose (derived primarily from liver glycogen and gluconeogenesis) [1]. Compared to fat stores, the capacity for humans to store carbohydrates is limited; >100,000 kcal stored as fat versus <3000 kcal stored as carbohydrate in a typical 75-kg person with 15% body fat [5]. Therefore, glycogen stores can be almost entirely depleted within 45–90 min of moderate- to high-intensity exercise [6,7], with the occurrence of fatigue strongly associated with the depletion of endogenous carbohydrate stores [8–10]. Nutritional strategies to complement or replace endogenous carbohydrate stores as a fuel during exercise have been studied for decades [9,11]. It is now well established that carbohydrate ingestion during exercise improves endurance performance and delays fatigue in events requiring a sustained moderate to high intensity for more than 45 min [12]. Due to the strong relationship between replenishment of liver and skeletal muscle glycogen stores with subsequent exercise tolerance [7,10], the main factor determining recovery time is the rate of glycogen repletion. This is especially relevant when optimal performance is required on more than one occasion with a limited interval between bouts, such as during intensive training periods, stage races (e.g., Tour de France) and tournament-style competitions. In the hours following exercise, carbohydrate ingestion is a requirement for substantial replenishment of skeletal muscle glycogen stores [13], and the appropriate dose of carbohydrate (or co-ingestion of protein with suboptimal carbohydrate intake) can accelerate the replenishment of skeletal muscle glycogen contents [14,15].

In recent years, there has been an increasing appreciation of the different types of carbohydrates that can be ingested during and after exercise. When large amounts of carbohydrate are ingested (>1.4 g·min^{-1}) the combined ingestion of glucose and fructose can improve performance by ~1–9% over the ingestion of glucose (polymers) alone [16]. The performance benefits of glucose–fructose co-ingestion are likely due to more rapid digestion and absorption of the carbohydrate, providing exogenous fuel at a faster rate than glucose ingestion alone. Faster digestion and absorption rates of carbohydrates during recovery from exercise may also have benefits for more rapid recovery of glycogen stores post-exercise [15,17]. With this in mind, this review provides an overview of dietary carbohydrates, glycogen stores and exercise capacity, before focussing on the role of glucose–fructose mixtures in post-exercise recovery of skeletal muscle and liver glycogen stores.

2. Dietary Carbohydrates for Sport Nutrition

Dietary carbohydrates come in many forms, comprising monosaccharides such as glucose, fructose and galactose; disaccharides such as maltose, sucrose and lactose; and polysaccharides such as maltodextrin and starch (Table 1). The rates of digestion, intestinal absorption and hepatic metabolism of carbohydrates are key determinants of carbohydrate delivery to skeletal muscle tissue. These factors are therefore important considerations when choosing a nutritional strategy to optimize carbohydrate delivery during and after exercise.

Table 1. Common dietary carbohydrates, their constituent monomers and major intestinal transport proteins.

Carbohydrate	Chain Length	Constituent Monomers	Bonds	Apical Membrane Intestinal Transport Protein(s)
Glucose	1	-	-	**SGLT1**; GLUT2; GLUT12
Fructose	1	-	-	**GLUT5**; GLUT2; GLUT7; GLUT8; GLUT12
Galactose	1	-	-	**SGLT1**; GLUT2
Maltose	2	Glucose + Glucose	α-1,4-glycosidic	**SGLT1**; GLUT2; GLUT8/12
Sucrose	2	Glucose + Fructose	α-1,2-glycosidic	**SGLT1; GLUT5**; GLUT2; GLUT7; GLUT8 GLUT12
Isomaltulose	2	Glucose + Fructose	α-1,6-glycosidic	**SGLT1; GLUT5**; GLUT2; GLUT7; GLUT8 GLUT12
Lactose	2	Glucose + Galactose	β-1,4-glycosidic	**SGLT1**; GLUT2; GLUT12
Maltodextrin	~3–9	Glucose + Glucose ...	α-1,4-glycosidic	**SGLT1**; GLUT2; GLUT12
Starch	>9 (typically >300)	Glucose + Glucose ...	α-1,4- and α-1,6-glycosidic	**SGLT1**; GLUT2; GLUT12

Major transport proteins are highlighted in bold. GLUT, glucose transporter; SGLT, sodium-dependent glucose transporter. Table comprised using information from references [18–23].

Glucose is a constituent of most disaccharides and polysaccharides and is therefore the most ubiquitous carbohydrate in most people's diets (Table 1). Glucose is also the primary cellular fuel source in almost all human tissues. Carbohydrates must first be hydrolysed into their constituent monomers before being absorbed across the intestine and entering the systemic circulation [23]. Therefore, most dietary carbohydrates are broken down into glucose, fructose and/or galactose prior to their subsequent absorption. The major intestinal absorption route of glucose involves sodium-dependent glucose transporter 1 (SGLT1), which transports glucose from the intestinal lumen into the enterocyte [23]. Other putative routes include transport by glucose transporter 2 (GLUT2) and GLUT12, although these are yet to be clearly established in humans [24], and are likely to play only minor roles in intestinal glucose absorption [23]. Whilst fructose has an identical chemical formula to glucose ($C_6H_{12}O_6$), glucose has an aldehyde group at position 1 of its carbon chain, whereas fructose possesses a keto group in position two of its carbon chain [25]. A notable difference in the handling of fructose compared to most other carbohydrates is the primary intestinal transport protein responsible for transporting fructose from the intestinal lumen to within the enterocyte: GLUT5 (Table 1). Other fructose transporters may also be involved in fructose absorption, but again are likely to play minor roles in comparison to GLUT5 [22].

When ingested alone, the hydrolysis of most carbohydrates is rapid and does not limit the rate of digestion and absorption. Therefore, the rate at which glucose polymers such as maltose, maltodextrin and starch can be digested, absorbed and used as a fuel source is not substantially slower than that of glucose [26–28]. Furthermore, the hydrolysis of sucrose (by sucrase) is also rapid and exceeds the rate of intestinal absorption of glucose and fructose [29]. An exception to this rule is isomaltulose. Due to the different bond linking glucose and fructose, the hydrolysis rate of isomaltulose (by isomaltase) is drastically slower than that of sucrose [20,30]. Isomaltulose thereby produces a lower glycaemic and insulinaemic response following ingestion, and suppresses fat oxidation to a lesser extent than sucrose [31]. However, presumably due to this slow rate of digestion and absorption, isomaltulose exacerbates gastrointestinal distress when consumed in large amounts during exercise [32].

After intestinal absorption, the metabolism of various dietary carbohydrates also differs. In contrast to glucose, which can bypass the liver and enter the systemic circulation, fructose and galactose are almost completely metabolised upon first pass of the liver [25,33]. This splanchnic sequestration appears to be enhanced by the co-ingestion of glucose [33]. Fructose and galactose are converted in the liver into glucose, lactate, glycogen and lipids, which subsequently appear in the circulation [25,33]. The energy cost of converting fructose into glucose and other substrates is likely to account for the greater postprandial thermogenesis seen with fructose versus glucose ingestion [34]. Because of this hepatic metabolism, the blood glucose and insulin responses to fructose or galactose ingestion are attenuated when compared to glucose ingestion [35,36]. This lower insulin response may have implications for glycogen storage in recovery from exercise.

Hepatic fructose metabolism also differs from hepatic glucose metabolism in its regulation by insulin. Both glucose and fructose enter the liver via the insulin-independent transporter, GLUT2. However, hepatic glucose metabolism is then regulated by insulin and the cellular energy status [5,25]. Insulin, ATP and citrate concentrations regulate glucose flux to pyruvate via modulating the activity of hexokinase IV and glycolytic enzymes [37]. Hepatic fructose metabolism on the other hand, is independent of insulin and does not display negative feedback inhibition by ATP nor citrate [25].

3. Endogenous Carbohydrate Stores and Exercise Performance

3.1. Muscle Glycogen

The reintroduction of the muscle biopsy technique to exercise physiology in the 1960s clearly demonstrated the heavy reliance on skeletal muscle glycogen as a fuel source during exercise [8,38]. There is a strong relationship between baseline skeletal muscle glycogen contents and subsequent endurance exercise capacity [8]. Furthermore, the capacity for exercise is severely compromised when skeletal muscle glycogen stores are depleted, even when other substrate sources are available in abundance [9]. The defined mechanisms that link skeletal muscle glycogen contents and exercise tolerance are incompletely understood. It is thought that skeletal muscle glycogen is more than just a fuel source, and that glycogen also acts as a signalling molecule to control skeletal muscle cell function and regulate exercise capacity [39].

Skeletal muscle glycogen provides a rapid and efficient (energy yield per unit oxygen) fuel source for energy expenditure, such that when skeletal muscle glycogen stores are depleted, the rate of energy production is severely compromised. Clear support for the important role of glycogen as a substrate in supporting energy requirements to allow intense exercise is provided by observations of individuals with McArdle's disease (glycogen storage disease type V; GSD5). These individuals display high skeletal muscle glycogen concentrations but an inability to utilise this glycogen as a substrate source [40], and subsequently can also display extreme intolerance to intense exercise [41]. This is partly due to glycogen oxidation resulting in maximal ATP re-synthesis rates that are >2-fold greater than fat or plasma glucose oxidation [42,43]. Therefore, when high rates of ATP re-synthesis are required over a prolonged duration, it would appear there is no substitute for glycogen as a fuel. Furthermore, the oxidation of carbohydrates is more oxygen efficient than that of fat, deriving more energy per litre of oxygen consumed [44]. Consequently, oxidising carbohydrates over fats provides an advantage in sports where the rate of oxygen delivery to active muscle is limiting to performance.

A reduced ability of glycogen to fuel metabolism may not fully account for the exercise intolerance with low skeletal muscle glycogen content. Low glycogen contents are still associated with impaired skeletal muscle function, even when ATP concentrations would be normalised [45]. Therefore, it has recently been proposed that glycogen is also an important signalling molecule that regulates sarcoplasmic reticulum calcium release rates and thus skeletal muscle function [39]. Accordingly, adequate skeletal muscle glycogen availability appears to be critically important (via multiple mechanisms) in maintaining optimal performance during prolonged bouts of moderate-to high-intensity exercise.

3.2. Liver Glycogen

Liver glycogen plays a central role in blood glucose homeostasis during conditions such as exercise, fasting and feeding [5]. After an overnight fast (e.g., 12 h), ~50% of plasma glucose appearance at rest is accounted for by liver glycogen utilisation, with the remainder provided by gluconeogenesis [46]. Even resting metabolic requirements can therefore deplete liver glycogen stores almost entirely within 48 h of carbohydrate restriction [47].

Plasma glucose is constantly utilised as a fuel source at rest and during almost all exercise intensities [1]. During exercise in a fasted state, plasma glucose that is taken up by skeletal muscle is continuously replaced by gluconeogenesis and glycogen degradation, predominantly derived from the liver [48]. In the absence of carbohydrate ingestion liver glycogen stores can be rapidly depleted (by ~40%–60%) within 90 min of moderate- to high-intensity (~70% VO_2 peak) exercise [6,7,49]. The rate of liver glycogen depletion during exercise in a fasted state will depend primarily on the intensity of exercise and the training status of the individual; higher exercise intensities are associated with higher rates of liver glycogen utilisation, particularly in untrained individuals [5]. Endurance-trained athletes do not appear to store more liver glycogen than untrained individuals but endurance-type exercise training is associated with a lower rate of liver glycogen utilisation during exercise (at the same absolute or relative intensity) [5]. Therefore, endurance athletes can exercise at a given exercise intensity for longer before liver glycogen contents will reach a critically low level [5].

Few studies have directly measured the relationship between liver glycogen contents and exercise tolerance in humans. One of the only studies to have performed concomitant measures of liver glycogen content and exercise capacity demonstrated a modest positive relationship between liver glycogen repletion after an initial bout of exercise, and subsequent endurance capacity [7]. Furthermore, in this study the correlation between muscle glycogen repletion and subsequent endurance capacity was weaker than that with liver glycogen repletion, and the addition of muscle glycogen repletion to liver glycogen repletion did not further improve the relationship between liver glycogen repletion and exercise capacity [7]. Consequently, post-exercise recovery of liver glycogen stores may be at least as important as muscle glycogen stores for subsequent endurance capacity. The mechanisms by which liver glycogen contents regulate exercise capacity currently remain unknown, but given the fundamental role of hepatic metabolism in glucose homeostasis, low liver glycogen stores are likely to inhibit exercise capacity (at least in part) via a reduction in blood glucose availability and premature hypoglycaemia [5]. Liver glycogen may also act as a biological signal to regulate metabolism (and potentially exercise capacity). Rodent data suggest that liver glycogen contents modulate fatty acid availability via a liver–brain–adipose tissue axis [50]. Therefore, brain sensing of liver glycogen contents could regulate metabolism (and theoretically fatigue) during exercise.

It has been suggested that it may take longer to recover liver, compared to muscle glycogen stores post-exercise, in humans [5], which is likely due to changes in splanchnic handling of glucose in the post-exercise period. Splanchnic glucose output of an oral glucose load is ~30% at rest, but can double to ~60% post-exercise [51]. This may be partly due to greater post-exercise increases in blood flow to muscle [52], compared to the liver, resulting in relatively more ingested glucose made available to the muscle. On this basis, nutritional strategies to optimise short-term recovery from prolonged exercise should focus on both liver and muscle glycogen repletion, since both display limitations in their capacity to replenish carbohydrate stores and either could be instrumental to optimizing subsequent performance.

4. Physiological Rationale for Glucose–Fructose Co-Ingestion in Post-Exercise Recovery

Alongside insulin concentrations, carbohydrate delivery to the liver and skeletal muscle can be a rate limiting step in post-exercise glycogen re-synthesis, as demonstrated by >2-fold higher glycogen repletion rates with glucose infusion [53,54] compared to the highest rates ever reported with oral carbohydrate ingestion [55]. During exercise, exogenous carbohydrate oxidation can differ depending on the type of carbohydrates ingested [56]. These differences may be attributable to differences in carbohydrate digestion and absorption kinetics during exercise [56,57]. It could be hypothesised that these differences are also evident during post-exercise recovery, implying that rapidly digested and absorbed carbohydrates may accelerate recovery of endogenous glycogen stores.

To obtain insight into the role of glucose–fructose co-ingestion on carbohydrate digestion, absorption and utilisation kinetics during exercise, we performed a literature search (PubMed, February 2017). This included the search terms "exogenous", "carbohydrate", "glucose", "fructose", "sucrose" and "oxidation". This search was complemented by a manual search of references within papers. In order to minimize the potential for inter-subject and inter-laboratory variability, studies were limited to peer-reviewed published articles to date that have directly compared glucose (polymer) ingestion alone with glucose–fructose (sucrose) co-ingestion and determined exogenous carbohydrate oxidation rates during exercise. When ingesting glucose(polymers) during exercise, the maximal rate of exogenous carbohydrate oxidation increases in a curvilinear fashion with carbohydrate ingestion rate, reaching a peak exogenous oxidation rate of ~1.2 g·min^{-1} (Figure 1) [26,27,58–69]. The primary limitation in the rate of exogenous carbohydrate oxidation is thought to be intestinal absorption, since gastric emptying rates of glucose during exercise have been reported to exceed 1.5 g·min^{-1} [70], and when the intestine and liver are bypassed with intravenous glucose infusion, exogenous oxidation rates of 2 g·min^{-1} can be achieved [57]. Furthermore, maximal intestinal glucose absorption rates at rest have been estimated to be ~1.3 g·min^{-1} [71]. Exercise up to an intensity of 70% VO$_2$ peak does not alter the intestinal absorption of glucose [72]. Therefore, it is reasonable to assume that this ~1.3 g·min^{-1} limit also applies during most exercise intensities, suggesting that intestinal absorption rather than liver glucose metabolism is the primary limitation to exogenous glucose oxidation during exercise (Figure 2) [73]. Nevertheless, this remains speculative in the absence of direct measures of intestinal absorption.

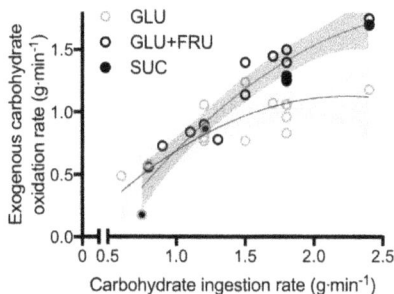

Figure 1. Peak exogenous carbohydrate oxidation rates during exercise in studies that directly compared glucose (polymer) ingestion alone (GLU), vs. either glucose plus fructose co-ingestion (GLU + FRU), or sucrose ingestion (SUC). Each symbol represents the mean from a single study. The light grey shaded area represents the 95% confidence intervals for GLU and the dark grey shaded area represents the 95% confidence intervals for GLU + FRU and SUC. Data extracted from references [22,23,55–66].

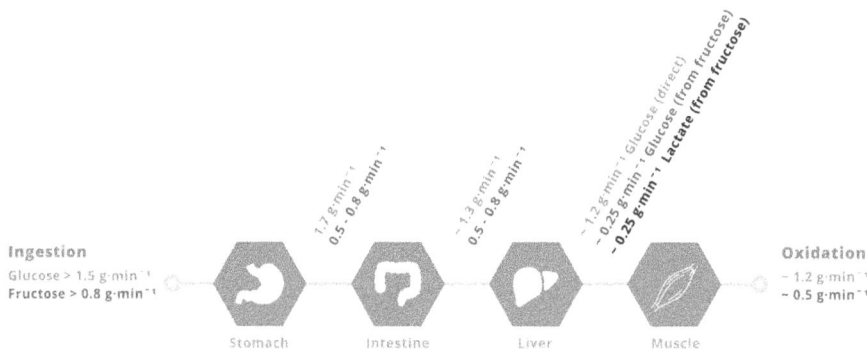

Figure 2. Putative limitations in carbohydrate delivery to skeletal muscle during exercise with glucose–fructose (or sucrose) co-ingestion. When large amounts of glucose (>1.5 g·min^{-1}) and fructose (>0.8 g·min^{-1}) are ingested during prolonged, moderate- to high-intensity (50%–70% VO$_2$ peak) exercise, the rate of gastric emptying is unlikely to be limiting, since gastric emptying rates of glucose are in the region of 1.7 g·min^{-1} [67]. Rates of intestinal glucose absorption are ~1.3 g·min^{-1} [68]. Rates of glucose appearance into the peripheral circulation and subsequently oxidised are ~1.2 g·min^{-1} [58,70]. Rates of fructose (and sucrose) gastric emptying and intestinal absorption must be at least 0.5 g·min^{-1} since the appearance rate into the peripheral circulation of fructose derived carbohydrate is ~0.5 g·min^{-1} [71], with ~50% in the form of glucose and 50% in the form of lactate, that are subsequently oxidised by skeletal muscle at a rate of ~0.5 g·min^{-1} [71].

When fructose is co-ingested with glucose during exercise, exogenous carbohydrate oxidation rates of ~1.7 g·min^{-1} can be achieved; substantially higher than that seen with glucose ingestion alone (Figure 1) [26,27,58–69]. Whether glucose and fructose are ingested as sucrose or as free monosaccharides does not appear to influence the rate of exogenous carbohydrate oxidation (Figure 1). This is consistent with observations that the rate of digestion and intestinal absorption of glucose and fructose does not differ when ingested as sucrose or as co-ingestion of free glucose and free fructose [29]. Therefore, the hydrolysis of sucrose does not appear to be rate limiting to absorption of its monosaccharide products and can be used as an alternative to free glucose and free fructose. In a systematic assessment of optimal fructose:glucose ratios using dual-isotope labelling, it is apparent that a fructose:glucose ratio of 0.8-1.0-1.0 (0.67 g·min^{-1} fructose plus 0.83 g·min^{-1} glucose (polymers)) provides the greatest exogenous carbohydrate oxidation efficiency and endurance performance [74].

Fructose metabolism differs markedly from glucose metabolism. Firstly, fructose is primarily absorbed across the apical membrane of the intestinal enterocytes by different transport proteins (GLUT5, as opposed to SGLT1). Secondly, plasma fructose concentrations remain relatively low (<0.5 mmol·L^{-1}) following fructose ingestion [75]. It is commonly reported that human skeletal muscle cannot directly oxidise fructose. This is based on human skeletal muscle lacking ketohexokinase (the enzyme responsible for catalysing the phosphorylation of fructose to fructose-1-phosphate). However, in addition to phosphorylating glucose, hexokinase is also able to phosphorylate fructose [76] and when fructose is infused (achieving plasma fructose concentrations of ~5.5 mmol·L^{-1}) during exercise, then quantitatively important amounts of fructose (0.3–0.4 g·min^{-1}) are likely to be directly oxidised by skeletal muscle [77]. Of course, this is of little relevance to sports nutrition because oral ingestion of fructose rarely results in plasma fructose concentrations exceeding ~0.4 mmol·L^{-1} and thus direct oxidation of fructose is negligible. The reason for a relatively low systemic fructose concentration after fructose ingestion is that fructose is rapidly converted in the intestine and liver to glucose and lactate, which then enter the systemic circulation and delivered to peripheral tissues [78] and/or contribute to liver glycogen synthesis.

When fructose is co-ingested with glucose in large amounts (>0.8 g·min^{-1} each) during exercise, systemic appearance of fructose derived carbohydrate is ~0.5 g·min^{-1} (equally split between fructose-derived glucose and fructose-derived lactate) [78], and the subsequent oxidation of this fructose derived glucose and lactate by skeletal muscle can thus fully account for the higher exogenous carbohydrate oxidation rates seen with glucose–fructose mixtures (sucrose) over glucose alone (Figures 1 and 2). It is unclear what the rate-limiting step in exogenous fructose oxidation is when co-ingested with glucose during exercise, although intestinal absorption is a probable factor. The capacity for humans to absorb dietary fructose is comparatively limited when ingested in isolation. Approximately 60% of individuals display fructose malabsorption after ingestion of large (50 g) fructose loads, with this proportion halved if co-ingested with glucose [79]. Similarly, only 11% of people exhibit fructose malabsorption when ingesting a lower dose of fructose (25 g), with appropriate absorption in almost all cases if that lower dose is ingested with glucose or as sucrose [79]. Therefore, not only does the addition of fructose to glucose ingestion takes advantage of an additional intestinal transport pathway, the ingestion of glucose alongside fructose enhances fructose absorption (via a currently unidentified mechanism) providing a dual mechanism for enhanced carbohydrate delivery. High-fructose diets have been shown to increase intestinal GLUT5 protein content in mice [80]. Therefore, it could be speculated that regularly consuming fructose may enhance the maximal capacity for intestinal fructose absorption, but this remains to be tested in humans.

For athletes, the primary benefit of ingesting glucose–fructose mixtures during exercise is an ability to absorb a greater amount of exogenous carbohydrate to the systemic circulation. This can then be used immediately as a fuel and/or to maintain endogenous carbohydrate stores. More rapid digestion and absorption is also a likely cause of the lower gastrointestinal distress observed with high ingestion rates of isocaloric glucose–fructose mixtures over glucose alone. Lower gastrointestinal distress could, in part, account for some of the performance benefits seen with glucose–fructose co-ingestion [16,81]. The high rates of carbohydrate absorption with glucose–fructose co-ingestion also raise the possibility of enhancing the rate of recovery of endogenous carbohydrate stores post-exercise.

5. Glucose–Fructose Co-Ingestion and Recovery from Exercise

5.1. Muscle Glycogen Repletion

Glucose and lactate are the primary substrates for muscle glycogen re-synthesis; the latter is able to account for at least 20% of total muscle glycogen re-synthesis following intense exhaustive exercise [82]. Therefore, the availability of carbohydrates (glucose and lactate) to muscle is an important factor in maximising the rate of muscle glycogen repletion and reducing recovery time. Alongside insulinotropic properties, the rate of digestion, intestinal absorption and hepatic metabolism of nutrients are thus important considerations for optimising sports nutrition for rapid post-exercise recovery. Insulin availability is also important for post-exercise glycogen re-synthesis. Insulin increases blood flow to muscle, GLUT4 translocation to the plasma membrane, hexokinase II and glycogen synthase activity [83–86], all of which contribute to enhanced muscle glucose uptake and glycogen synthesis. A further consideration in the post-exercise period is that elevated catecholamine concentrations may be inhibiting the rise in blood flow and some aspects of insulin signalling in muscle [85,87]. Based on the metabolism of glucose and fructose during exercise (Figures 1 and 2) it could be hypothesised that the greater carbohydrate availability to muscle with ingestion of large amounts of glucose–fructose (sucrose) mixtures could augment post-exercise muscle glycogen repletion rates over isocaloric glucose ingestion alone. In line with this, rates of post-exercise muscle glycogen repletion increase as the rate of carbohydrate ingestion increases, up until ~1 g carbohydrate·kgBM^{-1}·h^{-1}. This is equivalent to ~1.2 g·min^{-1} for a 72-kg athlete and is therefore in good agreement with the maximal rate of glucose (polymer) digestion and intestinal absorption during exercise (Figure 2). This provides further support for the rationale that carbohydrate delivery to muscle (controlled by digestion, absorption and hepatic metabolism) could be a limiting factor in post-exercise muscle glycogen repletion with carbohydrate feedings.

Studies that have directly compared the ingestion glucose–fructose mixtures (or sucrose) vs. glucose (polymers) alone on post-exercise muscle glycogen repletion, have employed carbohydrate ingestion rates ranging from 0.25 to 1.5 g·kgBM^{-1}·h^{-1}, across two to six hours of recovery [7,88–92]. Across this wide range of carbohydrate ingestion rates, post-exercise ingestion of glucose–fructose (sucrose) mixtures do not appear to accelerate muscle glycogen repletion when compared to glucose (polymer) ingestion alone (Figure 3A). However, lower insulinaemia was reported with glucose–fructose (sucrose) co-ingestion in most [7,88–90], but not all [91,92] studies. Therefore, similar muscle glycogen storage appears possible with glucose plus fructose ingestion, compared to glucose ingestion alone, even when insulin availability is lower. It has been suggested that due to the hepatic metabolism of fructose, less glucose may be retained in the liver with glucose–fructose (sucrose) mixtures and more glucose is made available for muscle to be utilised for glycogen re-synthesis, thus offsetting the lower insulin concentrations [89].

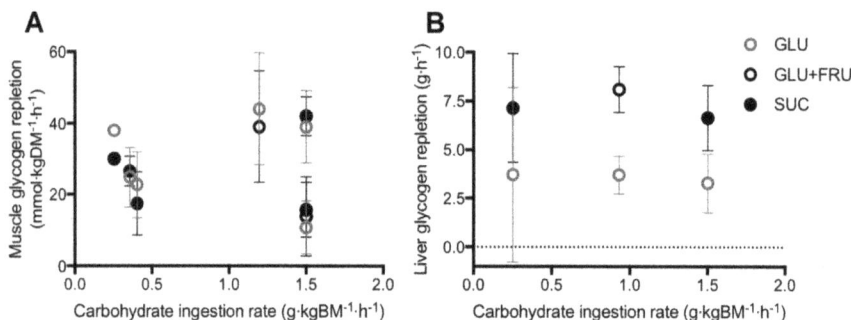

Figure 3. Post-exercise skeletal muscle (**A**) and liver (**B**) glycogen repletion rates in all published studies that have directly compared glucose (polymer) ingestion alone (GLU), vs. either glucose plus fructose co-ingestion (GLU+FRU), or sucrose ingestion (SUC). Bars represent means ± 95% confidence intervals (calculated when sufficient data were available). Data extracted from references [7,85–89,92].

A further addition to this hypothesis could be that fructose co-ingestion with glucose also provides lactate as an additional fuel source for muscle. Lactate can then be used for muscle glycogen synthesis and/or be oxidised [93], directing more glucose towards muscle glycogen synthesis. Consistent with this, plasma lactate concentrations are higher with glucose–fructose (sucrose) ingestion in post-exercise recovery, when compared to glucose alone, in all [88,90–92] but the lowest [7] carbohydrate ingestion rates. This raises the question as to whether providing additional substrate for liver glycogen synthesis (e.g., via galactose co-ingestion) and/or stimulating insulinaemia (e.g., via amino acid co-ingestion) can further accelerate muscle glycogen repletion rates with glucose–fructose mixtures over glucose (polymers) alone. One study has directly compared protein plus sucrose co-ingestion vs. sucrose ingestion alone with high carbohydrate ingestion rates (~1.25 g·kgBM^{-1}·h^{-1}) and found no difference in muscle glycogen repletion rates. However, arterial glucose concentrations were lower in the protein–sucrose co-ingestion trial [13]. This suggests that either gastric emptying was delayed, and/or splanchnic glucose retention was enhanced with protein co-ingestion. It is therefore currently unknown whether the addition of insulinotropic amino acids [that do not delay gastric emptying [94]] to glucose–fructose (sucrose) mixtures may augment muscle glycogen re-synthesis at high carbohydrate ingestion rates (1.5 g·kgBM^{-1}·h^{-1}). Combining amino acids with high ingestion rates of glucose–fructose mixtures could take better advantage of high rates of intestinal absorption and the capacity to deliver exogenous carbohydrate to the circulation in combination with higher insulin availability (Figure 2).

Whilst current evidence does not indicate that post-exercise muscle glycogen repletion is accelerated by glucose–fructose co-ingestion over glucose alone, this is achieved with lower gastrointestinal issues. Ingestion of large amounts of carbohydrates is associated with gastrointestinal distress. This could directly reduce the capacity to perform optimally in a subsequent bout of exercise and/or reduce the capacity to tolerate large amounts of carbohydrate ingestion to achieve a muscle glycogen repletion target. The ingestion of isocaloric amounts of glucose–fructose (or sucrose) mixtures, compared to glucose (polymers) alone, reduces ratings of gastrointestinal distress when large amounts of carbohydrate (1.5 g·kgBM^{-1}·h^{-1}) are ingested over a short-term recovery period (5 h) [90,92].

5.2. Liver Glycogen Repletion

In contrast to muscle, the liver is able to synthesize glucose in meaningful quantities from 3-carbon precursors such as glucogenic amino acids, galactose, fructose, glycerol, pyruvate and lactate, in addition to the direct pathway involving intact hexose units [5]. With this in mind, there is potentially a stronger hypothesis for glucose–fructose co-ingestion accelerating liver glycogen repletion over glucose ingestion alone. In addition to higher rates of carbohydrate digestion and absorption, the liver could make use of the ingested fructose for liver glycogen synthesis. Few studies have directly compared glucose plus fructose (sucrose) ingestion with glucose (polymer) ingestion alone, on post-exercise liver glycogen repletion (Figure 3B) [7,90,95]. From these studies, it is apparent that when glucose is ingested alone, the rate of post-exercise liver glycogen repletion is ~3.6 g·h^{-1}. Based on the limited number of studies available this does not appear to be dependent on the ingestion rate of glucose (Figure 3B). This may be due to differences in the degree of post-exercise liver glycogen depletion, which appears to be a major driver of liver glycogen synthesis rates [5]. Furthermore, there is large inter-individual variability in basal liver glycogen concentrations [49] and therefore it is recommended that within-subject designs are used to clearly establish the dose-response relationship between post-exercise carbohydrate ingestion and liver glycogen repletion.

When fructose is co-ingested with glucose (either as free glucose plus free fructose, or as sucrose), the rate of liver glycogen repletion is typically ~7.3 g·h^{-1}, approximately double the rate seen with glucose ingestion alone (Figure 3B). This effect is clearest when the carbohydrate ingestion rate exceeds 0.9 g·kg body mass^{-1}·h^{-1} (Figure 3B). Furthermore, the accelerated liver glycogen repletion rate is consistent when glucose and fructose are either co-ingested as their free monomers, or as the disaccharide sucrose (Figure 3B). The majority of these studies again report lower insulinaemia during post-exercise recovery with glucose–fructose co-ingestion vs. glucose ingestion alone [7,90,95]. It is currently unknown whether the addition of insulinotropic proteins to carbohydrate ingestion can augment post-exercise liver glycogen repletion. It has been speculated that the co-ingestion of protein and fat could also accelerate liver glycogen repletion by increasing gluconeogenic precursor availability [5]. However, on the basis that dietary fat can delay gastric emptying [96], rapidly absorbed amino acids/proteins would be preferable to fat as an option to explore in post-exercise recovery.

Only one study to date has determined post-exercise muscle *and* liver glycogen repletion with the ingestion of large amounts of carbohydrate (>1 g·kgBM^{-1}·h^{-1}) [90]. Over a five-hour recovery period, ~560 g of carbohydrate was consumed as either glucose (polymers) or sucrose. Based on the maximal rates of digestion, absorption and hepatic release (Figure 2) it could be expected that glucose ingestion would deliver ~360 g to the circulation over the recovery period, compared to ~510 g with sucrose ingestion. In spite of this theoretical 150 g surplus of carbohydrate, only an extra 17 g of glycogen was stored (net) in the liver, and no additional glycogen was stored (net) in muscle (numerical difference of <0.9 g·kg muscle^{-1}). It could be speculated that the additional carbohydrate was either oxidised, converted to lipid and/or stored in minor amounts in other glycogen containing tissues such as the kidneys, brain, heart and even adipose tissue [97–99]. Fructose plus glucose ingestion accelerates liver glycogen repletion rates over glucose ingestion alone. This acceleration is likely due to the preferential hepatic metabolism of fructose and/or faster digestion and absorption kinetics with glucose plus fructose ingestion, when compared to glucose ingestion.

6. Conclusions and Recommendations

The rapid recovery of both muscle and liver glycogen stores after prolonged exercise are important determinants of the capacity to perform a subsequent bout of moderate- to high- intensity exercise. The repletion of liver and muscle glycogen stores is limited by the systemic availability of carbohydrates and glucogenic precursors, along with insulinaemia, the balance of which varies depending on the scenario. The rate of appearance of ingested glucose in the circulation appears to be limited by the capacity of intestinal transporters. Since intestinal fructose absorption utilises a different transport mechanism, combining the ingestion of fructose and glucose takes advantage of both transport mechanisms, thereby increasing the total capacity to absorb carbohydrates. Post-exercise muscle glycogen repletion rates can be maximised by frequent ingestion of carbohydrate throughout recovery at a rate of $\geq$1.2 g·kg body mass^{-1} every hour, with no further acceleration of glycogen repletion rates if fructose (or sucrose) forms part of the ingested carbohydrate. However, when sufficient carbohydrate is consumed to maximise muscle glycogen replenishment after exercise, the ingestion of glucose plus fructose (sucrose) can minimise gastrointestinal distress. The combined ingestion of glucose plus fructose (or sucrose) during post-exercise recovery strongly enhances liver glycogen repletion rates, but there is currently insufficient evidence to provide guidelines on the carbohydrate ingestion rates required to specifically maximize liver glycogen repletion. When rapid recovery from prolonged exercise is a key objective, and maximal performance is required within 24 h, it is advised to consume more than 1 g carbohydrate^{-1}·kg body mass^{-1}·h^{-1}, starting as soon as possible after exercise and at frequent intervals thereafter (i.e., every 30 min). When ingested in the form of glucose–fructose mixtures (or sucrose), not only is this ingestion rate more tolerable due to lower gut discomfort but total body glycogen status can also be enhanced over glucose (polymer) ingestion alone, due to greater liver glycogen repletion.

Conflicts of Interest: The authors declare no conflicts of interest.

References

1. Van Loon, L.J.; Greenhaff, P.L.; Constantin-Teodosiu, D.; Saris, W.H.; Wagenmakers, A.J. The effects of increasing exercise intensity on muscle fuel utilisation in humans. *J. Physiol.* **2001**, *536*, 295–304. [CrossRef] [PubMed]
2. Romijn, J.A.; Coyle, E.F.; Sidossis, L.S.; Gastaldelli, A.; Horowitz, J.F.; Endert, E.; Wolfe, R.R. Regulation of endogenous fat and carbohydrate metabolism in relation to exercise intensity and duration. *Am. J. Physiol.* **1993**, *265*, E380–E391. [PubMed]

3. Gonzalez, J.T.; Veasey, R.C.; Rumbold, P.L.; Stevenson, E.J. Breakfast and exercise contingently affect postprandial metabolism and energy balance in physically active males. *Br. J. Nutr.* **2013**, *110*, 721–732. [CrossRef] [PubMed]

4. Van Loon, L.J.; Jeukendrup, A.E.; Saris, W.H.; Wagenmakers, A.J. Effect of training status on fuel selection during submaximal exercise with glucose ingestion. *J. Appl. Physiol.* **1999**, *87*, 1413–1420. [PubMed]

5. Gonzalez, J.T.; Fuchs, C.J.; Betts, J.A.; van Loon, L.J. Liver glycogen metabolism during and after prolonged endurance-type exercise. *Am. J. Physiol. Endocrinol. Metab.* **2016**, *311*, E543–E553. [CrossRef] [PubMed]

6. Stevenson, E.J.; Thelwall, P.E.; Thomas, K.; Smith, F.; Brand-Miller, J.; Trenell, M.I. Dietary glycemic index influences lipid oxidation but not muscle or liver glycogen oxidation during exercise. *Am. J. Physiol. Endocrinol. Metab.* **2009**, *296*, E1140–E1147. [CrossRef] [PubMed]

7. Casey, A.; Mann, R.; Banister, K.; Fox, J.; Morris, P.G.; Macdonald, I.A.; Greenhaff, P.L. Effect of carbohydrate ingestion on glycogen resynthesis in human liver and skeletal muscle, measured by (13)c mrs. *Am. J. Physiol. Endocrinol. Metab.* **2000**, *278*, E65–E75. [PubMed]

8. Bergstrom, J.; Hermansen, L.; Hultman, E.; Saltin, B. Diet, muscle glycogen and physical performance. *Acta. Physiol. Scand.* **1967**, *71*, 140–150. [CrossRef] [PubMed]

9. Coyle, E.F.; Coggan, A.R.; Hemmert, M.K.; Ivy, J.L. Muscle glycogen utilization during prolonged strenuous exercise when fed carbohydrate. *J. Appl. Physiol.* **1986**, *61*, 165–172. [PubMed]

10. Alghannam, A.F.; Jedrzejewski, D.; Tweddle, M.G.; Gribble, H.; Bilzon, J.; Thompson, D.; Tsintzas, K.; Betts, J.A. Impact of muscle glycogen availability on the capacity for repeated exercise in man. *Med. Sci. Sports Exerc.* **2016**, *48*, 123–131. [CrossRef] [PubMed]

11. Stellingwerff, T.; Boon, H.; Gijsen, A.P.; Stegen, J.H.; Kuipers, H.; van Loon, L.J. Carbohydrate supplementation during prolonged cycling exercise spares muscle glycogen but does not affect intramyocellular lipid use. *Med. Sci. Sports Exer.* **2007**, *454*, 635–647. [CrossRef]

12. Vandenbogaerde, T.J.; Hopkins, W.G. Effects of acute carbohydrate supplementation on endurance performance: A meta-analysis. *Sports Med.* **2011**, *41*, 773–792. [CrossRef] [PubMed]

13. Van Hall, G.; Shirreffs, S.M.; Calbet, J.A. Muscle glycogen resynthesis during recovery from cycle exercise: No effect of additional protein ingestion. *J. Appl. Physiol.* **2000**, *88*, 1631–1636. [PubMed]

14. Betts, J.A.; Williams, C. Short-term recovery from prolonged exercise: Exploring the potential for protein ingestion to accentuate the benefits of carbohydrate supplements. *Sports Med.* **2010**, *40*, 941–959. [CrossRef] [PubMed]

15. Burke, L.M.; van Loon, L.J.; Hawley, J.A. Post-exercise muscle glycogen resynthesis in humans. *J. Appl. Physiol.* **2016**. [CrossRef] [PubMed]

16. Rowlands, D.S.; Houltham, S.; Musa-Veloso, K.; Brown, F.; Paulionis, L.; Bailey, D. Fructose-glucose composite carbohydrates and endurance performance: Critical review and future perspectives. *Sports Med.* **2015**, *45*, 1561–1576. [CrossRef] [PubMed]

17. Burke, L.M.; Collier, G.R.; Hargreaves, M. Muscle glycogen storage after prolonged exercise: Effect of the glycemic index of carbohydrate feedings. *J. Appl. Physiol.* **1993**, *75*, 1019–1023. [PubMed]

18. Food and Agriculture Organization of the United Nations; The World Health Organization. Carbohydrates in Human Nutrition. Report of a joint FAO/WHO expert consultation. In *FAO Food and Nutrition Paper*; FAO: Rome, Italy, 1998; Volume 66.

19. Scientific Advisory Committee on Nutrition. *SACN Carbohydrates and Health Report*; Public Health England: London, UK, 2015.

20. Lina, B.A.; Jonker, D.; Kozianowski, G. Isomaltulose (palatinose): A review of biological and toxicological studies. *Food Chem. Toxicol.* **2002**, *40*, 1375–1381. [CrossRef]

21. Drozdowski, L.A.; Thomson, A.B. Intestinal sugar transport. *World J. Gastroenterol.* **2006**, *12*, 1657–1670. [CrossRef] [PubMed]

22. DeBosch, B.J.; Chi, M.; Moley, K.H. Glucose transporter 8 (glut8) regulates enterocyte fructose transport and global mammalian fructose utilization. *Endocrinology* **2012**, *153*, 4181–4191. [CrossRef] [PubMed]

23. Daniel, H.; Zietek, T. Taste and move: Glucose and peptide transporters in the gastrointestinal tract. *Exp. Physiol.* **2015**, *100*, 1441–1450. [CrossRef] [PubMed]

24. Rogers, S.; Chandler, J.D.; Clarke, A.L.; Petrou, S.; Best, J.D. Glucose transporter glut12-functional characterization in xenopus laevis oocytes. *Biochem. Biophys. Res. Commun.* **2003**, *308*, 422–426. [CrossRef]

25. Tappy, L.; Le, K.A. Metabolic effects of fructose and the worldwide increase in obesity. *Physiol Rev.* **2010**, *90*, 23–46. [CrossRef] [PubMed]

26. Jentjens, R.L.; Venables, M.C.; Jeukendrup, A.E. Oxidation of exogenous glucose, sucrose, and maltose during prolonged cycling exercise. *J. Appl. Physiol.* **2004**, *96*, 1285–1291. [CrossRef] [PubMed]

27. Moodley, D.; Noakes, T.D.; Bosch, A.N.; Hawley, J.A.; Schall, R.; Dennis, S.C. Oxidation of exogenous carbohydrate during prolonged exercise: The effects of the carbohydrate type and its concentration. *Eur. J. Appl. Physiol. Occup. Physiol.* **1992**, *64*, 328–334. [CrossRef] [PubMed]

28. Hawley, J.A.; Dennis, S.C.; Laidler, B.J.; Bosch, A.N.; Noakes, T.D.; Brouns, F. High rates of exogenous carbohydrate oxidation from starch ingested during prolonged exercise. *J. Appl. Physiol.* **1991**, *71*, 1801–1806. [PubMed]

29. Gray, G.M.; Ingelfinger, F.J. Intestinal absorption of sucrose in man: Interrelation of hydrolysis and monosaccharide product absorption. *J. Clin. Invest.* **1966**, *45*, 388–398. [CrossRef] [PubMed]

30. Dahlqvist, A.; Auricchio, S.; Semenza, G.; Prader, A. Human intestinal disaccharidases and hereditary disaccharide intolerance. The hydrolysis of sucrose, isomaltose, palatinose (isomaltulose), and a 1,6-alpha-oligosaccharide (isomalto-oligosaccharide) preparation. *J. Clin. Invest.* **1963**, *42*, 556–562. [CrossRef] [PubMed]

31. Van Can, J.G.; Ijzerman, T.H.; van Loon, L.J.; Brouns, F.; Blaak, E.E. Reduced glycaemic and insulinaemic responses following isomaltulose ingestion: Implications for postprandial substrate use. *Br. J. Nutr.* **2009**, *102*, 1408–1413. [CrossRef] [PubMed]

32. Oosthuyse, T.; Carstens, M.; Millen, A.M. Ingesting isomaltulose versus fructose-maltodextrin during prolonged moderate-heavy exercise increases fat oxidation but impairs gastrointestinal comfort and cycling performance. *Int. J. Sport Nutr. Exerc. Metab.* **2015**, *25*, 427–438. [CrossRef] [PubMed]

33. Sunehag, A.L.; Haymond, M.W. Splanchnic galactose extraction is regulated by coingestion of glucose in humans. *Metabolism* **2002**, *51*, 827–832. [CrossRef] [PubMed]

34. Tappy, L.; Egli, L.; Lecoultre, V.; Schneider, P. Effects of fructose-containing caloric sweeteners on resting energy expenditure and energy efficiency: A review of human trials. *Nutr. Metab.* **2013**, *10*, 54. [CrossRef] [PubMed]

35. Chong, M.F.; Fielding, B.A.; Frayn, K.N. Mechanisms for the acute effect of fructose on postprandial lipemia. *Am. J. Clin. Nutr.* **2007**, *85*, 1511–1520. [PubMed]

36. Jentjens, R.L.; Jeukendrup, A.E. Effects of pre-exercise ingestion of trehalose, galactose and glucose on subsequent metabolism and cycling performance. *Eur. J. Appl. Physiol.* **2003**, *88*, 459–465. [CrossRef] [PubMed]

37. Tornheim, K.; Lowenstein, J.M. Control of phosphofructokinase from rat skeletal muscle. Effects of fructose diphosphate, amp, atp, and citrate. *J. Biol. Chem.* **1976**, *251*, 7322–7328. [PubMed]

38. Bergstrom, J.; Hultman, E. Muscle glycogen synthesis after exercise: An enhancing factor localized to the muscle cells in man. *Nature* **1966**, *210*, 309–310. [CrossRef] [PubMed]

39. Ortenblad, N.; Westerblad, H.; Nielsen, J. Muscle glycogen stores and fatigue. *J. Physiol.* **2013**, *591*, 4405–4413. [CrossRef] [PubMed]

40. Nielsen, J.N.; Wojtaszewski, J.F.; Haller, R.G.; Hardie, D.G.; Kemp, B.E.; Richter, E.A.; Vissing, J. Role of 5'amp-activated protein kinase in glycogen synthase activity and glucose utilization: Insights from patients with mcardle's disease. *J. Physiol.* **2002**, *541*, 979–989. [CrossRef] [PubMed]

41. Lucia, A.; Ruiz, J.R.; Santalla, A.; Nogales-Gadea, G.; Rubio, J.C.; Garcia-Consuegra, I.; Cabello, A.; Perez, M.; Teijeira, S.; Vieitez, I.; et al. Genotypic and phenotypic features of mcardle disease: Insights from the spanish national registry. *J. Neurol. Neurosurg. Psychiatry* **2012**, *83*, 322–328. [CrossRef] [PubMed]

42. Walter, G.; Vandenborne, K.; Elliott, M.; Leigh, J.S. In vivo ATP synthesis rates in single human muscles during high intensity exercise. *J. Physiol.* **1999**, *519 Pt 3*, 901–910. [CrossRef] [PubMed]

43. Hultman, E.; Harris, R.C. Carbohydrate metabolism. In *Principles of Exercise Biochemistry*; Poortmans, J.R., Ed.; S.Karger: Basel, Switzerland, 1988.

44. Jeukendrup, A.E.; Wallis, G.A. Measurement of substrate oxidation during exercise by means of gas exchange measurements. *Int. J. Sports Med.* **2005**, *26*, S28–S37. [CrossRef] [PubMed]

45. Bangsbo, J.; Graham, T.E.; Kiens, B.; Saltin, B. Elevated muscle glycogen and anaerobic energy production during exhaustive exercise in man. *J. Physiol.* **1992**, *451*, 205–227. [CrossRef] [PubMed]

46. Petersen, K.F.; Price, T.; Cline, G.W.; Rothman, D.L.; Shulman, G.I. Contribution of net hepatic glycogenolysis to glucose production during the early postprandial period. *Am. J. Physiol.* **1996**, *270*, E186–E191. [PubMed]

47. Nilsson, L.H.; Hultman, E. Liver glycogen in man–the effect of total starvation or a carbohydrate-poor diet followed by carbohydrate refeeding. *Scand. J. Clin. Lab. Invest.* **1973**, *32*, 325–330. [CrossRef] [PubMed]

48. Bergman, B.C.; Horning, M.A.; Casazza, G.A.; Wolfel, E.E.; Butterfield, G.E.; Brooks, G.A. Endurance training increases gluconeogenesis during rest and exercise in men. *Am. J. Physiol. Endocrinol. Metab.* **2000**, *278*, E244–E251. [PubMed]

49. Gonzalez, J.T.; Fuchs, C.J.; Smith, F.E.; Thelwall, P.E.; Taylor, R.; Stevenson, E.J.; Trenell, M.I.; Cermak, N.M.; van Loon, L.J. Ingestion of glucose or sucrose prevents liver but not muscle glycogen depletion during prolonged endurance-type exercise in trained cyclists. *Am. J. Physiol. Endocrinol. Metab.* **2015**, *309*, E1032–E1039. [CrossRef] [PubMed]

50. Izumida, Y.; Yahagi, N.; Takeuchi, Y.; Nishi, M.; Shikama, A.; Takarada, A.; Masuda, Y.; Kubota, M.; Matsuzaka, T.; Nakagawa, Y.; et al. Glycogen shortage during fasting triggers liver-brain-adipose neurocircuitry to facilitate fat utilization. *Nat. Commun.* **2013**, *4*, 2316. [PubMed]

51. Maehlum, S.; Felig, P.; Wahren, J. Splanchnic glucose and muscle glycogen metabolism after glucose feeding during postexercise recovery. *Am. J. Physiol.* **1978**, *235*, E255–E260. [PubMed]

52. Hurren, N.M.; Balanos, G.M.; Blannin, A.K. Is the beneficial effect of prior exercise on postprandial lipaemia partly due to redistribution of blood flow? *Clin. Sci.* **2011**, *120*, 537–548. [CrossRef] [PubMed]

53. Bergstrom, J.; Hultman, E. Synthesis of muscle glycogen in man after glucose and fructose infusion. *Acta Med. Scand.* **1967**, *182*, 93–107. [CrossRef] [PubMed]

54. Roch-Norlund, A.E.; Bergstrom, J.; Hultman, E. Muscle glycogen and glycogen synthetase in normal subjects and in patients with diabetes mellitus. Effect of intravenous glucose and insulin administration. *Scand. J. Clin. Lab. Invest.* **1972**, *30*, 77–84. [CrossRef] [PubMed]

55. Pedersen, D.J.; Lessard, S.J.; Coffey, V.G.; Churchley, E.G.; Wootton, A.M.; Ng, T.; Watt, M.J.; Hawley, J.A. High rates of muscle glycogen resynthesis after exhaustive exercise when carbohydrate is coingested with caffeine. *J. Appl. Physiol.* **2008**, *105*, 7–13. [CrossRef] [PubMed]

56. Jeukendrup, A.E. Carbohydrate and exercise performance: The role of multiple transportable carbohydrates. *Curr. Opin. Clin. Nutr. Metab. Care* **2010**, *13*, 452–457. [CrossRef] [PubMed]

57. Hawley, J.A.; Bosch, A.N.; Weltan, S.M.; Dennis, S.C.; Noakes, T.D. Glucose kinetics during prolonged exercise in euglycaemic and hyperglycaemic subjects. *Pflugers Archiv. Eur. J. Physiol.* **1994**, *426*, 378–386. [CrossRef]

58. Hulston, C.J.; Wallis, G.A.; Jeukendrup, A.E. Exogenous cho oxidation with glucose plus fructose intake during exercise. *Med. Sci. Sports Exerc.* **2009**, *41*, 357–363. [CrossRef] [PubMed]

59. Jentjens, R.L.; Jeukendrup, A.E. High rates of exogenous carbohydrate oxidation from a mixture of glucose and fructose ingested during prolonged cycling exercise. *Br. J. Nutr.* **2005**, *93*, 485–492. [CrossRef] [PubMed]

60. Jentjens, R.L.; Shaw, C.; Birtles, T.; Waring, R.H.; Harding, L.K.; Jeukendrup, A.E. Oxidation of combined ingestion of glucose and sucrose during exercise. *Metabolism* **2005**, *54*, 610–618. [CrossRef] [PubMed]

61. Jentjens, R.L.; Achten, J.; Jeukendrup, A.E. High oxidation rates from combined carbohydrates ingested during exercise. *Med. Sci. Sports Exerc.* **2004**, *36*, 1551–1558. [CrossRef] [PubMed]

62. Jentjens, R.L.; Moseley, L.; Waring, R.H.; Harding, L.K.; Jeukendrup, A.E. Oxidation of combined ingestion of glucose and fructose during exercise. *J. Appl. Physiol.* **2004**, *96*, 1277–1284. [CrossRef] [PubMed]

63. Jentjens, R.L.; Underwood, K.; Achten, J.; Currell, K.; Mann, C.H.; Jeukendrup, A.E. Exogenous carbohydrate oxidation rates are elevated after combined ingestion of glucose and fructose during exercise in the heat. *J. Appl. Physiol.* **2006**, *100*, 807–816. [CrossRef] [PubMed]

64. Jeukendrup, A.E.; Moseley, L.; Mainwaring, G.I.; Samuels, S.; Perry, S.; Mann, C.H. Exogenous carbohydrate oxidation during ultraendurance exercise. *J. Appl. Physiol.* **2006**, *100*, 1134–1141. [CrossRef] [PubMed]

65. Rowlands, D.S.; Thorburn, M.S.; Thorp, R.M.; Broadbent, S.; Shi, X. Effect of graded fructose coingestion with maltodextrin on exogenous 14c-fructose and 13c-glucose oxidation efficiency and high-intensity cycling performance. *J. Appl. Physiol.* **2008**, *104*, 1709–1719. [CrossRef] [PubMed]

66. Roberts, J.D.; Tarpey, M.D.; Kass, L.S.; Tarpey, R.J.; Roberts, M.G. Assessing a commercially available sports drink on exogenous carbohydrate oxidation, fluid delivery and sustained exercise performance. *J. Int. Soc. Sports Nutr.* **2014**, *11*, 8. [CrossRef] [PubMed]

67. Wagenmakers, A.J.; Brouns, F.; Saris, W.H.; Halliday, D. Oxidation rates of orally ingested carbohydrates during prolonged exercise in men. *J. Appl. Physiol.* **1993**, *75*, 2774–2780. [PubMed]

68. Wallis, G.A.; Rowlands, D.S.; Shaw, C.; Jentjens, R.L.; Jeukendrup, A.E. Oxidation of combined ingestion of maltodextrins and fructose during exercise. *Med. Sci. Sports Exerc.* **2005**, *37*, 426–432. [CrossRef] [PubMed]

69. Trommelen, J.; Fuchs, C.J.; Beelen, M.; Lenaerts, K.; Jeukendrup, A.E.; Cermak, N.M.; van Loon, L.J. Fructose and sucrose intake increase exogenous carbohydrate oxidation during exercise. *Nutrients* **2017**, *9*, 167. [CrossRef] [PubMed]

70. Rehrer, N.J.; Wagenmakers, A.J.; Beckers, E.J.; Halliday, D.; Leiper, J.B.; Brouns, F.; Maughan, R.J.; Westerterp, K.; Saris, W.H. Gastric emptying, absorption, and carbohydrate oxidation during prolonged exercise. *J. Appl. Physiol.* **1992**, *72*, 468–475. [PubMed]

71. Duchman, S.M.; Ryan, A.J.; Schedl, H.P.; Summers, R.W.; Bleiler, T.L.; Gisolfi, C.V. Upper limit for intestinal absorption of a dilute glucose solution in men at rest. *Med. Sci. Sports Exerc.* **1997**, *29*, 482–488. [CrossRef] [PubMed]

72. Fordtran, J.S.; Saltin, B. Gastric emptying and intestinal absorption during prolonged severe exercise. *J. Appl. Physiol.* **1967**, *23*, 331–335. [PubMed]

73. Jeukendrup, A.E.; Jentjens, R. Oxidation of carbohydrate feedings during prolonged exercise: Current thoughts, guidelines and directions for future research. *Sports Med.* **2000**, *29*, 407–424. [CrossRef] [PubMed]

74. O'Brien, W.J.; Stannard, S.R.; Clarke, J.A.; Rowlands, D.S. Fructose-maltodextrin ratio governs exogenous and other cho oxidation and performance. *Med. Sci. Sports Exerc.* **2013**, *45*, 1814–1824. [CrossRef] [PubMed]

75. Rosset, R.; Lecoultre, V.; Egli, L.; Cros, J.; Dokumaci, A.S.; Zwygart, K.; Boesch, C.; Kreis, R.; Schneiter, P.; Tappy, L. Postexercise repletion of muscle energy stores with fructose or glucose in mixed meals. *Am. J. Clin. Nutr.* **2017**. [CrossRef] [PubMed]

76. Rikmenspoel, R.; Caputo, R. The michaelis-menten constant for fructose and for glucose of hexokinase in bull spermatozoa. *J. Reprod. Fertil.* **1966**, *12*, 437–444. [CrossRef] [PubMed]

77. Ahlborg, G.; Bjorkman, O. Splanchnic and muscle fructose metabolism during and after exercise. *J. Appl. Physiol.* **1990**, *69*, 1244–1251. [PubMed]

78. Lecoultre, V.; Benoit, R.; Carrel, G.; Schutz, Y.; Millet, G.P.; Tappy, L.; Schneiter, P. Fructose and glucose co-ingestion during prolonged exercise increases lactate and glucose fluxes and oxidation compared with an equimolar intake of glucose. *Am. J. Clin. Nutr.* **2010**, *92*, 1071–1079. [CrossRef] [PubMed]

79. Truswell, A.S.; Seach, J.M.; Thorburn, A.W. Incomplete absorption of pure fructose in healthy subjects and the facilitating effect of glucose. *Am. J. Clin. Nutr.* **1988**, *48*, 1424–1430. [PubMed]

80. Patel, C.; Douard, V.; Yu, S.; Gao, N.; Ferraris, R.P. Transport, metabolism, and endosomal trafficking-dependent regulation of intestinal fructose absorption. *FASEB J.* **2015**, *29*, 4046–4058. [CrossRef] [PubMed]

81. Stocks, B.; Betts, J.A.; McGawley, K. Effects of carbohydrate dose and frequency on metabolism, gastrointestinal discomfort, and cross-country skiing performance. *Scand. J. Med. Sci. Sports* **2016**, *26*, 1100–1108. [CrossRef] [PubMed]

82. Bangsbo, J.; Gollnick, P.D.; Graham, T.E.; Saltin, B. Substrates for muscle glycogen synthesis in recovery from intense exercise in man. *J. Physiol.* **1991**, *434*, 423–440. [CrossRef] [PubMed]

83. Kruszynska, Y.T.; Mulford, M.I.; Baloga, J.; Yu, J.G.; Olefsky, J.M. Regulation of skeletal muscle hexokinase ii by insulin in nondiabetic and niddm subjects. *Diabetes* **1998**, *47*, 1107–1113. [CrossRef] [PubMed]

84. Karlsson, H.K.; Chibalin, A.V.; Koistinen, H.A.; Yang, J.; Koumanov, F.; Wallberg-Henriksson, H.; Zierath, J.R.; Holman, G.D. Kinetics of glut4 trafficking in rat and human skeletal muscle. *Diabetes* **2009**, *58*, 847–854. [CrossRef] [PubMed]

85. Laakso, M.; Edelman, S.V.; Brechtel, G.; Baron, A.D. Effects of epinephrine on insulin-mediated glucose uptake in whole body and leg muscle in humans: Role of blood flow. *Am. J. Physiol.* **1992**, *263*, E199–E204. [PubMed]

86. Yki-Jarvinen, H.; Mott, D.; Young, A.A.; Stone, K.; Bogardus, C. Regulation of glycogen synthase and phosphorylase activities by glucose and insulin in human skeletal muscle. *J. Clin. Invest.* **1987**, *80*, 95–100. [CrossRef] [PubMed]

87. Jensen, J.; Ruge, T.; Lai, Y.C.; Svensson, M.K.; Eriksson, J.W. Effects of adrenaline on whole-body glucose metabolism and insulin-mediated regulation of glycogen synthase and pkb phosphorylation in human skeletal muscle. *Metabolism* **2011**, *60*, 215–226. [CrossRef] [PubMed]

88. Bowtell, J.L.; Gelly, K.; Jackman, M.L.; Patel, A.; Simeoni, M.; Rennie, M.J. Effect of different carbohydrate drinks on whole body carbohydrate storage after exhaustive exercise. *J. Appl. Physiol.* **2000**, *88*, 1529–1536. [PubMed]

89. Blom, P.C.; Hostmark, A.T.; Vaage, O.; Kardel, K.R.; Maehlum, S. Effect of different post-exercise sugar diets on the rate of muscle glycogen synthesis. *Med. Sci. Sports Exerc.* **1987**, *19*, 491–496. [CrossRef] [PubMed]

90. Fuchs, C.J.; Gonzalez, J.T.; Beelen, M.; Cermak, N.M.; Smith, F.E.; Thelwall, P.E.; Taylor, R.; Trenell, M.I.; Stevenson, E.J.; van Loon, L.J. Sucrose ingestion after exhaustive exercise accelerates liver, but not muscle glycogen repletion when compared to glucose ingestion in trained athletes. *J. Appl. Physiol.* **2016**, *120*, 1328–1334. [CrossRef] [PubMed]

91. Wallis, G.A.; Hulston, C.J.; Mann, C.H.; Roper, H.P.; Tipton, K.D.; Jeukendrup, A.E. Postexercise muscle glycogen synthesis with combined glucose and fructose ingestion. *Med. Sci. Sports Exerc.* **2008**, *40*, 1789–1794. [CrossRef] [PubMed]

92. Trommelen, J.; Beelen, M.; Pinckaers, P.J.; Senden, J.M.; Cermak, N.M.; van Loon, L.J. Fructose coingestion does not accelerate postexercise muscle glycogen repletion. *Med. Sci. Sports Exerc.* **2016**, *48*, 907–912. [CrossRef] [PubMed]

93. McLane, J.A.; Holloszy, J.O. Glycogen synthesis from lactate in the three types of skeletal muscle. *J. Biol. Chem.* **1979**, *254*, 6548–6553. [PubMed]

94. Ullrich, S.S.; Fitzgerald, P.C.; Schober, G.; Steinert, R.E.; Horowitz, M.; Feinle-Bisset, C. Intragastric administration of leucine or isoleucine lowers the blood glucose response to a mixed-nutrient drink by different mechanisms in healthy, lean volunteers. *Am. J. Clin. Nutr.* **2016**, *104*, 1274–1284. [CrossRef] [PubMed]

95. Decombaz, J.; Jentjens, R.; Ith, M.; Scheurer, E.; Buehler, T.; Jeukendrup, A.; Boesch, C. Fructose and galactose enhance postexercise human liver glycogen synthesis. *Med. Sci. Sports Exerc.* **2011**, *43*, 1964–1971. [PubMed]

96. Gentilcore, D.; Chaikomin, R.; Jones, K.L.; Russo, A.; Feinle-Bisset, C.; Wishart, J.M.; Rayner, C.K.; Horowitz, M. Effects of fat on gastric emptying of and the glycemic, insulin, and incretin responses to a carbohydrate meal in type 2 diabetes. *J. Clin. Endocrinol. Metab.* **2006**, *91*, 2062–2067. [CrossRef] [PubMed]

97. Rigden, D.J.; Jellyman, A.E.; Frayn, K.N.; Coppack, S.W. Human adipose tissue glycogen levels and responses to carbohydrate feeding. *Eur. J. Clin. Nutr.* **1990**, *44*, 689–692. [PubMed]

98. Oz, G.; Henry, P.G.; Seaquist, E.R.; Gruetter, R. Direct, noninvasive measurement of brain glycogen metabolism in humans. *Neurochem. Int.* **2003**, *43*, 323–329. [CrossRef]

99. Biava, C.; Grossman, A.; West, M. Ultrastructural observations on renal glycogen in normal and pathologic human kidneys. *Lab. Investig.* **1966**, *15*, 330–356. [PubMed]

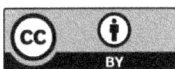

nutrients

MDPI

Article

Endurance Training with or without Glucose-Fructose Ingestion: Effects on Lactate Metabolism Assessed in a Randomized Clinical Trial on Sedentary Men

Robin Rosset [1], Virgile Lecoultre [1], Léonie Egli [1], Jérémy Cros [1], Valentine Rey [1], Nathalie Stefanoni [1], Valérie Sauvinet [2], Martine Laville [2], Philippe Schneiter [1] and Luc Tappy [1,*]

[1]   Department of Physiology, University of Lausanne, CH-1005 Lausanne, Switzerland;
      Robin.Rosset@unil.ch (R.R.); Virgile.Lecoultre@hibroye.ch (V.L.); Leonie.Egli@rdsg.nestle.com (L.E.);
      Jeremy.Cros@unil.ch (J.C.); Valentine.Rey@unil.ch (V.R.); Nathalie.Stefanoni@unil.ch (N.S.);
      Philippe.Schneiter@unil.ch (P.S.)
[2]   Centre for Research in Human Nutrition Rhône-Alpes and European Centre of Nutrition for Health,
      Lyon 1 University, INSERM, Hospices Civils de Lyon, F-69310 Pierre Bénite, France;
      Valerie.Sauvinet@chu-lyon.fr (V.S.); Martine.Laville@chu-lyon.fr (M.L.)
*   Correspondence: Luc.Tappy@unil.ch; Tel.: +41-21-692-5541

Received: 26 February 2017; Accepted: 18 April 2017; Published: 20 April 2017

Abstract: Glucose-fructose ingestion increases glucose and lactate oxidation during exercise. We hypothesized that training with glucose-fructose would induce key adaptations in lactate metabolism. Two groups of eight sedentary males were endurance-trained for three weeks while ingesting either glucose-fructose (GF) or water (C). Effects of glucose-fructose on lactate appearance, oxidation, and clearance were measured at rest and during exercise, pre-training, and post-training. Pre-training, resting lactate appearance was 3.6 ± 0.5 vs. 3.6 ± 0.4 mg·kg^{-1}·min^{-1} in GF and C, and was increased to 11.2 ± 1.4 vs. 8.8 ± 0.7 mg·kg^{-1}·min^{-1} by exercise (Exercise: $p < 0.01$). Lactate oxidation represented $20.6 \pm 1.0\%$ and $17.5 \pm 1.7\%$ of lactate appearance at rest, and $86.3 \pm 3.8\%$ and $86.8 \pm 6.6\%$ during exercise (Exercise: $p < 0.01$) in GF and C, respectively. Training with GF increased resting lactate appearance and oxidation (Training × Intervention: both $p < 0.05$), but not during exercise (Training × Intervention: both $p > 0.05$). Training with GF and C had similar effects to increase lactate clearance during exercise ($+15.5 \pm 9.2$ and $+10.1 \pm 5.9$ mL·kg^{-1}·min^{-1}; Training: $p < 0.01$; Training × Intervention: $p = 0.97$). The findings of this study show that in sedentary participants, glucose-fructose ingestion leads to high systemic lactate appearance, most of which is disposed non-oxidatively at rest and is oxidized during exercise. Training with or without glucose-fructose increases lactate clearance, without altering lactate appearance and oxidation during exercise.

Keywords: glucose; fructose; lactate; lactate metabolism; substrate oxidation; carbohydrate; exercise

1. Introduction

During moderate and high intensity exercise, muscle energy needs are essentially met by carbohydrate oxidation [1] and muscle performance is dependent on both muscle glycogen and plasma glucose concentrations [2–4]. Plasma glucose entry into skeletal muscle is activated by contraction [5] and depends on systemic glucose appearance, i.e., the sum of endogenous glucose production (hepatic glycogen breakdown and gluconeogenesis) and gut glucose absorption [1,6]. Accordingly, whole-body and muscle glucose oxidation can be enhanced by glucose ingestion that increases plasma glucose appearance and muscle glucose uptake [6]. A portion of glucose is actually made indirectly available through glycolytic lactate production in some muscle fibers, followed by lactate uptake and oxidation in other fibers [7]. These lactate "shuttles" may possibly increase muscle energy substrates provision when glucose transport and/or glycolytic capacity is saturated. Endurance training has also been well-established to increase the expression of proteins involved in lactate transport and metabolism [8], suggesting that lactate can be a major energy substrate for the trained muscle [7,9]. Alternatively, lactate can also be recycled into glucose (gluconeogenesis), with recent indications that this can be altered in trained subjects [10,11].

The oxidation rate of exogenous glucose increases dose-dependently up to ≈ 1 g·min^{-1}, but then plateaus at higher glucose ingestion rates [4]. Co-ingestion of glucose and fructose can further increase exogenous [12] and net carbohydrate oxidations [13], and can also improve exercise performance [14]. This has been attributed to glucose and fructose being absorbed through distinct transporter proteins in the apical membrane of enterocytes, thus allowing for a higher rate of total gut carbohydrate absorption [4]. In addition, a substantial portion of ingested fructose is converted into lactate in the liver, to increase plasma lactate concentration and lactate delivery as an energy substrate to working muscle [15,16].

Fructose absorption is poor when it is ingested alone, but is markedly enhanced by glucose co-ingestion [17]. Furthermore, gut fructose transport is potently induced by fructose itself, and fructose absorption increases within a few days upon chronic fructose ingestion [9]. One may therefore suspect that the beneficial effects of ingesting glucose and fructose mixtures during exercise may depend on their chronic use during training. In addition, hyperlactatemia is thought to be instrumental in training-induced increase in lactate clearance by the stimulation of muscle lactate transporters [9]. We therefore postulated that the combined, repeated effects of exercise and glucose-fructose ingestion may significantly impact training-induced adaptation of muscle lactate metabolism. To assess this hypothesis, we enrolled two groups of healthy sedentary males in a 3-week training program during which they consumed glucose-fructose drinks (GF intervention) or plain water as a control (C intervention) during training sessions.

2. Materials and Methods

2.1. Participants

Sixteen healthy young males (mean ± standard error (SEM) age: 25 ± 1 years; weight: 73.2 ± 2.0 kg; body mass index: 22.9 ± 0.4 kg·m^{-2}) completed this study. One additional volunteer dropped out prior to the interventions and was hence removed from all analyzes. At inclusion, all participants were sedentary and low-sugar consumers (exercise: <1 h·week^{-1} and sugar intake: <60 g·day^{-1}) and were asked to maintain their lifestyle with the exception of the supervised exercise sessions prescribed in the study protocol. They were fully informed of the nature and risks involved by the procedures, in accordance with the 1983 revision of the Declaration of Helsinki. All experiments were performed at the Clinical Research Center, Lausanne, Switzerland, after approbation by the local ethics committee. This study was registered at ClinicalTrials.gov database as NCT01610986.

2.2. Study Design

Prior to the 3-week exercise training program, participants underwent two pre-training visits to determine baseline characteristics. Maximal oxygen consumption (VO$_{2max}$), maximal aerobic workload (W$_{max}$), and workload eliciting the lactate turnpoint (W$_{LT}$) were assessed at the first visit. At a second visit 48 h later, plasma glucose and lactate metabolism were investigated at rest and during moderate-intensity exercise when fed glucose-fructose (metabolic evaluation). Participants were then separated into two parallel groups, and both groups performed 15 sessions of supervised moderate-intensity laboratory cycling on an ergometer (60 min each; 5 day·week^{-1}) either with glucose-fructose drinks in GF or water in C. Finally, preliminary visits were repeated post-training (beginning 48–72 h after the last training session) to assess the effect of exercise training with glucose-fructose ingestion on metabolic response to these drinks, at rest and during exercise (Figure 1).

To assume comparable glycogen concentrations between interventions, participants filled food diaries and were instructed to repeat dietary intake and physical activity patterns the 48 h prior to each visit.

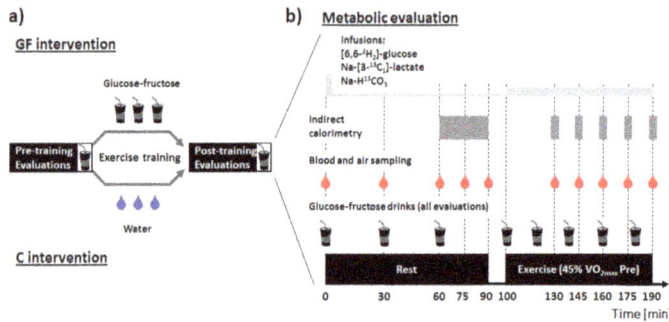

Figure 1. Study design (**a**) and description of the metabolic evaluations (**b**). Drinks containing 19 g glucose and 12 g fructose were administered at time 0, 30 and 60 min at rest, and at 20 min intervals during exercise. Primed-continuous infusions of $(6,6-^2H_2)$-D-(+)-glucose and Na-$(3-^{13}C_1)$-L-(+)-lactate were started at time 0, and resting measurements were obtained after 60 min equilibration. Continuous infusion rates were upgraded at the beginning of exercise at time 100 min (see methods for further details). GF: intervention in which glucose-fructose drinks were provided during training sessions; C: control intervention in which plain water was provided during training sessions.

2.3. Incremental Exercise-Testing

Overnight fasted participants performed an incremental test to exhaustion on a cycle ergometer (Ergoselect 100, Ergoline GmbH, Bitz, Germany) pre-training and post-training. Respiratory gas exchanges (SensorMedics Vmax; Sensormedics Corp., Yorba Linda, CA, USA) and heart-rate (Polar S810; Polar Electro Oy, Kempele, Finland) were continuously monitored throughout the test. Briefly, after a resting period of 5 min and a warm-up of 5 min at 40 W, ergometer workload was increased by 25 W every 3 min. As VCO_2 exceeded VO_2, ergometer workload was increased by 25 W every minute until volitional exhaustion. VO_{2max} and W_{max} were determined as previously described [13] and used to determine training intensities. Earlobe blood lactate concentration was measured at the end of each step (Lactate Pro, Arkray, Kyoto, Japan). Participants were then familiarized to the endurance capacity task (pre-training) or could leave the laboratory (post-training).

2.4. Metabolic Evaluations

Participants were instructed to remain sedentary, filled food diaries and had to avoid caffeine, alcohol and ^{13}C-rich foods the 48 h before metabolic evaluations. Overnight-fasted participants reported to the metabolic unit at 0700 h and, after a void, were weighed and installed on a bed. One indwelling venous cannula was then inserted into an antecubital vein for blood sampling. This forearm was then constantly placed under a heating pad to open arteriovenous anastomoses, allowing for accurate determination of substrate exchanges in arterialized venous blood [18]. Another cannula was inserted into a vein of the opposite forearm for the infusion of stable isotopes tracers (Cambridge Isotope Lab., Andover, MT, USA). After background sampling at 0800 h (time = 0 min), a labelled-bicarbonate bolus (Na-H$^{13}CO_3$: 3.05 g) and primed continuous infusions of glucose $((6,6-^2H_2)$-D-(+)-glucose; prime: 2 mg·kg^{-1}; continuous: 0.02 mg·kg^{-1}·min^{-1}) and sodium lactate (Na-$(3-^{13}C_1)$-L-(+)-lactate; prime: 0.4 mg·kg^{-1}; continuous: 0.02 mg·kg^{-1}·min^{-1}) were started. Infusion rates were tripled during exercise to account for increased substrate kinetics.

The metabolic evaluation consisted of a resting period (time = 0–90 min) in which participants remained in the supine position, followed by a continuous exercise session (time = 100–190 min) at 45% pre-training VO_{2max} (i.e., at the same workload pre-training and post-training). This intensity aimed to elicit the greatest effect of endurance-training on lactate metabolic clearance [19]. Glucose-fructose sweetened drinks (193 mL of a 9.8% glucose, 6.2% fructose drink flavored with 2% lemon juice and 1.17 $g \cdot L^{-1}$ NaCl) were provided at time = 0 then every 30 min at rest, and every 20 min during exercise. Blood and expired air samples were collected at time = 0, 30, 60, 75, and 90 min (rest), then 130, 145, 160, 175 and 190 min (exercise). Energy expenditure and substrate oxidation were measured by open-circuit indirect calorimetry (Quark RMR, Cosmed, Roma, Italia) in the last 30 min of rest and for 5 min intervals during exercise (SensorMedics Vmax; Sensormedics Corp, Yorba Linda, CA, USA). After 190 min, infusions were stopped and participants' urine was collected to estimate protein oxidation.

Twenty-five minutes later, ergometer workload was set at 85% of the current VO_{2max} and participants were asked to cycle at 60 rpm until exhaustion to measure endurance capacity.

2.5. Training Intervention

Starting 48–72 h after the pre-training evaluation, participants entered a supervised endurance-training program of 1 session·d^{-1}, 5 day·week^{-1} over 3 weeks. Each session consisted of 60 min cycling at a constant workload, with intensities set as 50% (sessions 1–3), 55% (sessions 4–6), 60% (sessions 7–9), and 65% (sessions 10–15) of pre-training VO_{2max}. Experimental interventions differed by the drinks provided during sessions: the GF group ingested three 163 mL doses of glucose-fructose drinks provided −20, 0, and +20 min referred to exercise onset, while the C group correspondingly received water. Participants were instructed to have their last meal at least two hours before exercise onset. Earlobe blood lactate concentration was measured at 0, 30 and 60 min (Lactate Pro, Arkray, Japan).

2.6. Analytical Procedures

Arterialized venous blood samples were collected on lithium heparin for measurement of glucose, lactate, fructose, and tracers, with ethylenediaminetetraacetic acid (EDTA)-coated tubes for free fatty acids, triglycerides and insulin or with trasylol-EDTA for glucagon. Plasma was immediately separated by centrifugation (10 min; 2800× g; 4 °C), and aliquots were stored at −20 °C until analyzed. Plasma glucose, lactate, free fatty acids, and urinary nitrogen concentrations were determined using a semi-automated clinical chemistry analyzer (RX Monza, Randox Laboratories Ltd., Crumlin, UK). Insulin and glucagon concentrations were obtained by radioimmunoassay using commercial kits (Merck Millipore, Billerica, MA, USA).

Expired air $^{13}CO_2$ isotopic enrichments were obtained by isotope-ratio mass spectrometry (IRMS) (SerCon Ltd., Crewe, UK), as previously described [13]. Gas chromatography-mass spectrometry (GCMS) (Hewlett-Packard Instruments, Palo Alto, CA, USA) was used to measure plasma fructose concentration [13] and plasma ($^{13}C_1$)lactate and ($^2H_2$)glucose isotopic enrichments [20,21]. Plasma (^{13}C)glucose enrichments were measured by GC/C/IRMS [22] (Thermo Scientific, Bremen, Germany).

2.7. Calculations

Energy expenditure and substrate oxidation were calculated from respiratory gas exchanges using standard equations [23]. When exceeding VO_2, VCO_2 values were set as corresponding to VO_2 to reflect aerobic metabolism, and $^{13}CO_2$ isotopic enrichment was corrected for bicarbonate retention [24]. Rates of plasma glucose and lactate appearance, disposal, and metabolic clearance were calculated using Steele's equations for non-steady state using a volume of distribution of 180 mL·kg^{-1} for both substrates [25]. Plasma lactate oxidation, non-oxidative lactate disposal (NOLD), and gluconeogenesis from lactate were calculated as:

$$\text{Lactate oxidation} = \frac{\text{lactate disposal} \cdot VCO_2 \cdot {}^{13}CO_2}{F \cdot k \cdot 89.08} \ (mg \cdot kg^{-1} \cdot min^{-1}) \tag{1}$$

$$\text{NOLD} = \text{lactate disposal} - \text{lactate oxidation} \ (mg \cdot kg^{-1} \cdot min^{-1}) \tag{2}$$

$$\text{Gluconeogenesis from lactate} = \frac{(^{13}C)\text{glucose} \cdot 6 \cdot \text{glucose appearance}}{(^{13}C)\text{lactate}} \quad (mg \cdot kg^{-1} \cdot min^{-1}) \qquad (3)$$

where $^{13}CO_2$ and (^{13}C)glucose represent ^{13}carbon isotopic enrichments in expired CO_2 (atom% excess) and plasma glucose (atom% excess), (^{13}C)lactate is (M+1)lactate isotopic enrichment (mol% excess), F is $(3-^{13}C_1)$lactate infusion rate, k is a correction factor for ^{13}C losses in body pools during substrate oxidation [24] (rest: k = 0.8; exercise: k = 1.0), 89.08 is the molar weight of lactate and 6 is the number of mole of CO_2 per mole of glucose. To minimize tracer assumptions, mean values of the last 30 min of rest (time = 60, 75 and 90 min) and exercise (time = 160, 175 and 190 min) are reported in figures (see results). Lactate turnpoint was obtained by the D-max method [18].

2.8. Statistics

Interventions allocation was determined by random generation of four-sequence blocks. A sample size of 16 participants was estimated (1-β: 90%; α = 0.05) to detect ≈15% difference in lactate clearance gain between GF and C. Normality and homoscedasticity were first checked visually, then using Shapiro-Wilk and Bartlett tests. Data were transformed in their square root when appropriate (plasma lactate, fructose, free fatty acids and insulin concentrations, carbohydrate and lipid oxidations, endurance capacity). Baseline values were compared using Student's *t*-tests. Evolving data were analyzed using mixed-models, with training (T) and intervention (I) as fixed effects and random effects for participant-specific intercepts and slopes. The training and intervention interaction (T × I), baseline (B) and exercise (E) effects were included in models whenever improving goodness of fit. Paired contrasts were used to determine differences between pre-training vs. post-training (symbol: #) and rest vs. exercise periods (symbol: $), and unpaired contrasts to compare GF vs. C interventions (symbol: *). Analyses were run on R version 3.1.3 (R Foundation for Statistical Computing, Vienna, Austria). $p < 0.05$ was considered significant. Data are presented as mean ± SEM.

3. Results

3.1. Participants Characteristics and Training Effectiveness

This study was completed between April 2012 and December 2014. All participants reported to have followed dietary instructions, completed every exercise session under investigators' supervision and remained weight-stable throughout the experiments (T effect: $p = 0.66$; T × I effect: $p = 0.54$). Plasma lactate concentration was monitored immediately before and during training sessions. Ingestion of GF increased pre-session lactate as compared to C. Lactate was then increased by exercise but, interestingly, mean concentrations after 30 and 60 min exercise were not different (Figure 2: rest: $p < 0.01$; exercise: both $p > 0.05$).

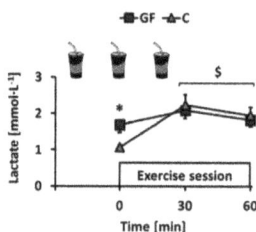

Figure 2. Changes over time of earlobe blood lactate concentration in GF and C groups during training sessions. GF received glucose-fructose drinks and C received water −20, 0, and +20 min relative to exercise onset. Effects of exercise (E) and intervention (I) were compared using a mixed-model analysis. Paired and unpaired contrasts were used to determine differences between rest and exercise (E effect: time = 0 min vs. time = 30–60 min: $: $p < 0.01$) and GF vs. C (I effect: *: $p < 0.05$). Mean ± SEM for $n = 8$ participants in all groups.

Training was effective in both GF and C and increased VO_{2max}, W_{max} and W_{LT} to similar extents (Table 1: all T effects: $p < 0.01$; T × I effects: $p > 0.05$). Consistent with improved conditioning, the fixed workload of the metabolic evaluation corresponded to lower relative exercise intensities post-training (GF and C, respectively 41% and 42% VO_{2max}) than pre-training (45% VO_{2max} by design). Heart rate was decreased similarly in GF and C (all T effects: $p < 0.01$; all T × I effects: $p > 0.05$).

Table 1. Participants' body weight and performance parameters.

	GF Pre	GF Post	C Pre	C Post
Body weight (kg)	73.7 ± 3.0	73.6 ± 2.8	72.9 ± 2.9	73.1 ± 3.0
VO_{2max} (mL·kg^{-1}·min^{-1})	44.3 ± 2.3	48.4 ± 2.0 #	46.4 ± 2.2	49.4 ± 2.1 #
W_{max} (W)	249 ± 20	281 ± 19 #	249 ± 16	287 ± 21 #
W_{LT} (W)	156 ± 15	180 ± 15 #	156 ± 12	181 ± 14 #
Endurance capacity (s)	663 ± 110	1134 ± 163 #	687 ± 177	1455 ± 293 #

Changes of participants' body weight and performance parameters. Baseline values were compared using an unpaired Student's *t*-test. Effects of training interventions were compared using a mixed-model analysis. Paired contrasts were used to determine differences between pre- vs. post-training (T effect: #: $p < 0.01$). GF: glucose-fructose intervention; C: control intervention; Pre: pre-training; Post: post-training; VO_{2max}: maximal oxygen consumption; W_{max}: maximal workload; W_{LT}: workload at lactate turnpoint. SEM: standard error of the mean; Mean $\pm$ SEM for $n = 8$ participants in all groups.

3.2. Metabolic Evaluation: Plasma Substrates and Hormones

In overnight-fasted participants, training increased fasting glucose similarly in GF and C (Figure 3a: T effect: $p < 0.01$; T × I effect: $p = 0.69$), but did not affect plasma fructose, lactate, insulin and glucagon concentrations (Figure 3b,c, Figure S1a,b for insulin and glucagon: all effects: $p > 0.05$). Fasting free fatty acids concentration was decreased after training only in C (Figure S1c: T × I effect: $p = 0.02$).

With repeated ingestion of glucose-fructose drinks, glucose, lactate and fructose concentrations (Figure 3a–c) rapidly increased to stabilize in the last part of the resting period (time = 60–90 min). Plasma insulin followed the same time course, whereas glucagon decreased and free fatty acids were decreased below detectable values (Figure S1a–c; all T effect: $p < 0.01$). Regarding the effects of the interventions, plasma glucose was not affected by training (Figure 3a: T effect: $p = 0.86$; T × I effect: $p = 0.56$), while plasma lactate was decreased post-training compared to pre-training in both GF and C (Figure 3b: T effect: $p = 0.02$; T × I effect: $p = 0.18$). Plasma fructose tended to be increased in GF and decreased in C (Figure 3c: T effect: $p = 0.39$; T × I effect: $p = 0.06$) and other parameters were not altered by the interventions (Figure S1a–c: all T and T × I effects: $p > 0.05$).

As compared to rest, exercise then decreased glucose, lactate and insulin and increased fructose and glucagon concentrations (all E effects: $p < 0.01$) to new steady-state values in the last part of the exercise period (time = 160–190 min). However, free fatty acids concentrations remained below the detection limit (Figure S1c: E effect: $p > 0.05$). Plasma lactate was decreased post-training compared to pre-training in both GF and C (Figure 3b: T effect: $p < 0.01$; T × I effect: $p = 0.13$), while plasma glucose, fructose, free fatty acids, insulin and glucagon were unaffected by the interventions (Figure 3a,b, Figure S1a–c for insulin, glucagon and free fatty acids: all effects: $p > 0.05$).

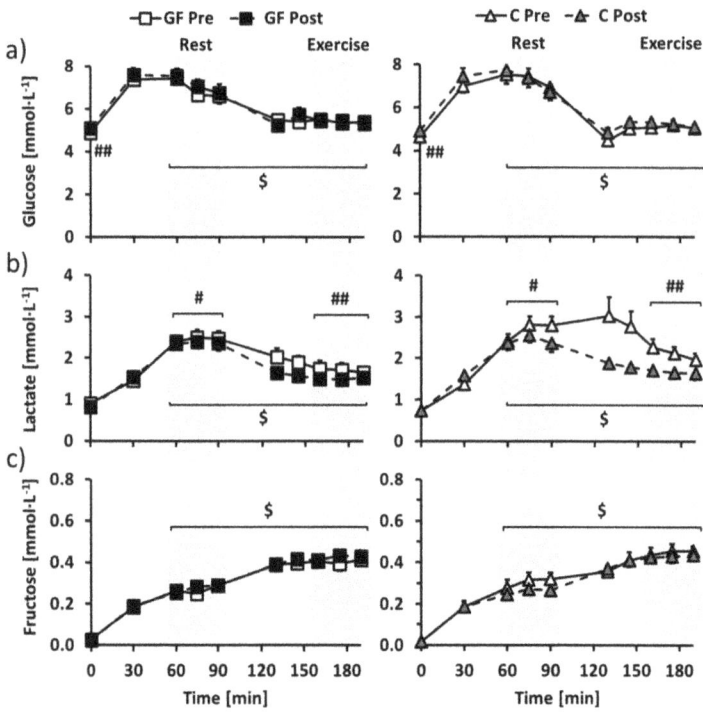

Figure 3. Changes over time of plasma (**a**) glucose, (**b**) lactate and (**c**) fructose concentrations in GF (**left**) and C (**right**) participants during metabolic evaluations. Glucose-fructose drinks were provided both at rest (time = 0–90 min) and during exercise (time = 100–190 min) in all tests. GF pre-training (GF Pre) and C pre-training (C Pre) is indicated in white, GF post-training (GF Post) in black and C post-training (C Post) in grey. Effects of exercise and interventions were compared using a mixed-model analysis. Paired contrasts were used for rest vs. exercise periods (E effect: $: $p < 0.01$) and pre- vs. post-training (T effect: #: $p < 0.05$; ##: $p < 0.01$). Dashed zones: Measures considered for tracer calculations. Mean ± SEM for $n = 8$ participants in all groups.

3.3. Metabolic Evaluation: Isotopic Enrichments

Glucose, lactate and CO_2 isotopic enrichments (Figure 4) of the last 30 min of rest (time = 60–90 min) and exercise (time = 160–190 min) were selected to determine glucose and lactate metabolisms at rest and during exercise. Mean ($^2H_2$)glucose and (^{13}C)glucose isotopic enrichments were increased from rest to exercise, but were not affected by both GF and C interventions (Figure 4a,b: E effects: $p < 0.01$; all T and T × I effects: $p > 0.05$). At rest, (^{13}C)lactate isotopic enrichment was distinctly affected after GF and C (Figure 4c: T effect: $p = 0.89$; T × I effect: $p = 0.02$), and the difference was no longer significant during exercise (Figure 4c: T effect: $p = 0.61$; T × I effect: $p = 0.18$). $^{13}CO_2$ isotopic enrichment was increased from rest to exercise, without being affected by GF or C (Figure 4d: E effect: $p < 0.01$; all T and T × I effects: $p > 0.05$).

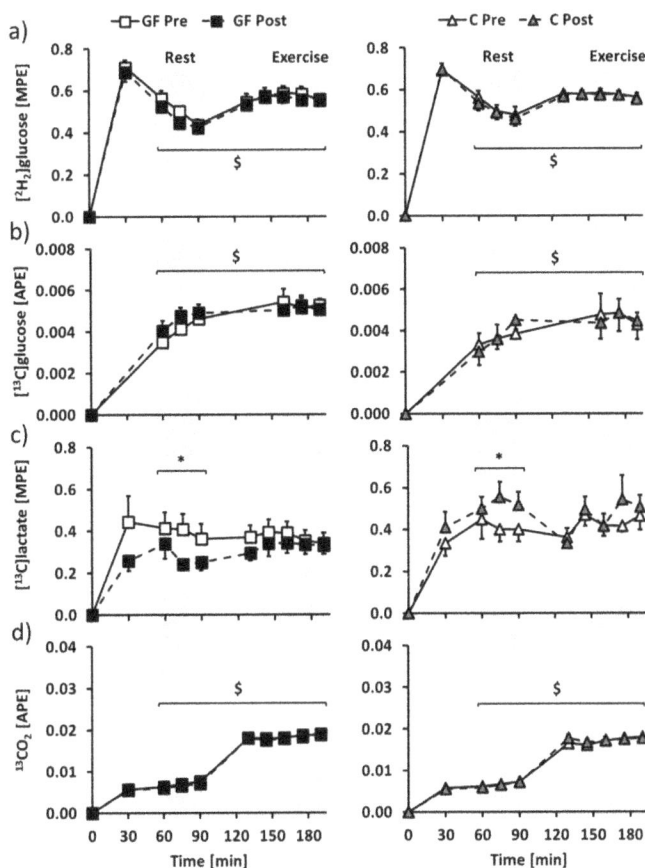

Figure 4. Changes over time of plasma (**a**) ($^2H_2$)glucose, (**b**) (^{13}C)glucose, (**c**) ($^{13}C_1$)lactate and (**d**) expired air $^{13}CO_2$ isotopic enrichments in GF (**left**) and C (**right**) participants during metabolic evaluations. Glucose-fructose drinks were provided in all tests, both during rest (time = 0–90 min) and exercise (time = 100–190 min) periods. GF pre-training (GF Pre) and C pre-training (C Pre) is indicated in white, GF post-training (GF Post) in black and C post-training (C Post) in grey. Effects of exercise and training interventions were compared using a mixed-model analysis. Paired contrasts were used for rest vs. exercise periods (E effect: \$: $p < 0.01$) and training × interventions (T × I effect: *: $p < 0.05$). Dashed zones: Measures considered for tracer calculations. Mean ± SEM for $n = 8$ participants in all groups.

3.4. Metabolic Evaluation: Glucose Metabolism

Summarized as mean values for selected periods of rest and exercise (Table 2), glucose appearance was similar in GF pre-training, GF post-training, C pre-training and C post-training at rest (T effect: $p = 0.19$; T × I effect: $p = 0.99$), then was increased to the same extent by exercise in all evaluations (E effect: $p < 0.01$; T effect: $p = 0.71$; T × I effect: $p = 0.98$). Glucose disposal was also similarly increased by exercise (rest: T effect: $p = 0.19$; T × I effect: $p = 0.62$; exercise: E effect: $p < 0.01$; T effect: $p = 0.38$; T × I effect: $p = 0.90$). Glucose clearance was also increased by exercise as compared to rest and remained constant after training in both GF and C (rest: T effect: $p = 0.70$; T × I effect: $p = 0.74$; exercise: E effect: $p < 0.01$; T effect: $p = 0.78$; T × I effect: $p = 0.86$).

Table 2. Glucose and lactate fluxes in the resting and exercise periods

		GF Pre	GF Post	C Pre	C Post
Glucose appearance	Rest	5.6 ± 0.3	5.8 ± 0.2	5.1 ± 0.4	5.4 ± 0.4
$(mg \cdot kg^{-1} \cdot min^{-1})$	Exercise	$10.8 \pm 0.6\,\$$	$10.9 \pm 0.5\,\$$	$10.5 \pm 0.3\,\$$	$10.7 \pm 0.3\,\$$
Lactate $(mg \cdot kg^{-1} \cdot min^{-1})$	Rest	0.5 ± 0.1	$0.7 \pm 0.1\,*$	0.3 ± 0.0	$0.3 \pm 0.1\,*$
	Exercise	$1.2 \pm 0.2\,\$$	$1.1 \pm 0.2\,\$$	$0.7 \pm 0.1\,\$$	$0.7 \pm 0.2\,\$$
Other $(mg \cdot kg^{-1} \cdot min^{-1})$	Rest	5.1 ± 0.3	5.1 ± 0.2	4.8 ± 0.5	5.1 ± 0.4
	Exercise	$9.6 \pm 0.6\,\$$	$9.8 \pm 0.6\,\$$	$9.8 \pm 0.3\,\$$	$9.9 \pm 0.3\,\$$
Glucose disposal	Rest	6.2 ± 0.5	6.4 ± 0.4	5.5 ± 0.6	6.0 ± 0.5
$(mg \cdot kg^{-1} \cdot min^{-1})$	Exercise	$10.8 \pm 0.7\,\$$	$11.2 \pm 0.5\,\$$	$10.5 \pm 0.3\,\$$	$10.8 \pm 0.3\,\$$
Glucose clearance	Rest	5.0 ± 0.5	5.0 ± 0.4	4.4 ± 0.6	4.7 ± 0.4
$(mL \cdot kg^{-1} \cdot min^{-1})$	Exercise	$11.2 \pm 0.9\,\$$	$11.5 \pm 0.7\,\$$	$11.5 \pm 0.6\,\$$	$11.5 \pm 0.3\,\$$
Lactate appearance	Rest	3.6 ± 0.5	$5.2 \pm 0.7\,**$	3.6 ± 0.4	$2.6 \pm 0.5\,**$
$(mg \cdot kg^{-1} \cdot min^{-1})$	Exercise	$11.2 \pm 1.4\,\$$	$12.1 \pm 1.5\,\$$	$8.8 \pm 0.7\,\$$	$8.3 \pm 0.9\,\$$
Lactate disposal	Rest	3.4 ± 0.5	$5.0 \pm 0.7\,**$	3.2 ± 0.4	$2.5 \pm 0.4\,**$
$(mg \cdot kg^{-1} \cdot min^{-1})$	Exercise	$11.3 \pm 1.4\,\$$	$12.1 \pm 1.5\,\$$	$9.1 \pm 0.7\,\$$	$8.4 \pm 1.0\,\$$
Oxidation $(mg \cdot kg^{-1} \cdot min^{-1})$	Rest	0.7 ± 0.1	$0.9 \pm 0.1\,*$	0.6 ± 0.1	$0.4 \pm 0.1\,*$
	Exercise	$9.7 \pm 1.4\,\$$	$10.6 \pm 1.7\,\$$	$7.9 \pm 1.0\,\$$	$7.3 \pm 1.1\,\$$
NOLD $(mg \cdot kg^{-1} \cdot min^{-1})$	Rest	2.7 ± 0.4	$4.1 \pm 0.6\,**$	2.7 ± 0.4	$2.0 \pm 0.4\,**$
	Exercise	$1.5 \pm 0.3\,\$$	$1.5 \pm 0.4\,\$$	$1.2 \pm 0.6\,\$$	$1.0 \pm 0.5\,\$$
Lactate clearance	Rest	17.8 ± 3.0	$26.9 \pm 4.9\,*$	16.0 ± 2.6	$13.1 \pm 2.6\,*$
$(mL \cdot kg^{-1} \cdot min^{-1})$	Exercise	$75.5 \pm 8.7\,\$$	$91.0 \pm 9.6\,\$\#$	$47.6 \pm 4.7\,\$$	$57.6 \pm 7.0\,\$\#$

Mean values during rest (time = 60–90 min) and exercise (time = 160–190 min) periods of metabolic evaluations performed pre-training (Pre) and post-training (Post). Effects of exercise and training interventions were compared using a mixed-model analysis. Paired and unpaired contrasts were used for rest vs. exercise periods (E effect: $\$: p < 0.01$), pre- vs. post-training (T effect: #: $p < 0.01$) and training × interventions (T × I effect: *: $p < 0.05$; **: $p < 0.01$). NOLD: non-oxidative lactate disposal. Mean $\pm$ SEM for $n = 8$ participants in all groups.

3.5. Metabolic Evaluation: Lactate Metabolism

Distinctly from glucose metabolism, lactate metabolism was affected by GF and C interventions. Post-training, mean lactate appearance was increased in GF and decreased in C at rest (T effect: $p = 0.56$; T × I effect: $p < 0.01$). Lactate appearance was then significantly increased by exercise and, interestingly, the difference between GF and C interventions was no longer significant during exercise (E effect: $p < 0.01$; T effect: $p = 0.68$; T × I effect: $p = 0.16$). Lactate disposal was also differently affected by GF and C interventions at rest (T effect: $p = 0.41$; T × I effect: $p < 0.01$) and was increased by exercise (E effect: $p < 0.01$) during which differences between interventions were no longer significant (T effect: $p = 0.91$; T × I effect: $p = 0.12$). Lactate clearance followed the same trend at rest in which it was also differently affected by GF and C (T effect: $p = 0.30$; T × I effect: $p = 0.02$) and was then increased by exercise as compared to rest (E effect: $p < 0.01$). During exercise, lactate clearance was interestingly enhanced post-training compared to pre-training, but to similar extents in both GF and C (T effect: $p < 0.01$; T × I effect: $p = 0.53$).

3.6. Metabolic Evaluation: Lactate Disposal

The use of $(^{13}C_1)$lactate allowed to investigate several of its fates. Consistent with the effects of interventions on lactate metabolism, lactate oxidation (T effect: $p = 0.60$; T × I effect: $p = 0.01$), NOLD (T effect: $p = 0.40$; T × I effect: $p < 0.01$) and gluconeogenesis from lactate (T effect: $p = 0.57$; T × I effect: $p = 0.01$) measured during the resting period were all distinctly affected by GF and C interventions. Despite absolute values being affected by the interventions, lactate oxidation still represented a stable proportion of lactate disposal at rest (GF: $20.6 \pm 1.0\%$ to $18.6 \pm 0.6\%$ vs. C: $17.5 \pm 1.7\%$ to $17.7 \pm 0.8\%$; T effect: $p = 0.20$; T × I effect: $p = 0.52$). In contrast, resting gluconeogenesis from lactate represented a larger part of glucose production after GF than after C (GF: $8.2 \pm 1.5\%$ to $11.9 \pm 1.6\%$ vs. C: $5.7 \pm 1.2\%$ to $5.0 \pm 1.0\%$: T effect: $p = 0.21$; T × I effect: $p = 0.01$).

Compared to rest, exercise increased lactate oxidation, decreased NOLD and increased gluconeogenesis from lactate (all: E effects: $p < 0.01$). There were no more significant differences between GF and C interventions for absolute values of lactate oxidation (T effect: $p = 0.74$; T × I effect: $p = 0.14$), NOLD (T effect: $p = 0.60$; T × I effect: $p = 0.77$) and gluconeogenesis from lactate (T effect: $p = 0.86$; T × I effect: $p = 0.99$). Lactate oxidation represented a significantly higher part (and NOLD a lower part) of lactate disposal during exercise than at rest, yet without effect of GF or C interventions (lactate oxidation: GF: 86.3 ± 3.8% to 87.6 ± 4.9% vs. C: 86.8 ± 6.6% to 87.6 ± 6.6%; E effect: $p < 0.01$; T effect: $p = 0.99$; T × I effect: $p = 0.83$). Similarly, no training effect was observed on fractional gluconeogenesis from lactate measured during exercise after both GF and C (GF: 10.7 ± 1.9% to 10.4 ± 1.6% vs. C: 7.0 ± 1.2% to 6.8 ± 1.5%; E effect: $p = 0.06$; T effect: $p = 0.87$; T × I effect: $p = 0.97$).

3.7. Metabolic Evaluation: Substrate Oxidation and Exercise Capacity

Carbohydrates provided most of the substrates to be oxidized throughout the evaluations (Table 3). Accordingly, lipid oxidation and protein oxidation (from urinary nitrogen collected during both periods) were low at rest and during exercise. In contrast, energy expenditure, total carbohydrate, lactate and other carbohydrate oxidations were all markedly increased during exercise as compared to the resting period (all E effects: $p < 0.01$).

Table 3. Fuel Selection in the Resting and Exercise Periods of Metabolic Evaluations.

		GF Pre	GF Post	C Pre	C Post
Energy expenditure (kcal·min^{-1})	Rest	1.5 ± 0.1	1.5 ± 0.0	1.4 ± 0.1	1.4 ± 0.1
	Exercise	8.3 ± 0.5 $	8.4 ± 0.6 $	8.9 ± 0.5 $	9.0 ± 0.6 $
Protein (mg·kg^{-1}·min^{-1})	Both	0.8 ± 0.0	0.8 ± 0.1	0.8 ± 0.1	0.8 ± 0.1
Lipid (mg·kg^{-1}·min^{-1})	Rest	0.8 ± 0.1	0.8 ± 0.1	0.6 ± 0.1	0.6 ± 0.2
	Exercise	0.8 ± 0.3	0.5 ± 0.3	0.4 ± 0.2	0.8 ± 0.3
Carbohydrate (mg·kg^{-1}·min^{-1})	Rest	2.8 ± 0.4	2.8 ± 0.3	2.9 ± 0.4	2.8 ± 0.4
	Exercise	27.6 ± 2.4 $	28.5 ± 2.6 $	30.6 ± 1.7 $	30.0 ± 1.7 $
Lactate (mg·kg^{-1}·min^{-1})	Rest	0.7 ± 0.1	0.9 ± 0.1 *	0.6 ± 0.1	0.4 ± 0.1 *
	Exercise	9.7 ± 1.4 $	10.6 ± 1.7 $	7.9 ± 1.0 $	7.3 ± 1.1 $
Other (mg·kg^{-1}·min^{-1})	Rest	2.1 ± 0.4	1.8 ± 0.4	2.4 ± 0.5	2.3 ± 0.4
	Exercise	17.8 ± 1.5 $	17.9 ± 1.4 $	22.7 ± 1.4 $	22.7 ± 1.8 $

Mean values during rest (time = 60–90 min) and exercise (time = 160–190 min) periods of metabolic evaluations performed pre-training (Pre) and post-training (Post). Effects of exercise and training interventions were compared using a mixed-model analysis. Paired and unpaired contrasts were used for rest vs. exercise periods (E effect: $: $p < 0.01$) and training × interventions (T × I effect: *: $p < 0.05$). Mean ± SEM for $n = 8$ participants in all groups.

As reported, at rest, lactate oxidation was increased post-training as compared to pre-training in GF, but not in C (T effect: $p = 0.55$; T × I effect: $p = 0.01$). Yet, this occurred within a stable total carbohydrate oxidation (T effect: $p = 0.75$; T × I effect: $p = 0.61$) and reflected an increasing proportion of carbohydrate oxidation coming from lactate oxidation after GF, but not after C (GF: 30 ± 6% to 38 ± 7% vs. C: 22 ± 4% to 15 ± 2%; T effect: $p = 0.89$; T × I effect: $p < 0.01$).

During exercise, there were no longer differences in lactate oxidation (T effect: $p = 0.73$; T × I effect: $p = 0.11$), total carbohydrate oxidation (T effect: $p = 0.15$; T × I effect: $p = 0.71$), or the fraction of total carbohydrate oxidation as lactate (GF: 35 ± 4% to 36 ± 4% vs. C: 26 ± 3% to 24 ± 3%; T effect: $p = 0.92$; T × I effect: $p = 0.22$) after interventions.

Finally, training with GF was hypothesized to specifically increase endurance capacity at 85% of current VO$_{2max}$. Yet, time-to-exhaustion was similarly improved by GF and C interventions (Table 1: T effect: $p < 0.01$; T × I effect: $p = 0.19$).

4. Discussion

4.1. Efficiency of the Training Programs

Pre-training, participants' VO$_{2max}$ were in the middle range of normal values [26]. The exercise training programs were effective, and produced a +8% VO$_{2max}$ increase similar to results from previous studies using a comparable training load [19,27]. Similar to other works comparing the effects of training with or without carbohydrate ingestion [27,28], no difference in performance gain was observed between GF and C.

4.2. Lactate Appearance and Energy Metabolism before Training

The initial metabolic evaluation involved the ingestion of repeated glucose-fructose drinks by both groups of participants at rest and during exercise. Since this visit was performed prior to intervention, results were expectedly similar in GF and C. In all participants, glucose-fructose ingestion increased blood lactate concentration compared to fasting values. Plasma lactate appearance, presumably from fructose in splanchnic tissues [29], but also resulting from glucose/glycogen degradation in various tissues including skeletal muscle, amounted to 3.6 mg·kg^{-1}·min^{-1} in both GF and C. We did not measure fasting lactate appearance, but it was previously estimated as ≈1.4 mg·kg^{-1}·min^{-1} in resting subjects [30]. This is consistent with GF being responsible for a substantial increase in lactate production. Our tracer approach does not allow the relative contributions of glucose and fructose to total lactate appearance to be estimated. Published human reports, however, indicate that intravenous fructose essentially stimulated splanchnic lactate release at rest [31] and during exercise [15], while animal studies suggest that glucose stimulated extra-splanchnic (presumably muscle) lactate production [32].

Gluconeogenesis from lactate was also minimal, most likely because it was inhibited by hyperinsulinemia induced by glucose ingestion [6]. Interestingly, lactate oxidation represented only ≈20% of lactate disposal, and the remaining ≈80% was metabolized non-oxidatively. Since there is no substantial lactate and glucose stores in the human body, this most likely corresponded to liver and/or muscle glycogen synthesis. In support of this hypothesis, we recently reported that post-exercise muscle glycogen resynthesis was quantitatively similar when subjects were fed glucose or fructose, and that lactate concentrations elicited by fructose ingestion were positively correlated with muscle glycogen resynthesis [33].

During exercise, lactate appearance increased to ≈10 mg·kg^{-1}·min^{-1}, of which ≈30% may have derived from fructose contribution, according to a previous study using comparable glucose-fructose drinks [13]. Relative to resting conditions, plasma lactate concentrations decreased, reflecting the effect of exercise to increase muscle lactate uptake and hence lactate clearance [30]. In addition, exercise directed ≈90% of lactate appearance toward oxidation, representing a much larger fraction than at rest. This is consistent with previous investigations of lactate metabolism in unfed individuals [10,11,34], confirming that lactate disposal between oxidative and non-oxidative fates is largely dictated by metabolic rate [7], also with glucose-fructose ingestion. We postulate that the transfer of lactate from splanchnic organs to working muscle after glucose-fructose ingestion (i.e., "reverse Cori cycle") is the result of two simultaneous processes: first, an increase of splanchnic lactate production pushed by fructose lacticogenesis increasing intrasplanchnic lactate concentration, and thus lactate efflux; second, an increased muscle lactate uptake pulled by low intramuscular lactate concentration due to continuous lactate removal toward oxidation.

4.3. Evolution of Plasma Lactate Concentration during Training Sessions

There was no detailed metabolic evaluation during training sessions. However, plasma lactate concentration was measured throughout the training program at rest and during exercise. At rest, plasma lactate concentration was higher in the GF group than in the C group, reflecting the well-known increase in plasma lactate induced by fructose ingestion [29,35]. During exercise, interestingly, plasma lactate concentration was similar in both groups, suggesting that the effect of glucose-fructose drinks was minor compared to that of exercise per se [30].

4.4. Lactate Appearance and Disposal after Training

All participants returned at the end of the training program for a second evaluation with glucose-fructose ingestion at rest and during exercise. The resting period revealed differences after GF and C interventions. Interestingly, unlike C that induced a decrease in lactate metabolism, confirming previous reports [19,34,36], GF differed by increasing lactate appearance. This may derive from an enhanced capacity to digest, absorb and metabolize fructose [29,37] or reflect the increased lactate appearance observed in fasted individuals after a few days of fructose exposure [38]. The mechanisms of such adaptations remain to be elucidated. Lactate clearance was increased in GF only, while lactate oxidative and non-oxidative disposal remained remarkably stable after training. Interestingly, resting lactate metabolism was increased by GF along with an unchanged glucose metabolism and carbohydrate oxidation, consistent with considerations that lactate may be preferred over other substrates for energy or glucose production [7].

In contrast to the resting period, lactate appearance measured during exercise was unaltered by training. Lactate clearance, however, increased by ≈20% in both GF and C, and plasma lactate concentration decreased. This can be attributed to an enhanced expression of muscle lactate transporters and lactate metabolizing enzymes [8]. However, and contrary to our hypothesis, training with glucose-fructose did not potentiate the effects of training alone. This observation is in line with the fact that lactate concentration was similar during training sessions with or without glucose-fructose drinks, and suggests that any additional effect of glucose-fructose ingestion during exercise was minimal compared to the effects of exercise training on lactate metabolism.

4.5. Limitations

First, glucose-fructose drinks were used as a tool to change lactate metabolism through effects on lactate concentration. While measuring blood lactate concentration during training sessions, our experimental protocol did not allow to assess intrasplanchnic and intramuscular lactate concentrations. Second, participants' diet was not entirely controlled during the training period and we cannot ascertain how glucose-fructose drinks modified total sugars intake in GF and C interventions. Third, our choice of tracers did not allow endogenous glucose appearance to be distinguished from exogenous glucose appearance, nor lactate appearance from fructose and from glucose-lactate shuttles. Four, the small sample size may have prevented the detection of still meaningful differences.

5. Conclusions

Ingestion of glucose-fructose drinks increase lactate appearance, metabolism and plasma lactate concentration above fasting values. This lactate is then mainly metabolized non-oxidatively at rest (presumably ending up in glycogen stores [33]) and oxidatively during exercise [13]. After having completed the 3-week training program, the ingestion at rest of glucose-fructose drinks increased lactate appearance and oxidation more in subjects who had received glucose-fructose during sessions than in those who had received water. This suggests that repeated glucose-fructose ingestion during training upregulated fructose absorption and splanchnic lacticogenesis from fructose. During exercise, however, lactate appearance and oxidation remained unchanged compared to pre-training conditions, indicating that neither training nor glucose-fructose consumption had a major impact on splanchnic lacticogenesis from fructose.

Supplementary Materials: The following are available online at www.mdpi.com/2072-6643/9/4/411/s1, Figure S1: Changes over time of plasma insulin, glucagon free fatty acids concentrations during metabolic evaluations.

Acknowledgments: The authors are thankful to Christiane Pellet and Françoise Secretan from the Clinical Research Center, Lausanne University Hospital for their memorable assistance. They also express a sincere gratitude to all study participants. This project was funded by a research grant to Luc Tappy from the Bundesamt fur Sport, Macolin, Switzerland, also covering open access publishing (grant 11-06). Part of this work was presented at the European College of Sport Science annual congress 2016, Vienna, Austria.

Author Contributions: L.T., V.L. and L.E. designed the study; R.R., L.E., V.L. and J.C. recruited participants and performed metabolic evaluations; V.R., N.S., R.R., V.S., M.L. and P.S. performed analyzes; R.R. and L.T. analyzed data and interpreted results; R.R. and L.T. drafted the manuscript, which was revised by all authors.

Conflicts of Interest: L.T. received support from Nestlé SA and Ajinomoto Co., Inc., for research unrelated to this trial. L.E. and V.L. were employed at the University of Lausanne during their involvement in this work. The other authors declare no conflict of interest. The founding sponsors had no role in the design of the study, in the collection, analyses or data interpretation, in the writing of the manuscript and in decision for publication.

Abbreviations

C	Control intervention in which plain water was provided during training sessions
GF	Intervention in which glucose-fructose drinks were provided during training sessions
VO_{2max}	Maximal oxygen consumption during incremental tests
W_{max}	Maximal workload during incremental tests
W_{LT}	Workload eliciting lactate turnpoint during incremental tests
VO_2	Oxygen consumption
VCO_2	Carbon dioxide production
$Na\text{-}H^{13}CO_3$	Sodium bicarbonate with its carbon being a carbon-13
NOLD	Non-oxidative lactate disposal
$(6,6\text{-}^2H_2)\text{-}D\text{-}(+)\text{-glucose}$	D-(+)-glucose deuterated twice on 6th carbon
$(3\text{-}^{13}C_1)\text{-}L\text{-}(+)\text{-lactate}$	L-(+)-lactate with its 3rd carbon being a carbon-13
NaCl	Sodium chloride
EDTA	Ethylenediaminetetraacetic acid

References

1. Romijn, J.A.; Coyle, E.F.; Sidossis, L.S.; Gastaldelli, A.; Horowitz, J.F.; Endert, E.; Wolfe, R.R. Regulation of endogenous fat and carbohydrate metabolism in relation to exercise intensity and duration. *Am. J. Physiol.* **1993**, *265*, E380–E391. [PubMed]
2. Coyle, E.F.; Coggan, A.R.; Hemmert, M.K.; Ivy, J.L. Muscle glycogen utilization during prolonged strenuous exercise when fed carbohydrate. *J. Appl. Physiol. (1985)* **1986**, *61*, 165–172.
3. Cermak, N.M.; van Loon, L.J. The use of carbohydrates during exercise as an ergogenic aid. *Sports Med.* **2013**, *43*, 1139–1155. [CrossRef] [PubMed]
4. Jeukendrup, A.E.; Jentjens, R. Oxidation of carbohydrate feedings during prolonged exercise: Current thoughts, guidelines and directions for future research. *Sports Med.* **2000**, *29*, 407–424. [CrossRef] [PubMed]
5. Ploug, T.; van Deurs, B.; Ai, H.; Cushman, S.W.; Ralston, E. Analysis of glut4 distribution in whole skeletal muscle fibers: Identification of distinct storage compartments that are recruited by insulin and muscle contractions. *J. Cell Biol.* **1998**, *142*, 1429–1446. [CrossRef] [PubMed]
6. Jeukendrup, A.E.; Raben, A.; Gijsen, A.; Stegen, J.H.; Brouns, F.; Saris, W.H.; Wagenmakers, A.J. Glucose kinetics during prolonged exercise in highly trained human subjects: Effect of glucose ingestion. *J. Physiol.* **1999**, *515 Pt 2*, 579–589. [CrossRef] [PubMed]
7. Brooks, G.A. Cell-cell and intracellular lactate shuttles. *J. Physiol.* **2009**, *587*, 5591–5600. [CrossRef] [PubMed]
8. Dubouchaud, H.; Butterfield, G.E.; Wolfel, E.E.; Bergman, B.C.; Brooks, G.A. Endurance training, expression, and physiology of ldh, mct1, and mct4 in human skeletal muscle. *Am. J. Physiol. Endocrinol. Metab.* **2000**, *278*, E571–E579. [PubMed]
9. Thomas, C.; Bishop, D.J.; Lambert, K.; Mercier, J.; Brooks, G.A. Effects of acute and chronic exercise on sarcolemmal mct1 and mct4 contents in human skeletal muscles: Current status. *Am. J. Physiol. Regul. Integr. Comp. Physiol.* **2012**, *302*, R1–R14. [CrossRef] [PubMed]

10. Emhoff, C.A.; Messonnier, L.A.; Horning, M.A.; Fattor, J.A.; Carlson, T.J.; Brooks, G.A. Gluconeogenesis and hepatic glycogenolysis during exercise at the lactate threshold. *J. Appl. Physiol. (1985)* **2013**, *114*, 297–306. [CrossRef] [PubMed]

11. Emhoff, C.A.; Messonnier, L.A.; Horning, M.A.; Fattor, J.A.; Carlson, T.J.; Brooks, G.A. Direct and indirect lactate oxidation in trained and untrained men. *J. Appl. Physiol. (1985)* **2013**, *115*, 829–838. [CrossRef] [PubMed]

12. Jentjens, R.L.; Jeukendrup, A.E. High rates of exogenous carbohydrate oxidation from a mixture of glucose and fructose ingested during prolonged cycling exercise. *Br. J. Nutr.* **2005**, *93*, 485–492. [CrossRef] [PubMed]

13. Lecoultre, V.; Benoit, R.; Carrel, G.; Schutz, Y.; Millet, G.P.; Tappy, L.; Schneiter, P. Fructose and glucose co-ingestion during prolonged exercise increases lactate and glucose fluxes and oxidation compared with an equimolar intake of glucose. *Am. J. Clin. Nutr.* **2010**, *92*, 1071–1079. [CrossRef] [PubMed]

14. Currell, K.; Jeukendrup, A.E. Superior endurance performance with ingestion of multiple transportable carbohydrates. *Med. Sci. Sports Exerc.* **2008**, *40*, 275–281. [CrossRef] [PubMed]

15. Ahlborg, G.; Bjorkman, O. Splanchnic and muscle fructose metabolism during and after exercise. *J. Appl. Physiol. (1985)* **1990**, *69*, 1244–1251.

16. Tappy, L.; Rosset, R. Fructose metabolism from a functional perspective: Implications for athletes. *Sports Med.* **2017**, *47*, 23–32. [CrossRef] [PubMed]

17. Truswell, A.S.; Seach, J.M.; Thorburn, A.W. Incomplete absorption of pure fructose in healthy subjects and the facilitating effect of glucose. *Am. J. Clin. Nutr.* **1988**, *48*, 1424–1430. [PubMed]

18. Goodwin, M.L.; Harris, J.E.; Hernandez, A.; Gladden, L.B. Blood lactate measurements and analysis during exercise: A guide for clinicians. *J. Diabetes Sci. Technol.* **2007**, *1*, 558–569. [CrossRef] [PubMed]

19. MacRae, H.S.; Dennis, S.C.; Bosch, A.N.; Noakes, T.D. Effects of training on lactate production and removal during progressive exercise in humans. *J. Appl. Physiol. (1985)* **1992**, *72*, 1649–1656.

20. Tounian, P.; Schneiter, P.; Henry, S.; Delarue, J.; Tappy, L. Effects of dexamethasone on hepatic glucose production and fructose metabolism in healthy humans. *Am. J. Physiol.* **1997**, *273*, E315–E320. [PubMed]

21. Novel-Chate, V.; Rey, V.; Chiolero, R.; Schneiter, P.; Leverve, X.; Jequier, E.; Tappy, L. Role of Na$^+$-K$^+$-Atpase in insulin-induced lactate release by skeletal muscle. *Am. J. Physiol. Endocrinol. Metab.* **2001**, *280*, E296–E300. [PubMed]

22. Sauvinet, V.; Gabert, L.; Qin, D.; Louche-Pelissier, C.; Laville, M.; Desage, M. Validation of pentaacetylaldononitrile derivative for dual ^{2}H gas chromatography/mass spectrometry and ^{13}C gas chromatography/combustion/isotope ratio mass spectrometry analysis of glucose. *Rapid Commun. Mass Spectrom.* **2009**, *23*, 3855–3867. [CrossRef] [PubMed]

23. Frayn, K.N. Calculation of substrate oxidation rates in vivo from gaseous exchange. *J. Appl. Physiol. Respir. Environ. Exerc. Physiol.* **1983**, *55*, 628–634. [PubMed]

24. Van Hall, G. Correction factors for ^{13}C-labelled substrate oxidation at whole-body and muscle level. *Proc. Nutr. Soc.* **1999**, *58*, 979–986. [CrossRef] [PubMed]

25. Steele, R.; Wall, J.S.; De Bodo, R.C.; Altszuler, N. Measurement of size and turnover rate of body glucose pool by the isotope dilution method. *Am. J. Physiol.* **1956**, *187*, 15–24. [PubMed]

26. Schneider, J. Age dependency of oxygen uptake and related parameters in exercise testing: An expert opinion on reference values suitable for adults. *Lung* **2013**, *191*, 449–458. [CrossRef] [PubMed]

27. Cox, G.R.; Clark, S.A.; Cox, A.J.; Halson, S.L.; Hargreaves, M.; Hawley, J.A.; Jeacocke, N.; Snow, R.J.; Yeo, W.K.; Burke, L.M. Daily training with high carbohydrate availability increases exogenous carbohydrate oxidation during endurance cycling. *J. Appl. Physiol. (1985)* **2010**, *109*, 126–134. [CrossRef] [PubMed]

28. De Bock, K.; Derave, W.; Eijnde, B.O.; Hesselink, M.K.; Koninckx, E.; Rose, A.J.; Schrauwen, P.; Bonen, A.; Richter, E.A.; Hespel, P. Effect of training in the fasted state on metabolic responses during exercise with carbohydrate intake. *J. Appl. Physiol. (1985)* **2008**, *104*, 1045–1055. [CrossRef] [PubMed]

29. Sun, S.Z.; Empie, M.W. Fructose metabolism in humans—What isotopic tracer studies tell us. *Nutr. Metab.* **2012**, *9*, 89. [CrossRef] [PubMed]

30. Van Hall, G. Lactate kinetics in human tissues at rest and during exercise. *Acta Physiol.* **2010**, *199*, 499–508. [CrossRef] [PubMed]

31. Bjorkman, O.; Gunnarsson, R.; Hagstrom, E.; Felig, P.; Wahren, J. Splanchnic and renal exchange of infused fructose in insulin-deficient type 1 diabetic patients and healthy controls. *J. Clin. Investig.* **1989**, *83*, 52–59. [CrossRef] [PubMed]

32. Youn, J.H.; Bergman, R.N. Conversion of oral glucose to lactate in dogs. Primary site and relative contribution to blood lactate. *Diabetes* **1991**, *40*, 738–747. [CrossRef] [PubMed]

33. Rosset, R.; Lecoultre, V.; Egli, L.; Cros, J.; Dokumaci, A.S.; Zwygart, K.; Boesch, C.; Kreis, R.; Schneiter, P.; Tappy, L. Postexercise repletion of muscle energy stores with fructose or glucose in mixed meals. *Am. J. Clin. Nutr.* **2017**, *105*, 609–617. [CrossRef] [PubMed]

34. Bergman, B.C.; Wolfel, E.E.; Butterfield, G.E.; Lopaschuk, G.D.; Casazza, G.A.; Horning, M.A.; Brooks, G.A. Active muscle and whole body lactate kinetics after endurance training in men. *J. Appl. Physiol. (1985)* **1999**, *87*, 1684–1696.

35. Mayes, P.A. Intermediary metabolism of fructose. *Am. J. Clin. Nutr.* **1993**, *58*, 754S–765S. [PubMed]

36. Holloszy, J.O. Muscle metabolism during exercise. *Arch. Phys. Med. Rehabil.* **1982**, *63*, 231–234. [PubMed]

37. Douard, V.; Ferraris, R.P. The role of fructose transporters in diseases linked to excessive fructose intake. *J. Physiol.* **2013**, *591*, 401–414. [CrossRef] [PubMed]

38. Abdel-Sayed, A.; Binnert, C.; Le, K.A.; Bortolotti, M.; Schneiter, P.; Tappy, L. A high-fructose diet impairs basal and stress-mediated lipid metabolism in healthy male subjects. *Br. J. Nutr.* **2008**, *100*, 393–399. [CrossRef] [PubMed]

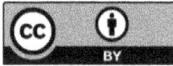

nutrients

MDPI

Review

Chronic Fructose Ingestion as a Major Health Concern: Is a Sedentary Lifestyle Making It Worse? A Review

Amy J. Bidwell

Department of Health Promotion and Wellness, State University of New York at Oswego, 105G Park Hall, Oswego, NY 13027, USA; Amy.bidwell@oswego.edu; Tel.: +1-315-569-3543

Received: 21 March 2017; Accepted: 25 May 2017; Published: 28 May 2017

Abstract: Obesity contributes to metabolic abnormalities such as insulin resistance, dyslipidemia, hypertension, and glucose intolerance, all of which are risk factors associated with metabolic syndrome. The growing prevelance of metabolic syndrome seems to be an end result of our current lifestyle which promotes high caloric, high-fat foods and minimal physical activity, resulting in a state of positive energy balance. Increased adiposity and physical inactivity may represent the beginning of the appearance of these risk factors. Understanding the metabolic and cardiovascular disturbances associated with diet and exercise habits is a crucial step towards reducing the risk factors for metabolic syndrome. Although considerable research has been conducted linking chronic fructose ingestion to the increased prevalence of obesity and metabolic syndrome risk factors, these studies have mainly been performed on animals, and/or in a post-absorptive state. Further, the magnitude of the effect of fructose may depend on other aspects of the diet, including the total amount of carbohydrates and fats in the diet and the overall consumption of meals. Therefore, the overall aim of this review paper is to examine the effects of a diet high in fructose on postprandial lipidemia, inflammatory markers and glucose tolerance, all risk factors for diabetes and cardiovascular disease. Moreover, an objective is to investigate whether increased physical activity can alter such effects.

Keywords: fructose; physical activity; metabolic syndrome; inflammation; insulin resistance; hyperlipidemia

1. Introduction

The prevalence of obesity and obesity-related diseases in the United State and worldwide is increasing rapidly, with 67% of the population considered overweight and 33% obese [1]. Moderate obesity can contribute to chronic metabolic abnormalities characteristic of metabolic syndrome which include insulin resistance, dyslipidemia and hypertension [2]. Increased consumption of added sugar, specifically in the form of high-fructose corn syrup (HFCS) and sucrose, has paralleled the increased prevalence of metabolic abnormalities, and may be a contributing factor to the rise in the incidence of such disease-related risk factors [2].

The addition of fructose in the food supply became popular in the 1970s when fructose was used to produce high fructose corn syrup HFCS. HFCS can contain up to 90% fructose, however, most of the HFCS that is commercially sold contains 55% fructose and 45% glucose [2]. HFCS is frequently used as a sweetener in the food industry because it is cheaper to produce, has a long shelf-life, maintains long-lasting moisturization in industrial bakeries, and is sweeter than most other sugars [3].

There has been an increased interest in the potential role of these added sugars as a contributing factor to metabolic syndrome. When consumed in elevated concentrations, fructose can promote metabolic changes that may contribute to risk factors associated with metabolic syndrome as well as hyperuricemia, inflammation, and alterations in various metabolic hormones [4]. Today, the average

American consumes ~94 g of added sugar per day. These values are significantly higher than the new dietary guidelines that state that no more than 25 g of added sugar should be consumed per day. The following review of literature will present evidence that fructose, either in the form of sucrose or HFCS, may cause substantial alterations in the risk factors associated with metabolic syndrome. Furthermore, partaking in an inactive lifestyle will also be addressed as increased physical inactivity may attenuate such risk factors.

2. Fructose Intake, Absorption and Metabolism

2.1. Fructose Intake

In recent years, manufacturers have been replacing HFCS with sucrose or other types of sugars, which is sometimes confusing the consumer, as one may think the product is somehow healthier than it really is. Sucrose, or table sugar, is a disaccharide composed of one glucose molecule and one fructose molecule, making it 50% fructose and 50% glucose [5]. Because sucrose has slightly lower concentrations of fructose compared to the 55/45 ratio of fructose to glucose in HFCS, often manufacturers will put more sucrose in the product in order to have it taste similar to products containing HFCS. Added sugar can be disguised as cane juice, evaporated cane juice, cane juice solids, cane juice crystals, or dehydrated cane juice, all made from sugar cane, therefore making them potentially as harmful as the now frowned upon HFCS.

2.2. Fructose Absorption

Fructose enters the brush border of the stomach in the form of either pure fructose, HFCS or as sucrose [6]. When fructose is ingested as a disaccharide in the form of sucrose, the sucrose must first be cleaved, via sucrose, into one molecule of glucose and one molecule of fructose before being metabolized. Fructose is then absorbed and transported through the enterocytes to the portal bloodstream by a fructose-specific hexose transporter, glucose transporter 5 (GLUT 5). Unlike glucose, which uses a sodium- and protein-based transporter molecule to assist the glucose with transport out of the enterocytes, the activation of GLUT 5 transporters is sodium–independent and does not require ATP hydrolysis [6]. Once inside the enterocytes, fructose diffuses across the basolateral pole of the enterocytes and into the portal circulation via glucose transporter 2 (GLUT 2) transporters [7].

Unlike glucose, fructose is incompletely absorbed in the enterocytes. The absorption capacity of fructose is limited to approximately 5–50 g at one time before some individuals suffer from symptoms of diarrhea and flatulence [8]. Ushijima et al. [9] showed that 80% of healthy adults experienced incomplete absorption when given 50 g of fructose, yet when fructose is consumed with glucose, the rate of absorption is increased [10]. Thus, when fructose is consumed as sucrose or as HFCS, more fructose is absorbed through the enterocytes. The improved absorption of fructose in conjunction with glucose may be due to the up-regulation of GLUT 5 receptors which is stimulated by elevated glucose absorption [8]. Once within the enterocytes, fructose can be easily converted into triglycerides (TGs). Specifically, intestinal TGs, in the form of chylomicrons, have been apparent in hamsters fed a high-fructose diet in as little as three weeks [11]. Moreover, chronic fructose feeding seems to be associated with increases in intracellular apoprotein-B48 (apoB-48) and enhanced intestinal enterocyte de novo lipogenesis (DNL) [11]. The intestinal overproduction of apoB-48-containing lipoproteins may be an important contributor to the elevation of circulating TG-rich lipoproteins, which may potentially lead to atherosclerosis.

2.3. Fructose Metabolism

Although fructose can be lipogenic within the enterocytes, fructose is also readily absorbed and stimulates lipogenesis within the hepatocytes [6]. Once fructose travels through the enterocytes and into the portal vein, it is readily absorbed by the liver via GLUT 2 transporters. Due to the high concentration of GLUT 2 transporters and fructokinase, there is a high affinity for fructose uptake in the liver [6]. Within the liver, fructose is rapidly converted to fructose-1-phospate via fructokinase. Fructokinase has a low affinity for fructose, resulting in rapid metabolism of fructose by the liver cells. Fructose is further metabolized into triose phosphates, glyceraldehyde and dihydroxyacetone phosphate [12]. The triose phosphate that is produced can then be converted to pyruvate and oxidized into carbon dioxide and water in the citric acid cycle or a portion of the triose phosphate can be converted to lactate and released into the systemic circulation [6]. A portion of the carbon derived from the triose phosphates can also enter the gluconeogenic pathway where it can be stored as glycogen to be later released as glucose [12]. This gluconeogenic process results in a small but measurable increase in systemic glucose concentrations [6].

Within the liver, fructose metabolism differs substantially from glucose metabolism in that entry of glucose into the glycolytic pathway is under the control of glucokinase which has a low affinity for glucose within the hepatocytes, and is dependent on the concentration of glucose [6]. Therefore, the rate of glucose phosphorylation varies with changes in glucose concentrations. Moreover, downstream, when fructose-6-phosphate is converted to fructose 1,6-bisphosphate, this reaction is catalyzed by phosphofructokinase (PFK), an enzyme regulated by the energy status of the cell. In particular, PFK is inhibited by elevations in ATP and citrate. This inhibition allows for a close regulation of glycolysis based on the energy status of the cell [12]. On the contrary, fructose is phosphorylated to fructose-1-phoshpate by fructokinase, but this rate-limiting enzyme does not have the tight regulation as seen with PFK [3]. Figure 1 depicts the metabolic fate of fructose within the hepatocytes. When acetyl-CoA combines with oxaloacetate to form citrate in the mitochondria, the carbon atoms can be used for DNL and then form long-chained fatty acids that are eventually esterified into TGs [12]. This large source of unregulated TG formation is unlike that of glucose metabolism which has a rate-limiting step to regulate it, preventing such effects.

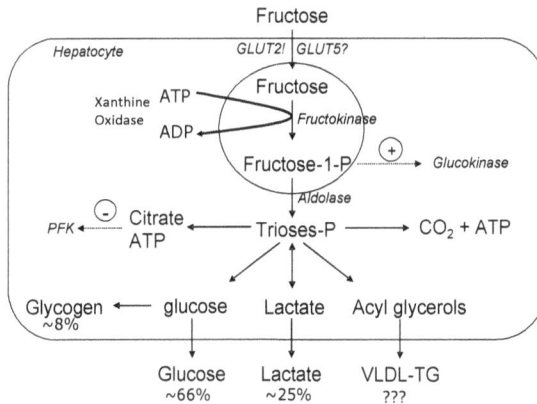

Figure 1. Metabolic fate of hepatic fructose. Fructose provides a high concentration of unregulated acetyl-CoA which can be converted to very-low density lipoprotein-triglyceride (VLDL-TG), glucose and/or lactate. (Figure adapted from Le and Tappy, 2006 [13]). GLUT: glucose transporter; PFK: phosphofructokinase.

3. Fructose-Induced Lipogenesis

The most detrimental aspect of fructose is its ability to be converted to fatty acids within the hepatocytes via DNL, as pictured in Figure 1. In rodents, a high-fructose diet (60% fructose) has been shown to increase intra-hepatocellular lipids as well as stimulate hepatic DNL within a few days [14]. When such diets are sustained over a prolonged period of time, high fructose or sucrose diets will induce hepatic stenosis and whole-body insulin resistance with a concomitant accumulation of intramyocellular lipids [15].

To date there is an abundance of research indicating that acute and/or chronic ingestion of fructose causes hyperlipidemia in rats [14,16,17] and in humans [18–21]. Faeh et al. [21] discovered that after six days of fructose loading, subjects' plasma triglyceride concentrations were increased by 79% from baseline values, possibly due to the six-fold increase in fractional DNL [21]. It should be noted that the fructose load that was given (~210 g/day) in this study was an extremely high load and therefore may not be clinically relevant. Using a more clinically relevant fructose load, Swanson et al. [22] discovered that serum total and low-density lipoprotein (LDL) cholesterol levels were 9% and 11% higher, respectively, when consuming a high fructose diet compared to an isocaloric starch diet [22]. Furthermore, within the first 24 h, serum triglyceride levels in the fructose-fed group were significantly higher than the starch group, indicating that fructose induced hyperlipidemia can occur in as little as 24 h after the first fructose load [22]. In a slightly longer intervention, Bantle et al. [23] compared similar effects and found that a diet consisting of either 17% of energy from fructose or 17% glucose for six weeks was associated with elevations in fasting and postprandial TG concentrations [23]. These results were similar to those obtained by Schwarz et al. [24] in which elevated liver DNL was apparent in eight healthy men consuming 25% fructose/25% glucose mixture compared to a 50% complex carbohydrate mixture. It is important to mention that the above-mentioned study was one of the first studies to indicate an increase in DNL during a weight-neutral period, therefore demonstrating that the changes in DNL are not the result of increased weight but are from increased fructose consumption [24].

Although the research regarding fructose ingestion and fasting and postprandial lipogenesis is apparent in normal weight individuals, research is more limited in the obese population. Swarbrick et al. [18] investigated the metabolic effects of a high-fructose diet in seven overweight, post-menopausal women who consumed standardized, energy-balanced meals for 14 weeks. After two weeks on the diet, triglyceride area under the curve (AUC) was unchanged, however after week ten, triglyceride AUC values were 141% higher than at baseline. Additionally, fasting apolipoprotein B concentrations were increased by 19% compared to baseline. The authors speculated that the increases in fasting and postprandial TG concentrations were most likely due to stimulation of TG synthesis [18]. Likewise, Stanhope et al. [19] also investigated the overweight/obese population. After studying 18 post-menopausal women for 12 weeks, the high fructose group had elevated fasting and 24-h postprandial TG concentrations compared to the isocaloric glucose group [19]. Post-intervention, fasting apolipoprotein B, low-density lipoproteins (LDLs), small-dense LDLs, and oxidized LDLs were significantly higher in the fructose group compared to the glucose group. This study reiterates the fact that long-term consumption of fructose of ≥ 2 weeks negatively alters lipid remodeling in obese, post-menopausal women [19]. It seems that the mechanism by which fructose-induced lipemia occurs is a result of the carbon atoms from fructose being converted to fatty acids, skipping the rate-limiting step in glycolysis. Fructose increases DNL by increasing hepatic TG formation, however, fructose-induced hepatic DNL may also limit fatty acid oxidation as well. Fructose increases acetyl-CoA concentrations in the liver, subsequently leading to increased production of malonyl CoA, which inhibits the entry of fatty acids into the mitochondria [3]. Taken together, fructose indirectly inhibits fatty acid oxidation by increasing production of malonyl CoA, which decreases fatty acid transport into the mitochondria [3]. Malonyl CoA is an important intermediate to fructose-induced lipogenesis because acetyl CoA is added to long-chained fatty acids via malonyl CoA, therefore allowing fructose to provide carbon atoms for both glycerol, and the acyl portion of the acylglycerol molecule [3].

To better understand the hypothesis that fructose ingestion may also inhibit fat oxidation, Abdel-Sayed et al. [25] investigated whether a high-fructose diet (234 g) impaired lipid metabolism. After seven days on the high fructose diet, basal non-esterified fatty acid (NEFA) concentrations significantly decreased by 19.5%, net lipid oxidation by 21.3% and plasma β-hydroxybutyrate concentrations by 78.2%. After a period of lipid loading, the increase in net lipid oxidation and exogenous lipid oxidation were comparable between the two groups. However, after the mental stress, there was a markedly blunted stimulation of plasma NEFA and β-hydroxybutyrate release in the fructose group. The lower basal plasma NEFA concentrations indicated that an inhibition of adipose tissue lipolysis occurred after the high fructose diet. This phenomenon suggests that the decreased NEFA seen with the high-fructose diet was likely related to fructose-induced stimulation of hepatic DNL lipogenesis, and not secondary to an increased hepatic re-esterification. Additionally, the inhibition of lipolysis may, in turn, be directly responsible for lower whole-body net lipid oxidation following fructose loading since NEFA concentrations are the main determinant in this process [25].

4. Fructose and Postprandial Lipemia

Although research regarding fasting hyperlipidemia and fructose consumption has been well established, high postprandial triglyceride levels have been associated with the risk of coronary artery disease [26]. Hence, there is growing evidence linking increased postprandial TG concentrations with a pro-atherogenic state. This link may be due to lipoprotein remodeling induced by increased levels of very-low density lipoproteins (VLDLs) and mediated by cholesteryl ester transfer protein (CETP) and hepatic lipase. Both increased VLDLs and CEPT resulted in increased concentrations of small-dense lipoproteins and remnant-like lipoproteins [26].

When in the blood, TGs can be referred to as "triglyceride-rich lipoproteins" (TRLs) and consist of two main components: very-low density lipoproteins (VLDL) and chylomicrons. Very low-density lipoproteins are a result of hepatic synthesis and chylomicrons are produced by the gut postprandially in order to transport dietary lipids from the intestines to other locations in the body [26]. Therefore, TRLs can be produced exogenously from the diet or endogenously from the liver. Chylomicrons and VLDLs can then form intermediate-density lipoproteins catalyzed by lipoprotein lipase (LPL), an enzyme released from the capillary beds of adipose tissue and skeletal muscle [26]. Lipoprotein lipase, situated in the capillary endothelial, is responsible for hydrolyzing the TG into NEFA [27]. This pathway is up-regulated by insulin, which increases rapidly in response to a carbohydrate meal. In a fructose-rich diet, due to the suppression of insulin, reduced insulin concentrations may contribute to lower postprandial LPL activity. Research has indicated that glucose has a significantly greater postprandial LPL response than fructose [19], signifying that reduced TG clearance with chronic fructose ingestion might also contribute to the fructose-induced postprandial hypertriglyceridemia that is often evident in fructose-fed individuals [19]. Other studies have shown similar results in that fructose, not glucose, leads to an attenuated LPL response which potentiated postprandial lipidemia as the TG-VLDL and TG-rich chylomicron levels were significantly higher than in the glucose group [28]. The lower insulin concentrations seen with the fructose load led to a decreased production of LPL, resulting in impaired triacylglycerol clearance [28].

Often, consumption of fructose occurs in a postprandial state as the average Western diet is consumed every 3–6 h. Previous research has shown that a bolus of fructose in the morning with a subsequent meal at lunch stimulates lipogenesis and seems to be dose-dependent [20]. This same study found TG incremental AUC to be higher after a fructose bolus than a glucose bolus, signifying that fructose acutely and significantly increases lipogenesis in the morning and meals thereafter. The fructose-induced increase in lipogenesis displaced the use of stored TG for VLDL synthesis and the stimulation of lipogenesis represents an intracellular signal for the liver to esterify fatty acids from any source into TGs [20]. Similar results can be found in overweight and obese individuals [19]. Based on these findings, DNL and decreased lipoprotein lipase-mediated clearance may be a contributing factor to fructose-induced postprandial hypertriglyceridemia [19,20]. Although more research needs to be conducted in the postprandial state, when fructose is consumed in the morning, the succeeding meal will augment the postprandial lipidemia induced during the prior meal [20]. Possible mechanisms involved in the stimulation of fructose-induced postprandial lipidemia are: (1) the liver being the main site of fructose metabolism; (2) fructose bypassing the main rate limiting step of glycolysis, thus providing unregulated amounts of lipogenic substrates such as acetyl-CoA and glycerol-3-phosphate; and (3) fructose enhancing DNL when subsequent meals were ingested [19,20].

5. Fructose and Insulin Resistance

Type 2 diabetes is a progressive disorder that begins with the development of insulin resistance and potentially ends with pancreatic β-cell failure [29]. A dietary recommendation often proposed for patients suffering from type 2 diabetes is to ingest foods that do not cause an acute rise in insulin levels, therefore preventing over-stimulation of insulin secretion from the pancreas. Initially, fructose was a popular macronutrient choice for individuals with type 2 diabetes because fructose does not cause an acute rise in insulin due to the low glycemic index related to fructose. Although there is a blunted insulin response, fructose consumption has been associated with increased hepatic VLDL triglyceride secretion, and possibly decreased extra-hepatic clearance of very-low density lipoprotein-triglyceride (VLDL-TG), both of which are associated with the development of hepatic and adipose tissue insulin resistance. The VLDL-TG formed from fructose-induced hepatic DNL can be released into the systemic circulation, consequently leading to an increase in the levels of fatty acids in the circulation. Signaling abnormalities in adipocytes can also trigger lipolysis of TG stores and efflux of NEFA into the bloodstream, augmenting the problem [30]. NEFA in the bloodstream as a result of increased fructose-induced lipidemia may be a key mechanistic link between fructose consumption and insulin resistance, type 2 diabetes and metabolic dyslipidemia. These conditions are a result of increased ectopic storage of NEFA by non-adipose tissues such as liver and skeletal muscle where they are stored as TG or diacylglycerol. The exposure of these organs to increased concentrations of NEFA from fructose ingestion may reduce insulin sensitivity by increasing the intramyocellular lipid content [31]. Once stored as ectopic lipids, the fatty acids can interfere with the metabolic pathways of that tissue, resulting in fructose-induced insulin resistance [30].

In a healthy adult, insulin suppresses hepatic gluconeogenesis and glycogenolysis, however, in the insulin-resistant state, this suppression no longer occurs, causing a subsequent increase in glucose output from the liver [29]. Insulin resistance in fat cells reduces the normal effects of insulin on lipids and results in reduced uptake of circulating lipids and increased hydrolysis of stored TG. Increased mobilization of stored lipids in these cells elevates free fatty acids in the blood plasma, leading to reduced muscle glucose uptake and increased liver glucose production, all of which contribute to elevated blood glucose levels [32]. This chronic state of excess fatty acid release into the circulation can induce lipotoxicity, or pancreatic β-cell death. To compensate for the increased peripheral insulin resistance, the pancreatic β-cells increase in mass and secrete more insulin, resulting in hyperinsulinemia. Since the β-cells cannot compensate for the resistant state, hyperglycemia occurs. Hyperglycemia further damages the β-cells, resulting in glycotoxicity, leading to a progressive loss of the pancreatic islet β-cells manifesting into type 2 diabetes [29].

The molecular mechanisms underlying fructose-induced insulin resistance are not completely understood but may be similar to that of a high-fat diet. Both high-fructose and high-fat diets interfere with insulin signaling at common steps in skeletal muscle [13]. In liver cells, both high fructose and high-fat diets elicit hepatic stress responses and activation of pro-inflammatory cascades that lead to insulin resistance. Sucrose-fed rats demonstrate an early alteration of hepatic VLDL-TG secretion, leading to impaired insulin-mediated suppression of glucose production in hepatic tissues after 1–2 weeks, but show no changes in extra-hepatic insulin sensitivity after this time period [33]. After 4–6 weeks, impaired extra-hepatic insulin sensitivity, in conjunction with muscle lipids occurs [33].

The mechanism by which intercellular lipids cause insulin resistance in both liver and muscle is through diacylclycerol (DAG)-induced activation of novel protein kinase C (nPKC) [34]. DAG is a known activator of nPKC, and both DAG and nPKC are associated with lipid-induced insulin resistance in humans [34]. Activation of nPKC causes a decrease in insulin receptors or insulin receptor substrate 1 (IRS1) tyrosine phosphorylation [13]. This IRS-1 inhibition decreases insulin-stimulated glucose transporter (GLUT 4) activity resulting in reduced glucose uptake into the cell [35]. Increases in DAG also activate several other serine/threonine kinases such as inhibitory κβ kinase β (IKKβ) and nuclear factor κB (NF-κB). These inflammatory markers are also activated by tumor necrosis factor-α (TNF-α) and interleukin 6 (IL-6), both known to down-regulate IRS-1 phosphorylation [35]. This is in contrast to a healthy cell in which case insulin binds to its receptor, and causes auto-phosphorylation of the receptors. The phosphorylated receptor then phosphorylates the IRS on the tyrosine residues. The phosphorylated IRS recruits a variety of second messenger proteins, initiating a complex signaling cascade which involves Akt/PKB (protein kinase B) stimulation of glucose uptake into the cell. Insulin sensitivity is thus maintained as a result of enhanced glycogen synthesis, suppression of hepatic gluconeogenesis, increased fatty acid and triglyceride synthesis and suppression of lipolysis in adipose tissue [36]. Cortright et al. [37] found in isolated human skeletal muscles strips and adipocytes that activation of PKC reduced insulin-stimulated glucose uptake; whereas pharmacological inhibition of PKC activity increased insulin-stimulated glucose uptake by 2-fold. This increase was associated with elevated insulin receptor tyrosine phosphorylation of (phosphatidylinositide 3-kinases (PI 3-kinase) activity. Hence, inappropriate activation of PKC may interfere with insulin action by promoting serine/threonine phosphorylation of IRS-1, resulting in prevention of tyrosine phosphorylation of these proteins that is necessary for adequate function on the insulin-signaling pathway [37].

Human research investigating the effects of fructose on insulin sensitivity is limited but the animal literature is more extensive. Specifically, when rats consumed 35% energy as fructose for four weeks, reduced insulin sensitivity associated with impaired hepatic insulin action and whole-body glucose disposal occurred [38]. Although fructose does not increase insulin acutely, the long-term consumption of fructose seems to result in insulin resistance [38,39]. Similarly, rats fed 15% energy from fructose for 15 months displayed elevated fasting serum insulin and glucose concentrations. These results were in conjunction with a more recent animal study in which mice were fed an isocaloric, standard diet; a 60% glucose diet; or a 60% fructose diet for twelve weeks. Glucose disposal was reduced in the fructose fed animals, which resulted in a 1.3-fold lower glucose-stimulated increase in insulin. From these results, and more recent research by Yoo et al [39], a high-fructose diet results in a reduced glucose-stimulated insulin release and impaired glucose disposal [39,40].

In humans, there is limited research confirming the negative effects of fructose on insulin sensitivity and glucose intolerance in adults and adolescents. Sunehag et al. [41] discovered no change in insulin sensitivity or secretion in obese subjects on a high fructose diet, however, the subjects were insulin resistant to start with. In order to maintain substrate homeostasis, normal rates of glucose production, gluconeogenesis, lipolysis and appropriate substrate oxidation, the obese subjects required a more than 2-fold increase in their insulin secretion as compared to what would have been needed had lean adolescents been studied [41]. Similarly, Le et al. [15] found that moderate fructose (1.5 g/kg of body weight) intake for four weeks in seven male subjects induced significant increases in plasma TGs, and VLDL-TG with no change in insulin sensitivity or ectopic fat deposition. The authors speculated that the duration of fructose consumption may need to be longer than 4 weeks in order for the increases in plasma TGs and VLDL-TGs to affect insulin sensitivity [15]. In contrast, Dirlewanger et al. [42] investigated the effects of an acute fructose infusion on hepatic insulin sensitivity during moderate hyperglycemic conditions in ten healthy adults. The infusion with fructose resulted in alterations in endogenous glucose production such that insulin requirements increased 2.3-fold above the two other infusions in order to maintain blood glucose levels [42]. The increased total glucose output indicated that the absolute rate of glucose-6-phosphate hydrolysis and release of free glucose from the liver cells was increased during fructose infusion. Simultaneously, glucose cycling was increased, indicating enhanced reuptake and phosphorylation of glucose by the liver cells. Therefore, an acute fructose infusion induces both extrahepatic and hepatic insulin resistance, with the latter being secondary to an increased intrahepatic glucose 6-phosphate synthesis [42]. Researchers have proposed that the increased hepatic lipid accumulation resulting from fructose-induced DNL would lead to hepatic insulin resistance by increasing levels of DAG. Increases in both DAG and novel PKC are associated with lipid-induced insulin resistance [19,42]. After assessing insulin sensitivity with deuterated glucose disposal prior to and after the 10-week intervention, Stanhope et al. [19] determined that the fructose group had significantly higher fasting insulin and glucose levels as well as increased insulin excursions and endogenous glucose production as compared to the glucose group. Additionally, DNL was significantly higher in the fructose-fed group than the glucose-fed group after the 10-week intervention. These results indicated that hepatic insulin resistance was most likely due to increased DNL from increased DAG and novel PKC [19].

The most commonly proposed mechanism for the fructose-induced insulin resistance appears to be the diminished ability of insulin to suppress hepatic glucose output and decrease insulin receptor density apparent in skeletal muscle and liver [43]. Catena et al. [43] found that insulin receptor number and messenger RNA (mRNA) levels were significantly decreased in skeletal muscle and liver of fructose-fed rats (66% fructose) after two weeks when compared to control rats. These findings suggested that a down-regulation of insulin receptor gene expression is a possible molecular mechanism for insulin resistance. Moreover, abnormalities in insulin action at a post-receptor level in muscles and liver with fructose consumption may also occur, such as decreased phosphorylation of IRS-1 and decreased associated of IRS-1 with PI 3-kinase [44]. This evidence shows that these early steps in insulin signaling are important for insulin's metabolic effect [43,44]. Therefore, it is concluded that the mechanisms behind fructose-induced insulin resistance are possibly due to the combination of various factors such as a reduction in the number of insulin receptors in skeletal muscle and liver as well as decreased phosphorylation, both caused by increased fat production [43–45].

6. Fructose and Inflammation

Tumor necrosis factor (TNF)-α, interleukin (IL)-6 and c-reactive protein (CRP), are important pro-inflammatory cytokines induced by elevated triglyceride concentrations which have been linked to insulin resistance [46]. Increases in postprandial TGs and glucose stimulate the activation of neutrophils, leading to an increase in pro-inflammatory cytokines such as IL-6 and TNF-α [47]. IL-6 leads to increased insulin resistance by blocking the IRS-mediated insulin signaling in hepatocytes and muscle cells causing impaired insulin-stimulated glucose uptake into muscle cells [48]. Although the exact mechanism as to how IL-6 affects IRS receptors is not completely understood, it could involve the activation of tyrosine phosphatase or an interaction between suppressor of cytokine signaling (SOCS) proteins and the insulin receptor itself [49]. One of the primary effects of IL-6 is to induce the production of hepatic CRP, which is a known independent risk factor of cardiovascular disease [46]. CRP is an acute phase reactant inflammatory protein which reflects systemic low-grade inflammation [50]. Elevated levels of IL-6 and CRP levels among individuals with features of the insulin resistance and type 2 diabetes have been apparent [51]. Given IL-6's position in the cytokine cascade as a key mediator of downstream inflammatory processes including activation of coagulation, hepatic release of acute phase reactant proteins, IL-6 may have a potential causal role in metabolic risk factors associated with type 2 diabetes and cardiovascular disease.

Previous studies have shown that increased consumption of fructose results in hyperlipidemia accompanied by insulin resistance and elevated plasma TGs, all leading to increased inflammation [21,52,53]. Specifically, rats fed a diet of 30% fructose for eight weeks experienced increased lipid peroxidation and elevated hepatic TNF-α mRNA expression when compared to all other conditions [53]. Lipid peroxidation led to induction of nitric oxide synthase (NOS) and TNF-α expression in the liver when exposed to high levels of fructose. Moreover, the chronic intake of fructose, and to a lesser extent sucrose, caused significant liver stenosis and increased neutrophil production [53]. Additionally, phosphorylation status of Akt in the liver was altered in mice fed the fructose solution; however, a similar effect of fructose feeding was not found in the TNF-α knockout mice. This implies that TNF-α may be critical in mediating insulin resistance in mice chronically fed fructose [53]. It has been suggested that an induction of TNF-α may suppress the activation of AMP-activated protein kinase (AMPK) in the liver [54]. Kanuri et al. [52] found similar results when wild-type mice or TNF-α knockout mice were fed a 30% fructose solution or tap water for eight weeks. The fructose-fed, wild-type mice had significantly higher TG accumulation, which resulted in a 5-fold increase from baseline values. Moreover, the fructose-fed mice had significantly higher neutrophil infiltration; whereas in the fructose-fed TNF-α knockout mice, the neutrophil infiltration was similar to in the water-fed controls [52]. In the fructose-fed TNF-α knockout mice, hepatic stenosis and neutrophil infiltration was attenuated, which resulted in increased phosphorylation of AMPK and Akt, similar to the water-fed controls. Since phosphorylation status of Akt in the liver was altered in the fructose-fed mice wild-type mice and not the TNF-α knockout mice, it was concluded that TNF-α and its receptor 1 may be critical in mediating insulin resistance in the mice chronically fed fructose [52,55]. In a longer duration study, Sanchez-Lozada et al. [56] investigated whether a drink containing 30% glucose with 30% fructose or 60% sucrose induced fatty liver when compared to rats fed a standard chow diet for 16 weeks [56]. Liver inflammation was induced as a result of elevated TNF-α with both the fructose + glucose diet as well as the sucrose diet when compared to the control group (standard chow). The increases in inflammatory markers significantly correlated with increases TG levels as well [56].

The aforementioned studies [52–56] have indicated that increases in inflammatory markers such as TNF-α can create changes in insulin signaling which can be exacerbated with fructose ingestion. Although there is a lack of direct experimental evidence linking fructose and inflammation, the process of lipid accumulation within the liver may induce a sub-acute inflammatory response that is similar to that seen in obesity-related inflammation within adipocytes. TNF-α, IL-6 and IL-1β, all pro-inflammatory markers, are overproduced in fatty liver and participate in the development of insulin resistance and activate hepatic macrophages called Kupffer cells [57]. Unlike adipose tissue in which macrophages are relatively sparse in a basal state and increase with increased adiposity, the liver is densely populated with Kupffer cells. Toll-like receptor 4 (TLR4) and cluster of differentiation 14 (CD14, receptors on the Kupffer cell that internalize endotoxins activate the transcription of pro-inflammatory cytokines such as TNFα and interleukins [57]. More research needs to be conducted to fully elucidate the impact that fructose has on inflammation.

7. Physical Inactivity and Fructose Consumption

7.1. Physical Inactivity

Physical inactivity and poor cardiovascular fitness has been consistently associated with an increased risk of chronic diseases such as type 2 diabetes and cardiovascular disease [58]. Being physically inactive and/or unfit is associated with many health consequences and is an important component of a comprehensive approach to disease prevention and health promotion [59]. Observational studies have demonstrated that the most unfit individuals are at the greatest risk of chronic diseases and all-cause mortality regardless of their gender, race, ethnic background or weight [60]. Therefore, preventing metabolic risk factors such as coronary artery disease, type 2 diabetes and hyperlipidemia can be accomplished by incorporating moderate activity into a person's daily routine in order to avoid the ill effects of physical inactivity [61,62].

In 1953, Morris et al. [63] determined that workers who were seated most of the day, such as bus drivers and telephonists, were twice as likely to develop cardiovascular disease than workers who stand or are ambulatory most of the work day such as mail carriers. This study was reproduced more recently in 2005 [64] in an epidemiologic study of 73,743 postmenopausal women from the Woman's Health Initiative Study in which those who were inactive had increased risk of cardiovascular disease, and this was reversed with increased physical activity [64]. The Australian Diabetes, Obesity and Lifestyle Study also reported that sitting time and self-reported television viewing was positively correlated with undiagnosed abnormal glucose metabolism [65]. These results persisted after adjustment for sustained and moderate-intensity leisure-time physical activity. A subsequent study from the same Australian cohort found that individuals who reported having participated in the required dose of weekly physical activity (30 min/day, 5 times/week) still had detrimental waist circumference, systolic blood pressure, and 2-hour plasma glucose after correcting for such variables with television viewing time [66]. Clearly, this indicates that focusing on acquiring the recommended dose of exercise is not a strong enough of a stimulant to completely protect the body from physical inactivity the other 23+

h/day. In this same cohort, 1958 adults over the age of 60 years who reported high levels of sedentary behavior, had a greater prevalence of developing metabolic syndrome [67]. This data provides evidence that reducing prolonged overall sitting time may reduce metabolic disturbances. Hence, there is a need for more specific sedentary behavior recommendations and health guidelines for adults in addition to the current recommendations on physical activity [66]. Data from the Medical Expenditure Panel Survey indicated that both physical inactivity and obesity are strongly and independently correlated with diabetes and cardiovascular disease [68]. According to the survey, the likelihood of having diabetes increases with physical inactivity regardless of body mass index (BMI), indicating that it is better to be active than inactive. Hence, both physical inactivity and obesity seem to be independently associated with diabetes and diabetes-related risk factors [68]. Moreover, Healy et al. [61] discovered that adults participating in minimal physical activity had higher glucose concentrations compared to more active individuals, reiterating the findings that physical inactivity alters glucose homeostasis [61].

Not only does prolonged inactivity decrease the opportunity for cumulative energy expenditure resulting from numerous muscle contractions [60], physical inactivity also induces molecular changes. Within six to eight hours of physical inactivity, the suppression of skeletal muscle LPL activity and reduced muscle glucose uptake occur, resulting in elevated plasma TG and reduced high density lipoprotein (HDL)levels [60]. Lipoprotein lipase is an important enzyme involved in the molecular alterations, affecting physical inactivity [69]. LPL is the main enzyme responsible for the breakdown of VLDL-TGs and chylomicrons on the endothelial. LPL also enhances the removal of VLDL by the VLDL receptor and indirectly plays a role in maintaining high levels of plasma HDL cholesterol. Hence, low LPL is associated with blunted plasma TG uptake as well as reduced HDL levels [60]. Local regulation of LPL provides a means of generating a concentrated source of fatty acids as well as other lipoprotein-derived lipids [69]. Moreover, LPL is involved in the regulation of gene expression of inflammatory markers which lead to cardiovascular disease [69]. Because physical inactivity regulates LPL activity in the vasculature and skeletal muscle, reduced physical activity can decrease LPL activity 10–20 fold [62]. However, such decreases can be reversed within several hours of ambulatory contractions, implying that a reduction in contractile activity is a potent physiological factor determining LPL activity [69]. Lipoprotein lipase response to physical inactivity and plasma lipid in the microvasculature of skeletal muscle can best be described by first understanding the mechanisms behind the LPL response during ambulation [70]. During ambulation, the vascular endothelial cells are at the interface with plasma TG and fatty acids bound to albumin. During standing or ambulation, there is high LPL activity in the microvasculature of the skeletal muscle. Physically active muscles have greater rates of TG-derived fatty acid uptake, albumin-bound fatty acid transport, fatty acid oxidation, and intracellular TG synthesis. Moreover, there are reduced concentrations of intramuscular fatty acids and fatty acetyl-CoA [70]. In contrast, during inactivity when normal metabolic processes have slowed down, there is a removal of the local energy demands of physical activity, leading to an elevation in TGs and fatty acids. Plasma fatty acids and TGs accumulate as a result of a lower rate of LPL-induced fatty acid oxidation.

Regulation of LPL activity may be different during states of inactivity versus activity [62]. Normally, high activity of LPL in oxidative muscle significantly decreases with physical inactivity and increased physical activity restores such effects. In conjunction with the changes seen with LPL, the uptake of TGs and high density lipoprotein cholesterol decreases with physical inactivity. Therefore, the steps involved in muscle LPL regulation, which are sensitive to inactivity, can be prevented and even reversed with minimal, non-fatiguing contractions (ex: slow treadmill walking) [62]. Zderic and Hamilton [69] found that inactivity causes a 47% decrease in LPL activity within eight hours and an additional 13% after 12 h of inactivity. Moreover, plasma TG concentrations increase after twelve hours, resulting in significant decreases in LPL activity [69]. They too concluded that decreased physical activity depresses LPL activity and that increased fat intake with ambulation suppresses LPL activity, similar to that of inactivity. These results parallel the previously stated concept that there is an inverse relationship between TG concentrations and LPL activity and that decreased activity amplifies the response.

In the Studies of Targeted Risk Reduction Intervention through Defined Exercise (STRIDDE), the researchers investigated whether the training-induced benefits in serum lipids and lipoproteins are sustained over five and/or fifteen days of exercise detraining [71]. Subjects were randomized into one of four groups: (1) high amount/vigorous intensity (caloric equivalent to approximately 20 minutes per week at 65–80% peak oxygen consumption; (2) low amount/vigorous intensity equivalent to approximately 12 m per week at 65% to 80% peak oxygen consumption; and (3) low amount/moderate intensity with a caloric equivalent of approximately 12 m per week at 40–55% peak oxygen consumption and (4) a control non-exercising group for six months. The modest-intensity training group reduced total TGs and VLDL-TG at 24-h post-exercise training by twice the magnitude of the two more vigorous exercise-training groups. In the two vigorous-intensity training groups, total TGs and VLDL-TGs had returned to baseline after only 5 days, indicating that there was no sustained TG-lowering effect in those two groups. While the mechanisms for the aforementioned effects were unclear, the authors speculated that exercise of different intensities may have tissue-specific effects on the LPL bound to the endothelial cells, resulting in differential effects of exercise of varying intensities on TG, VLDL and HDL metabolism [71]. Subsequently, endurance athletes are also not protected from physical in activity. Herd et al. [72] put endurance-trained subjects on a detraining program and discovered that within 60 h after the last training session, the runners' lipidemic response to a fat load was 37% higher than baseline, and 46% higher after 9 days of detraining. These changes correlated with a reciprocal decrease in LPL activity [72]. This data supported the previous hypothesis that hydrolysis at the endothelial surface of capillaries by LPL is the rate-limiting step in TG clearance, and changes in LPL activity with changes in exercise or training status are most likely the cause of the above findings [72].

As seen in the previous research, physical inactivity creates a significant deleterious metabolic state in which insulin sensitivity is decreased within a few hours of detraining. Physical activity improves insulin sensitivity both acutely and chronically as a result of changes in insulin signaling. This process is not mediated by the insulin-dependent rapid phosphorylation of the insulin receptors [69,73,74]. In contrast, exercise stimulates an insulin-independent pathway. With muscle contraction, glucose uptake is mediated by multiple signaling pathways such as protein kinase-C, Ca^{+2}/calmodulin-dependent protein kinase (CaMKK) and AMPK [69]. The translocation of glucose receptors (GLUT 4) to the cell membrane occur because of increased Akt activity and phosphorylation within the cell [75]. This effect is short-lived, lasting 48–72 h; therefore, to maximize the benefits of physical activity on insulin sensitivity exercise should be repeated within this timeframe.

7.2. Physical Activity and Inflammation

Although exercise causes an acute inflammatory response [76], physical activity and improved cardiovascular fitness decreases low-grade inflammation by decreasing body fat, decreasing chronic production of pro-inflammatory cytokines and increasing production of anti-inflammatory cytokines. Moreover, exercise reduces expression of adhesion molecules, up-regulates antioxidant and other cellular defenses and improves endothelial function [77]. Although low-grade inflammation, characteristic of elevated IL-6 levels, has been associated with obesity and insulin resistance, it is markedly produced and released after an acute bout of exercise. However, IL-6 may actually help to prevent or reduce risk factors associated with metabolic syndrome and type 2 diabetes in the long-term [75]. During exercise, the magnitude of the increase in IL-6 is relative to the duration, intensity of exercise and amount of muscle mass involved. Muscle biopsies from humans and rats have demonstrated increases in IL-6 after exercise up to 100 times that of resting values [78]. In response to muscle contraction, both type I and type II muscle fibers express IL-6, which exerts its effects both locally and peripherally in several organs of the body when released into circulation. IL-6 may also work in an endocrine manner to increase hepatic glucose production during exercise or during lipolysis in adipose tissue [79]. The anti-inflammatory effects of IL-6 have been demonstrated by the ability of IL-6 to stimulate the release of classical anti-inflammatory cytokines such as IL-1ra (receptor antagonist) and IL-10 [78]. Hence, IL-6 has both pro- and anti-inflammatory properties. When IL-6 is signaling monocytes or macrophages, the activation of nuclear factor (NF-κB) and TNF-α occurs, leading to an inflammatory state but when IL-6 is released from muscle, it creates an anti-inflammatory state [75]. Therefore, the possibility exists that the long-term effect of exercise may be a result of the anti-inflammatory process of an acute bout of exercise. For that reason, acute exercise will protect against chronic systemic low-grade inflammation, and thereby offer protection against insulin resistance and atherosclerosis.

7.3. Fructose Ingestion and Physical Activity

For athletes, fructose provides a beneficial aid in training due to its ability to stimulate rapid nutrient absorption in the small intestine and help increase exogenous carbohydrate oxidation during exercise [6]. When fructose is mixed with glucose in sports drinks, carbohydrate oxidation is enhanced by 40%. This dramatic increase in oxidation can be explained by the different transport systems used for intestinal absorption. Moreover, fructose has been shown to reduce the perception of fatigue and stress during exercise, and improve exercise performance during cycling exercises [80].

Although fructose consumption may pose an advantage in an athletic environment, it does not seem to be warranted for the general public. To date, there are only two reports of fructose and physical activity. Botezelli et al. [27] studied 48 Wister rats to determine whether aerobic exercise alters markers of fatty liver disease when fed a diet high in fructose. Thirty days of aerobic exercise resulted in the fructose-fed rats having altered metabolic profiles which included elevated plasma TG as a result of the fructose diet. However, they had improved insulin sensitivity and decreased cholesterol levels, resulting from the exercise regimen. The changes in TG levels were most likely due to the improved lipid oxidation and availability of circulation TG as a result of exercise [27]. In a more recent study in young, healthy individuals, consumption of an additional 75 g of fructose per day in conjunction with physical inactivity (~4200 steps/day) resulted in increased postprandial lipidemia and precursors to low-grade inflammation, whereas when physical activity was increased to ~12,000 steps/day, these effects were ameliorated [81]. Hence, increased physical activity may improve features of fructose-induced metabolic syndrome. More studies on humans still need to be conducted to determine the interaction between fructose consumption and physical activity, however, preliminary research indicates that increasing ones' physical activity may counteract the adverse effects of a fructose-rich diet.

8. Conclusions

Although it seems apparent that increased intake of fructose leads to various risk factors associated with metabolic syndrome such as hypertension, hyperlipidemia, insulin resistance, inflammation and hyperuricemia, there is still numerous contradictory evidence which states that as long as fructose is consumed in moderate doses, fructose may not augment these risk factors. The quantities of fructose administered in many of the studies used concentrations that were well above the average fructose intake of 60–70 g/day, and with increased daily caloric intake, which may have differing results. Hence, there is a need for future research investigating the effects of fructose when using quantities that more closely match that of the average population. Moreover, there is very limited research indicating how physical inactivity may confound these risks. Although fructose consumption cannot be completely to blame for the increased rates of obesity and metabolic syndrome, fructose is often associated with additional detrimental behaviors such as a hypercaloric diet, or a diet rich in saturated fats, as well as low physical activity [6]. These behaviors lead to risk factors of metabolic syndrome, and as such could be prevented and/or reduced.

The above review of literature summarizes the proposed mechanisms associated with the fructose-induced metabolic alterations related to metabolic syndrome. These risk factors, such as postprandial hyperlipidemia, insulin resistance, and hyperuricemia, seem to be exacerbated with fructose ingestion in a dose-dependent manner; hence continued research must be conducted to completely elucidate the importance of decreasing fructose consumption. Specifically, this includes research into whether ingesting large amounts of fructose, with an ab libitum diet, will cause changes in circulation LPL concentrations. Furthermore, compounding the increased fructose consumption with a sedentary lifestyle may be exacerbating the fructose-induced metabolic disturbances, therefore, more research should be conducted to determine whether increasing physical activity will improve LPL activity in a fructose-fed individual. Although there is still too little data to suggest, at this point, that increased physical activity can attenuate these metabolic disturbances, increasing one's physical activity, regardless of the amount of structured exercise that is performed, should be a national priority, as the minimal amount of research regarding fructose and physical activity is positive.

Conflicts of Interest: The author declare no conflict of interest.

References

1. U.S. Department of Health and Human Services. National Institute of Diabetes and Digestive and Kidney Diseases (NIDDK). Overweight and Obesity Statistics. Updated October 2012. Available online: https://www.niddk.nih.gov/health-information/health-statistics/overweight-obesity (accessed on 4 April 2017).
2. Elliott, S.S.; Keim, N.L.; Stern, J.S.; Teff, K.; Havel, P.J. Fructose, weight gain, and the insulin resistance syndrome. *Am. J. Clin. Nutr.* **2002**, *76*, 911–922. [PubMed]
3. Mayes, P.A. Intermediary metabolism of fructose. *Am. J. Clin. Nutr.* **1993**, *58*, 754S–765S. [PubMed]
4. Miller, A.; Adeli, K. Dietary fructose and the metabolic syndrome. *Curr. Opin. Gastroenterol.* **2008**, *24*, 204–209. [CrossRef] [PubMed]
5. Malik, V.; Hu, F. Fructose and cardiometabolic health. What the Evidence from sugar-sweetened Beverages Tells Us. *J. Am. Coll. Cardiol.* **2015**, *66*, 1615–1624. [CrossRef] [PubMed]
6. Tappy, L.; Le, K.A. Metabolic effects of fructose and the worldwide increase in obesity. *Physiol. Rev.* **2010**, *90*, 23–46. [CrossRef] [PubMed]
7. Douard, V.; Ferraris, R. Regulation of the fructose transporter GLUT5 in health and disease. *Am. J. Physiol. Endocrinol. Metab.* **2008**, *295*, E227–E237. [CrossRef] [PubMed]
8. Kneepkens, C.M.; Vonk, R.J.; Fernandes, J. Incomplete intestinal absorption of fructose. *Arch. Dis Child.* **1984**, *59*, 735–738. [CrossRef] [PubMed]
9. Ushijima, K.; Riby, J.E.; Fujisawa, T.; Kretchmer, N. Absorption of fructose by isolated small intestine of rats is via a specific saturable carrier in the absence of glucose and by the disaccharidase-related transport system in the presence of glucose. *J. Nutr.* **1995**, *125*, 2156–2164. [PubMed]
10. Truswell, A.S.; Seach, J.M.; Thorburn, A.W. Incomplete absorption of pure fructose in healthy subjects and the facilitating effect of glucose. *Am. J. Clin. Nutr.* **1988**, *48*, 1424–1430. [PubMed]
11. Haidari, M.; Leung, N.; Mahbub, F.; Uffelman, K.D.; Kohen-Avramoglu, R.; Lewis, G.F.; Adeli, K. Fasting and postprandial overproduction of intestinally derived lipoproteins in an animal model of insulin resistance. Evidence that chronic fructose feeding in the hamster is accompanied by enhanced intestinal de novo lipogenesis and ApoB48-containing lipoprotein overproduction. *J. Biol. Chem.* **2002**, *277*, 31646–31655. [PubMed]
12. Havel, P.J. Dietary fructose: Implications for dysregulation of energy homeostasis and lipid/carbohydrate metabolism. *Nutr. Rev.* **2005**, *63*, 133–157. [CrossRef] [PubMed]
13. Le, K.A.; Tappy, L. Metabolic effects of fructose. *Curr. Opin. Clin. Nutr. Metab. Care* **2006**, *9*, 469–475. [CrossRef] [PubMed]
14. Carmona, A.; Freedland, R.A. Comparison among the lipogenic potential of various substrates in rat hepatocytes: The differential effects of fructose-containing diets on hepatic lipogenesis. *J. Nutr.* **1989**, *119*, 1304–1310. [PubMed]
15. Lê, K.A.; Faeh, D.; Stettler, R.; Ith, M.; Kreis, R.; Vermathen, P.; Boesch, C.; Ravussin, E.; Tappy, L. A 4-wk high-fructose diet alters lipid metabolism without affecting insulin sensitivity or ectopic lipids in healthy humans. *Am. J. Clin. Nutr.* **2006**, *84*, 1374–1379. [PubMed]
16. Dai, S.; Todd, M.E.; Lee, S.; McNeill, J.H. Fructose loading induces cardiovascular and metabolic changes in non-diabetic and diabetic rats. *Can. J. Physiol. Pharmacol.* **1994**, *72*, 771–781. [CrossRef] [PubMed]
17. Luo, J.; Rizkalla, S.W.; Lerer-Metzger, M.; Boillot, J. A fructose-rich diet decreases insulin-stimulated glucose incorporation into lipids but not glucose transport in adipocytes of normal and diabetic rats. *J. Nutr.* **1995**, *125*, 164–171. [PubMed]

18. Swarbrick, M.M.; Stanhope, K.L.; Elliott, S.S.; Graham, J.L.; Krauss, R.M.; Christiansen, M.P.; Griffen, S.C.; Keim, N.L.; Havel, P.J. Consumption of fructose-sweetened beverages for 10 weeks increases postprandial triacylglycerol and apolipoprotein-B concentrations in overweight and obese women. *Br. J. Nutr.* **2008**, *100*, 947–952. [CrossRef] [PubMed]

19. Stanhope, K.L.; Schwarz, J.M.; Keim, N.L.; Griffen, S.C.; Bremer, A.A.; Graham, J.L.; Hatcher, B.; Cox, C.L.; Dyachenko, A.; Zhang, W.; et al. Consuming fructose-sweetened, not glucose-sweetened, beverages increases visceral adiposity and lipids and decreases insulin sensitivity in overweight/obese humans. *J. Clin. Investig.* **2009**, *119*, 1322–1334. [CrossRef] [PubMed]

20. Parks, E.J.; Skokan, L.E.; Timlin, M.T.; Dingfelder, C.S. Dietary sugars stimulate fatty acid synthesis in adults. *J. Nutr.* **2008**, *138*, 1039–1046. [PubMed]

21. Faeh, D.; Minehira, K.; Schwarz, J.M.; Periasamy, R.; Park, S.; Tappy, L. Effect of fructose overfeeding and fish oil administration on hepatic de novo lipogenesis and insulin sensitivity in healthy men. *Diabetes* **2005**, *54*, 1907–1913. [CrossRef] [PubMed]

22. Swanson, J.E.; Laine, D.C.; Thomas, W.; Bantle, J.P. Metabolic effects of dietary fructose in healthy subjects. *Am. J. Clin. Nutr.* **1992**, *55*, 851–856. [PubMed]

23. Bantle, J.P.; Raatz, S.K.; Thomas, W.; Georgopoulos, A. Effects of dietary fructose on plasma lipids in healthy subjects. *Am. J. Clin. Nutr.* **2000**, *72*, 1128–1134. [PubMed]

24. Schwarz, J.; Noworolski, S.; Wen, M.; Dyachenko, A.; Prior, J.; Weinberg, M.; Herraiz, L.; Tai, V.; Bergeron, N.; Bersot, T.; et al. Effect of a High-Fructose Weight-Maintaining Diet on Lipogenesis and Liver Fat. *J. Clin. Endocrinol. Metab.* **2015**, *100*, 2434–2442. [CrossRef] [PubMed]

25. Abdel-Sayed, A.; Binnert, C.; Le, K.A.; Bortolotti, M.; Schneiter, P.; Tappy, L. A high-fructose diet impairs basal and stress-mediated lipid metabolism in healthy male subjects. *Br. J. Nutr.* **2008**, *100*, 393–399. [CrossRef] [PubMed]

26. Kannel, W.B.; Vasan, R.S. Triglycerides as vascular risk factors: New epidemiologic insights. *Curr. Opin. Cardiol.* **2009**, *24*, 345–350. [CrossRef] [PubMed]

27. Alipour, A.; Elte, J.W.; van Zaanen, H.C.; Rietveld, A.P.; Cabezas, M.C. Postprandial inflammation and endothelial dysfuction. *Biochem. Soc. Trans.* **2007**, *35*, 466–469. [CrossRef] [PubMed]

28. Chong, M.F.; Fielding, B.A.; Frayn, K.N. Mechanisms for the acute effect of fructose on postprandial lipemia. *Am. J. Clin. Nutr.* **2007**, *85*, 1511–1520. [PubMed]

29. Chang, Y.C.; Chuang, L.M. The role of oxidative stress in the pathogenesis of type 2 diabetes: From molecular mechanism to clinical implication. *Am. J. Transl. Res.* **2010**, *2*, 316–331. [PubMed]

30. Rutledge, A.C.; Adeli, K. Fructose and the metabolic syndrome: Pathophysiology and molecular mechanisms. *Nutr. Rev.* **2007**, *65*, S13–S23. [CrossRef] [PubMed]

31. Rebrin, K.; Steil, G.M.; Getty, L.; Bergman, R.N. Free fatty acid as a link in the regulation of hepatic glucose output by peripheral insulin. *Diabetes* **1995**, *44*, 1038–1045. [CrossRef] [PubMed]

32. LDL Cholesterol. New measurements of risk. *Mayo Clin. Health Lett.* **2011**, *29*, 1–3.

33. Pagliassotti, M.J.; Prach, P.A. Quantity of sucrose alters the tissue pattern and time course of insulin resistance in young rats. *Am. J. Physiol.* **1995**, *269*, R641–R646. [PubMed]

34. Morino, K.; Petersen, K.F.; Shulman, G.I. Molecular mechanisms of insulin resistance in humans and their potential links with mitochondrial dysfunction. *Diabetes* **2006**, *55*, S9–S15. [CrossRef] [PubMed]

35. Delarue, J.; Magnan, C. Free fatty acids and insulin resistance. *Curr. Opin. Clin. Nutr. Metab. Care* **2007**, *10*, 142–148. [CrossRef] [PubMed]

36. Saltiel, A.R.; Kahn, C.R. Insulin signaling and the regulation of glucose and lipid metabolism. *Nature* **2001**, *414*, 799–806. [CrossRef] [PubMed]

37. Cortright, R.N.; Azevedo, J.L., Jr.; Zhou, Q.; Sinha, M.; Pories, W.J.; Itani, S.I.; Dohm, G.L. Protein kinase C modulates insulin action in human skeletal muscle. *Am. J. Physiol. Endocrinol. Metab.* **2000**, *278*, E553–E562. [PubMed]

38. Thorburn, A.W.; Storlien, L.H.; Jenkins, A.B.; Khouri, S.; Kraegen, E.W. Fructose-induced in vivo insulin resistance and elevated plasma triglyceride levels in rats. *Am. J. Clin. Nutr.* **1989**, *49*, 1155–1163. [PubMed]

39. Yoo, S.; Ahn, H.; Park, Y.K. High Dietary Fructose Intake on Cardiovascular Disease Related Parameters in Growing Rats. *Nutrients* **2017**, *9*, 11. [CrossRef] [PubMed]

40. Huang, D.; Dhawan, T.; Young, S.; Yong, W.H.; Boros, L.G.; Heaney, A.P. Fructose impairs glucose-induced hepatic triglyceride synthesis. *Lipids Health Dis.* **2011**, *10*. [CrossRef] [PubMed]

41. Sunehag, A.L.; Toffolo, G.; Campioni, M.; Bier, D.M.; Haymond, M.W. Short-term high dietary fructose intake had no effects on insulin sensitivity and secretion or glucose and lipid metabolism in healthy, obese adolescents. *J. Pediatr. Endocrinol. Metab.* **2008**, *21*, 225–235. [CrossRef] [PubMed]

42. Dirlewanger, M.; Schneiter, P.; Jequier, E.; Tappy, L. Effects of fructose on hepatic glucose metabolism in humans. *Am. J. Physiol. Endocrinol. Metab.* **2000**, *279*, E907–E911. [PubMed]

43. Catena, C.; Giacchetti, G.; Novello, M.; Colussi, G.; Cavarape, A.; Sechi, L.A. Cellular mechanisms of insulin resistance in rats with fructose-induced hypertension. *Am. J. Hypertens.* **2003**, *16*, 973–978. [CrossRef]

44. Ueno, M.; Bezerra, R.M.; Silva, M.S.; Tavares, D.Q.; Carvalho, C.R.; Saad, M.J. A high-fructose diet induces changes in pp185 phosphorylation in muscle and liver of rats. *Braz. J. Med. Biol. Res.* **2000**, *33*, 1421–1427. [CrossRef] [PubMed]

45. Dupas, J.; Goanvec, C.; Guernec, A.; Feray, A.; Goanvec, C.; Samson, N.; Bougaran, P.; Guerrero, F.; Mansourati, J. Metabolic Syndrome and Hypertension Resulting from Fructose Enriched Diet in Wistar Rats. *Biomed. Res. Int.* **2017**, *2017*, 1–10. [CrossRef] [PubMed]

46. Hotamisligil, G.S.; Shargill, N.S.; Spiegelman, B.M. Adipose expression of tumor necrosis factor-alpha: Direct role in obesity-linked insulin resistance. *Science* **1993**, *259*, 87–91. [CrossRef] [PubMed]

47. Alipour, A.; van Oostrom, A.J.; Izraeljan, A.; Verseyden, C.; Collins, J.M.; Frayn, K.N.; Plokker, T.W.M.; Elte, J.W.F.; Cabezas, M.C. Leukocyte activation by triglyceride-rich lipoproteins. *Arterioscler. Thromb. Vasc. Biol.* **2008**, *28*, 792–797. [CrossRef] [PubMed]

48. Zeyda, M.; Stulnig, T.M. Obesity, inflammation, and insulin resistance—A mini-review. *Gerontology* **2009**, *55*, 379–386. [CrossRef] [PubMed]

49. Bastard, J.P.; Maachi, M.; Lagathu, C.; Kim, M.J.; Caron, M.; Vidal, H.; Capeau, J.; Feve, B. Recent advances in the relationship between obesity, inflammation, and insulin resistance. *Eur. Cytokine Netw.* **2006**, *17*, 4–12. [PubMed]

50. Pradhan, A.D.; Ridker, P.M. Do atherosclerosis and type 2 diabetes share a common inflammatory basis? *Eur. Heart J.* **2002**, *23*, 831–834. [CrossRef] [PubMed]

51. Pickup, J.C.; Mattock, M.B.; Chusney, G.D.; Burt, D. NIDDM as a disease of the innate immune system: Association of acute-phase reactants and interleukin-6 with metabolic syndrome X. *Diabetologia* **1997**, *40*, 1286–1292. [CrossRef] [PubMed]

52. Kanuri, G.; Spruss, A.; Wagnerberger, S.; Bischoff, S.C.; Bergheim, I. Role of tumor necrosis factor alpha (TNFalpha) in the onset of fructose-induced nonalcoholic fatty liver disease in mice. *J. Nutr. Biochem.* **2011**, *22*, 527–534. [CrossRef] [PubMed]

53. Bergheim, I.; Weber, S.; Vos, M.; Krämer, S.; Volynets, V.; Kaserouni, S.; McClain, C.J.; Bischoff, S.C. Antibiotics protect against fructose-induced hepatic lipid accumulation in mice: Role of endotoxin. *J. Hepatol.* **2008**, *48*, 983–992. [CrossRef] [PubMed]

54. Shimano, H. SREBP-1c and TFE3, energy transcription factors that regulate hepatic insulin signaling. *J. Mol. Med.* **2007**, *85*, 437–444. [CrossRef] [PubMed]

55. Spruss, A.; Kanuri, G.; Wagnerberger, S.; Haub, S.; Bischoff, S.C.; Bergheim, I. Toll-like receptor 4 is involved in the development of fructose-induced hepatic steatosis in mice. *Hepatology* **2009**, *50*, 1094–1104. [CrossRef] [PubMed]

56. Sánchez-Lozada, L.G.; Mu, W.; Roncal, C.; Sautin, Y.Y.; Abdelmalek, M.; Reungjui, S.; Le, M.; Nakagawa, T.; Lan, H.Y.; Yu, X.; et al. Comparison of free fructose and glucose to sucrose in the ability to cause fatty liver. *Eur. J. Nutr.* **2010**, *49*, 1–9. [CrossRef] [PubMed]

57. Shoelson, S.E.; Lee, J.; Goldfine, A.B. Inflammation and insulin resistance. *J. Clin. Investig.* **2006**, *116*, 1793–1801. [CrossRef] [PubMed]

58. Lakka, T.A.; Laaksonen, D.E.; Lakka, H.M.; Männikkö, N.I.K.O.; Niskanen, L.K.; Rauramaa, R.A.I.N.E.R.; Salonen, J.T. Sedentary lifestyle, poor cardiorespiratory fitness, and the metabolic syndrome. *Med. Sci. Sports Exerc.* **2003**, *35*, 1279–1286. [CrossRef] [PubMed]

59. Haskell, W.L.; Lee, I.M.; Pate, R.R.; Powell, K.E.; Blair, S.N.; Franklin, B.A.; Macera, C.A.; Heatg, G.W.; Thompson, P.D.; Bauman, A. Physical activity and public health: Updated recommendation for adults from the American College of Sports Medicine and the American Heart Association. *Med. Sci. Sports Exerc.* **2007**, *39*, 1423–1434. [CrossRef] [PubMed]

60. Hamilton, M.T.; Hamilton, D.G.; Zderic, T.W. Role of low energy expenditure and sitting in obesity, metabolic syndrome, type 2 diabetes, and cardiovascular disease. *Diabetes* **2007**, *56*, 2655–2667. [CrossRef] [PubMed]

61. Healy, G.N.; Dunstan, D.W.; Salmon, J.; Cerin, E.; Shaw, J.E.; Zimmet, P.Z.; Owen, N. Objectively measured light-intensity physical activity is independently associated with 2-h plasma glucose. *Diabetes Care* **2007**, *30*, 1384–1389. [CrossRef] [PubMed]

62. Bey, L.; Hamilton, M.T. Suppression of skeletal muscle lipoprotein lipase activity during physical inactivity: A molecular reason to maintain daily low-intensity activity. *J. Physiol.* **2003**, *551*, 673–682. [CrossRef] [PubMed]

63. Morris, J.N.; Heady, J.A.; Raffle, P.A.; Roberts, C.G.; Parks, J.W. Coronary heart-disease and physical activity of work. *Lancet* **1953**, *265*, 1111–1120. [CrossRef]

64. Hsia, J.; Wu, L.; Allen, C.; Oberman, A.; Lawson, W.E.; Torréns, J.; Safford, M.; Limacher, M.C. Physical activity and diabetes risk in postmenopausal women. *Am. J. Prev. Med.* **2005**, *28*, 19–25. [CrossRef] [PubMed]

65. Wijndaele, K.; Healy, G.N.; Dunstan, D.W.; Barnett, A.G.; Salmon, J.; Shaw, J.E.; Zimmet, P.Z.; Owen, N. Increased cardiometabolic risk is associated with increased TV viewing time. *Med. Sci. Sports Exerc.* **2010**, *42*, 1511–1518. [CrossRef] [PubMed]

66. Healy, G.N.; Dunstan, D.W.; Salmon, J.; Shaw, J.E.; Zimmet, P.Z.; Owen, N. Television time and continuous metabolic risk in physically active adults. *Med. Sci. Sports Exerc.* **2008**, *40*, 639–645. [CrossRef] [PubMed]

67. Gardiner, P.A.; Healy, G.N.; Eakin, E.G.; Clark, B.K.; Dunstan, D.W.; Shaw, J.E.; Zimmet, P.Z.; Owen, N. Associations between television viewing time and overall sitting time with the metabolic syndrome in older men and women: The Australian diabetes, obesity and lifestyle study. *J. Am. Geriatr. Soc.* **2011**, *59*, 788–796. [CrossRef] [PubMed]

68. Sullivan, P.W.; Morrato, E.H.; Ghushchyan, V.; Wyatt, H.R.; Hill, J.O. Obesity, inactivity, and the prevalence of diabetes and diabetes-related cardiovascular comorbidities in the U.S., 2000–2002. *Diabetes Care* **2005**, *28*, 1599–1603. [CrossRef] [PubMed]

69. Zderic, T.W.; Hamilton, M.T. Physical inactivity amplifies the sensitivity of skeletal muscle to the lipid-induced downregulation of lipoprotein lipase activity. *J. Appl. Physiol.* **2006**, *100*, 249–257. [CrossRef] [PubMed]

70. Peterson, J.; Bihain, B.E.; Bengtsson-Olivecrona, G.; Deckelbaum, R.J.; Carpentier, Y.A.; Olivecrona, T. Fatty acid control of lipoprotein lipase: A link between energy metabolism and lipid transport. *Proc. Natl. Acad. Sci. USA* **1990**, *87*, 909–913. [CrossRef] [PubMed]

71. Slentz, C.A.; Houmard, J.A.; Johnson, J.L.; Bateman, L.A.; Tanner, C.J.; McCartney, J.S.; Duscha, B.D.; Kraus, W.E. Inactivity, exercise training and detraining, and plasma lipoproteins. STRRIDE: A randomized, controlled study of exercise intensity and amount. *J. Appl. Physiol.* **2007**, *103*, 432–442. [CrossRef] [PubMed]

72. Herd, S.L.; Hardman, A.E.; Boobis, L.H.; Cairns, C.J. The effect of 13 weeks of running training followed by 9 d of detraining on postprandial lipaemia. *Br. J. Nutr.* **1998**, *80*, 57–66. [CrossRef] [PubMed]

73. Rockl, K.S.; Witczak, C.A.; Goodyear, L.J. Signaling mechanisms in skeletal muscle: Acute responses and chronic adaptations to exercise. *IUBMB Life* **2008**, *60*, 145–153. [CrossRef] [PubMed]

74. Jessen, N.; Goodyear, L.J. Contraction signaling to glucose transport in skeletal muscle. *J. Appl. Physiol.* **2005**, *99*, 330–337. [CrossRef] [PubMed]

75. Brandt, C.; Pedersen, B.K. The role of exercise-induced myokines in muscle homeostasis and the defense against chronic diseases. *J. Biomed. Biotechnol.* **2010**, *2010*. [CrossRef] [PubMed]

76. Vider, J.; Laaksonen, D.E.; Kilk, A.; Atalay, M.; Lehtmaa, J.; Zilmer, M.; Sen, C.K. Physical exercise induces activation of NF-kappaB in human peripheral blood lymphocytes. *Antioxid. Redox Signal.* **2001**, *3*, 1131–1137. [CrossRef] [PubMed]

77. Lakka, T.A.; Laaksonen, D.E. Physical activity in prevention and treatment of the metabolic syndrome. *Appl. Physiol. Nutr. Metab.* **2007**, *32*, 76–88. [CrossRef] [PubMed]

78. Pedersen, B.K.; Steensberg, A.; Fischer, C.; Keller, C.; Keller, P.; Plomgaard, P.; Febbraio, M.; Saltin, B. Searching for the exercise factor: Is IL-6 a candidate? *J. Muscle Res. Cell. Motil.* **2003**, *24*, 113–119. [CrossRef] [PubMed]

79. Pedersen, B.K.; Febbraio, M.A. Muscle as an endocrine organ: Focus on muscle-derived interleukin-6. *Physiol. Rev.* **2008**, *88*, 1379–1406. [CrossRef] [PubMed]

80. Currell, K.; Jeukendrup, A.E. Superior endurance performance with ingestion of multiple transportable carbohydrates. *Med. Sci. Sports Exerc.* **2008**, *40*, 275–281. [CrossRef] [PubMed]

81. Bidwell, A.J.; Fairchild, T.J.; Redmond, J.; Wang, L.; Keslacy, S.; Kanaley, J.A. Physical Activity Offsets the Negative Effects of a High Fructose Diet. *Med. Sci. Sports Exerc.* **2014**, *46*, 2091–2098. [CrossRef] [PubMed]

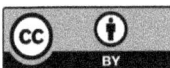

nutrients

MDPI

Review

Sugar Metabolism in Hummingbirds and Nectar Bats

Raul K. Suarez [1],* and Kenneth C. Welch Jr. [2]

1   Department of Zoology, University of British Columbia, #4200-6270 University Blvd., Vancouver,
    BC V6T 1Z4, Canada
2   Department of Biological Sciences, University of Toronto, 1265 Military Trail, Scarborough,
    ON M1C 1A4, Canada; kwelch@utsc.utoronto.ca
*   Correspondence: rksuarez@zoology.ubc.ca; Tel.: +1-604-961-8153

Received: 22 April 2017; Accepted: 4 July 2017; Published: 12 July 2017

Abstract: Hummingbirds and nectar bats coevolved with the plants they visit to feed on floral nectars rich in sugars. The extremely high metabolic costs imposed by small size and hovering flight in combination with reliance upon sugars as their main source of dietary calories resulted in convergent evolution of a suite of structural and functional traits. These allow high rates of aerobic energy metabolism in the flight muscles, fueled almost entirely by the oxidation of dietary sugars, during flight. High intestinal sucrase activities enable high rates of sucrose hydrolysis. Intestinal absorption of glucose and fructose occurs mainly through a paracellular pathway. In the fasted state, energy metabolism during flight relies on the oxidation of fat synthesized from previously-ingested sugar. During repeated bouts of hover-feeding, the enhanced digestive capacities, in combination with high capacities for sugar transport and oxidation in the flight muscles, allow the operation of the "sugar oxidation cascade", the pathway by which dietary sugars are directly oxidized by flight muscles during exercise. It is suggested that the potentially harmful effects of nectar diets are prevented by locomotory exercise, just as in human hunter-gatherers who consume large quantities of honey.

Keywords: sugar; glucose transport; hexokinase; metabolism; muscle; energetics; evolution; foraging behavior

1. Introduction

Hummingbirds and nectar bats became nectarivorous animals in a process that involved coevolution with the flowering plants offering them nectar [1]. As their diets, foraging and feeding modes evolved, so did the suite of morphological, physiological and biochemical traits that made them adapted for "aerial refueling" [2–4]. Hummingbirds rely mainly on the sugars in floral nectar to fuel their high metabolic rates [5]. Perhaps less widely known is that nectar bats also derive most of their dietary calories from sugars [4]. Some nectar bat species can hover while feeding [6], behaving as "hummingbirds of the night". The features allowing hover-feeding in hummingbirds and nectar bats are remarkable examples of convergent evolution. This review serves as a primer on their sugar metabolism. As such, the intention is not a comprehensive review of the literature but, rather, a more focused introduction to aspects of their sugar metabolism, particularly in relation to exercise, presented in an evolutionary and ecological framework. Most of the discussion shall be based on data obtained from hummingbird species of between 3 to 5 g in body mass and from 10 g Pallas' long-tongued nectar bats (*Glossophaga soricina*). The findings summarized here offer opportunities for comparison with *Homo sapiens*, a species that is unable to rely to the same extent on the direct oxidation of dietary sugar to fuel exercise and that suffers from the adverse effects of excessive sugar ingestion.

2. Diet and Digestion

The flowering plants visited by hummingbirds and nectar bats evolved as "prey that want to be eaten" [7,8] that benefit from the pollination services provided by these animals in exchange for the sugars they produce. In the course of their coevolution with flowering plants, three major groups of birds (hummingbirds, honeyeaters and sunbirds) [9] and two groups of phyllostomid bats (Lonchophyllinae and Glossophaginae) [10] adopted nectarivorous diets. While frugivorous birds generally ingest fruits rich in glucose and fructose, but not in sucrose [11], hummingbirds preferentially ingest sucrose-rich nectars that contain less glucose and fructose [8]. Nectar bats ingest sugar mixtures in fruits and nectars that are rich in these monosaccharides, but low in sucrose [11]. However, nectar bats are able to vary their degree of reliance on fruit pulp and floral nectar according to availability [12]. The dietary specialization of hummingbirds is made possible by expression of high levels of intestinal sucrase [13], a trait not found in many species of frugivorous birds. In addition, hummingbird intestines in vitro display the highest known rates of intestinal active transport of glucose [14,15]. However, the maximum capacity for active transport of glucose is far below the physiological rate at which sucrose is assimilated in vivo [5,14]. Instead, a paracellular transport mechanism accounts for most of the movement of sugar across the intestinal epithelium [16] (Figure 1). Nectar bats also have high levels of intestinal sucrase, allowing hydrolysis of sucrose contained in nectars and fruits [17], and make use of a predominantly paracellular pathway for intestinal sugar absorption [18]. Hummingbirds and nectar bats ingesting sugars display digestive efficiencies close to 100% [12,15].

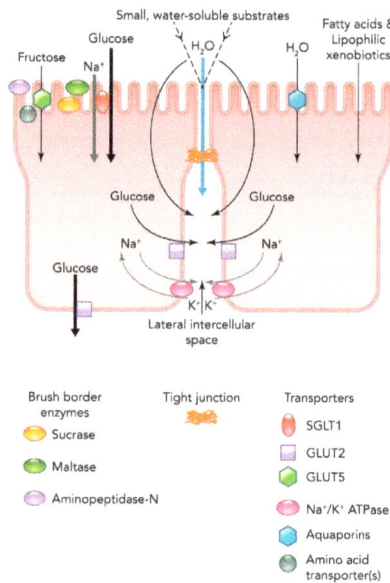

Figure 1. A model of the principal mechanisms by which nutrients are absorbed across the avian and chiropteran intestinal border. While both fructose and glucose are absorbed at high rates across the brush border via carrier-mediated pathways, as occurs in humans and other terrestrial mammals, substantial flux occurs via paracellular (diffusion or solvent drag) pathways in flying vertebrates [1]. Among small nectarivore species, like hummingbirds and nectar bats, brush border enzyme and glucose transporter (GLUT) and Na^+-dependent glucose transporter (SGLT)-mediated transport activity per unit of intestinal area is high. However, paracellular absorption must also occur at especially high rates in the intestines of these nectarivores in order to satisfy overall energy budget (and thus absorptive) demands. Figure reprinted with permission from Price et al. [19].

Feeding on floral nectar while hovering requires extremely high rates of energy expenditure. These are most commonly measured under laboratory conditions and in the field using mask-respirometry [6,20] (Figure 2). Small hummingbirds in routine hovering flight display wingbeat frequencies of 30–60 Hz [21,22] and, in the process, sustain the highest mass-specific rates of aerobic metabolism among vertebrates that are about tenfold higher than the maximum rates measured in human athletes [2]. Ten-gram nectar bats (*Glossophaga soricina*) beat their wings at lower frequencies (9 Hz) [23] and display hovering mass-specific metabolic rates [6,24] about half those of hummingbirds. Nevertheless, these approximate the mass-specific metabolic rates of shrews exposed to low ambient temperature [25] and are among the highest values recorded among mammals.

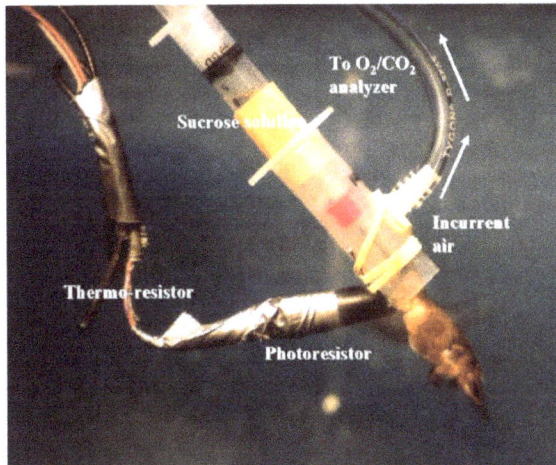

Figure 2. Hummingbird mask respirometry. The bird is freely hovering while feeding on a sucrose solution with its head in feeder modified to function as a mask for flow-through respirometry. Air is drawn into the mask at a known flow rate. The air, depleted of O_2 and enriched with CO_2, is analyzed downstream using O_2 and CO_2 analyzers. See [20,26] for detailed description of the method.

The need to fuel such high metabolic rates raises interesting and important questions concerning the fate of ingested sugars. At high exercise intensities, 90% or more of whole body O_2 consumption rates are accounted for by mitochondrial respiration in exercising muscles [2,27]. Decades ago, recognition of the importance of fat as the main fuel stored before and depleted during avian migration led to the idea that bird flight muscles use mainly fatty acid oxidation as their source of ATP during exercise [28]. The nectarivorous diet of hummingbirds and nectar bats therefore raises the question of whether their energy metabolism during flight might be fueled primarily by ingested sugar or, alternatively, by fat previously synthesized from ingested sugar. A third possibility is that ingested sugar is used for the synthesis of glycogen, which is then broken down to fuel metabolism during flight.

3. Biochemical Capacities for Substrate Oxidation

In their invasion of a niche previously occupied by insects, hummingbirds and hovering nectar bats evolved large pectoral muscles relative to total body mass. These consist exclusively of fast-twitch, oxidative fibers [29–31] that possess high mitochondrial content [30,32]. The high O_2 requirements during exercise are supported by high lung O_2 transport capacities [33,34], large hearts [35,36] and high muscle capillary densities [37]. In rufous hummingbird (*Selasphorus rufus*) flight muscle fibers, mitochondria occupy 35% of cell volume and respiratory capacities are further enhanced by cristae surface densities (cristae surface area/mitochondrial volume) about twofold higher than those found in mammalian muscle mitochondria [30]. Enzymatic capacities for substrate oxidation are enhanced, as indicated by V_{max} values ($=k_{cat} \times [E]$, where k_{cat} is catalytic efficiency and $[E]$ is enzyme concentration), measured in vitro (Table 1). Consistent with the high mitochondrial content of these muscles are their high V_{max} values for the Krebs cycle enzyme, citrate synthase. High capacities for glucose phosphorylation and fatty acid oxidation are indicated by high V_{max} values for hexokinase and carnitine palmitoyl transferase, respectively. It is important to point out that, although V_{max} values establish upper limits to flux [38,39], they do not serve as measures of physiological rates through metabolic pathways in vivo. Which fuels are oxidized, at what rates and under what circumstances are empirical questions that must be addressed using other approaches [39,40].

Table 1. Comparison of enzyme V_{max} values in locomotory muscles. Data are expressed as μmole substrate converted to product per g, wet mass per minute and temperature-corrected to allow comparison across species. V_{max} values serve as measures of maximum capacities of flux [38,39] and indicate much higher capacities for glycogen, glucose and long chain fatty acid oxidation in nectar bat and hummingbird pectoralis muscles than in shrew and rat leg muscles. Citrate synthase V_{max} values serve as relative measures of mitochondrial content [41] and show that nectar bat and hummingbird flight muscles have much higher mitochondrial oxidative capacities than shrew and rat leg muscles.

Enzyme	Nectar Bat [1] Pectoralis	Hummingbird [2] Pectoralis	Shrew [3] Quadriceps	Rat [4] Soleus
Glycogen phosphorylase	46.0	59.0	n.a.	10.08
Hexokinase	15.9	18.4	1.10	2.20
Citrate synthase	204.7	448.4	37.0	45.1
Carnitine palmitoyl transferase	6.0	7.2	2.7	0.28

[1] *Glossophaga soricina*, [2] *Selasphorus rufus*, [3] *Blarina brevicauda*, [4] *Rattus norvegicus*. Data from [32] and references cited therein; n.a. = not available.

4. Substrate Oxidation during Foraging Flights

Reaction to the suggestion that nectarivorous animals might directly fuel their metabolism during exercise using dietary sugar is often, "Of course—what else would one expect?" On the contrary, it is well known among exercise physiologists and biochemists that rates of glucose phosphorylation in most vertebrate skeletal muscles are insufficient to account for the metabolic rates required during high-intensity exercise [40,42]. Hexokinase V_{max} values in vertebrate muscles are generally low [43] (Table 1). In most species during exercise, hexokinase operates at very low fractional velocities (v/V_{max}) [40], limiting entry of glucose into the glycolytic pathway in muscles [44]. Fell [45] goes as far as to disqualify hexokinase as a glycolytic enzyme but, rather, considers the reaction it catalyzes to be primarily involved in the synthesis of glycogen. As exercise intensities increase, the reliance on fatty acid oxidation in mammalian muscles declines and carbohydrate oxidation becomes the greater contributor to the fueling of energy metabolism [46,47]. Since, under these conditions, glucose phosphorylation rates are insufficient to match the rates of carbohydrate oxidation observed, glycogenolysis provides most of the carbon oxidized during exercise as maximum aerobic metabolic rates ($V_{O_2 max}$ values) are approached [42,47]. What might seem so obviously true to some would therefore appear highly unlikely to those familiar with metabolism during exercise in mice, rats and humans. The contrast between preconceived notions and these empirical results makes the subject of sugar metabolism in hummingbirds and nectar bats all the more interesting.

Respiratory Exchange Ratios (RER = V_{CO_2}/V_{O_2}), measured using mask respirometry [20] (Figure 2), in these animals are considered to closely reflect cellular Respiratory Quotients (RQ = V_{CO_2}/V_{O_2}). This is likely to be the case: a 4-g hummingbird with a blood volume of 0.4 mL, carrying 0.088 mL O_2 [48], respires at a rate of about 2 mL O_2 per minute [30]. At this metabolic rate, blood O_2 stores would be completely depleted in 2.6 s if whole-body O_2 uptake and mitochondrial respiration were not tightly linked. The rate of mitochondrial respiration in the flight muscles during hovering is so high and so closely coupled to whole-body gas exchange rate that even substrate-dependent differences in moles of ATP synthesized per mole of O atom consumed [49,50] can be detected using respirometry [51]. Measured V_{CO_2}/V_{O_2} values shall henceforth be referred to as RQs to facilitate biochemical interpretation. Fasted hummingbirds and nectar bats, perched or hanging upside down, display RQ values of about 0.7, indicating that fatty acid oxidation fuels their whole-body resting metabolic rates [52–54]. Under resting conditions, energetically expensive internal organs account for most of the whole-body metabolic rate while skeletal muscles account for only a small fraction. When they fly to forage for food, whole-body metabolic rates increase dramatically and the high V_{O_2} values, measured using mask respirometry, are mainly due to the flight muscles. Repeated hover-feeding bouts and ingestion of sugar solutions result in progressive increases in RQ values to about 1.0 [52–54] (Figure 3). This indicates that the flight muscles progressively rely more on carbohydrate oxidation as sugar is repeatedly ingested.

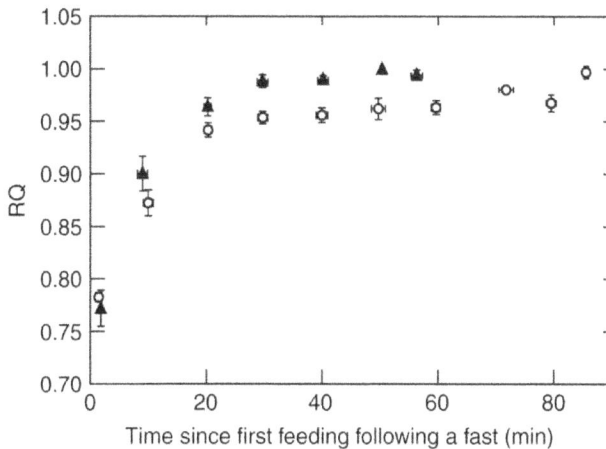

Figure 3. Respiratory quotients (RQ) during hover-feeding over time after fasting in rufous hummingbirds (*Selasphorus rufus*) (triangles) and nectar bats (*Glossophaga soricina*) (circles) (From [3]). Flight muscles oxidize mainly fat (RQ values close to 0.7) in fasted animals during hovering. RQs rise to about 1.0, indicating that flight muscles shift to carbohydrate oxidation as a result of repeated hover-feeding on sucrose solutions.

The nature of the carbohydrate oxidized during hover-feeding flights was revealed by combining the use of carbon stable isotopes with mask respirometry. Beet-derived sucrose, produced by C3 photosynthesis, is relatively more ^{13}C-depleted than cane-derived sucrose, the product of C4 photosynthesis [55]. Measured as $\delta^{13}C$, where

$$\delta^{13}C = \frac{[^{13}C]/[^{12}C]}{R_{std}} \tag{1}$$

and R_{std} is a standard [56], a more negative $\delta^{13}C$ value would be expected upon analysis of CO_2 expired by animals maintained on beet-derived sucrose compared with the CO_2 produced by animals maintained on cane-derived sucrose. In these experiments, animals were first maintained on diets containing beet-derived sucrose until they expired CO_2 with $\delta^{13}C$ values similar to that of beets. Animals were then fasted until RQ = 0.7, then given free access to feeders fitted with masks to allow sampling of expired CO_2 as well as measurement of V_{O_2} and Vc_{O_2} during hovering flight. Figure 4 shows that as the hummingbirds and nectar bats engaged in the first feeding bouts, RQ values were close to 0.7, indicating that their flight muscles oxidized mainly fat. As they made repeated hovering visits to the feeder and fed on sucrose solutions, the RQ values rapidly approached 1.0, while the $\delta^{13}C$ of their expired CO_2 rose from the more negative values characteristic of beet sucrose to less negative values characteristic of cane sucrose. It can be inferred from these results that the increase in RQ, i.e., the switch from fat oxidation to carbohydrate oxidation, represents a transition from the oxidation of endogenous fat to dietary sucrose by the flight muscles. Fasted animals that oxidize fat (synthesized from beet sucrose) rapidly switch to oxidizing cane sucrose to fuel their energetically expensive hovering flight soon after they start feeding on cane sucrose. While humans can directly fuel about 30%, at most, of exercise metabolism with ingested glucose and fructose [57], in hummingbirds and nectar bats, the contributions of recently-ingested sucrose to energy metabolism during hovering are about 95% and 80%, respectively [3]. The carbon stable isotope results obtained using the protocol outlined here are in general agreement with those obtained independently by Voigt and colleagues using a different approach [58].

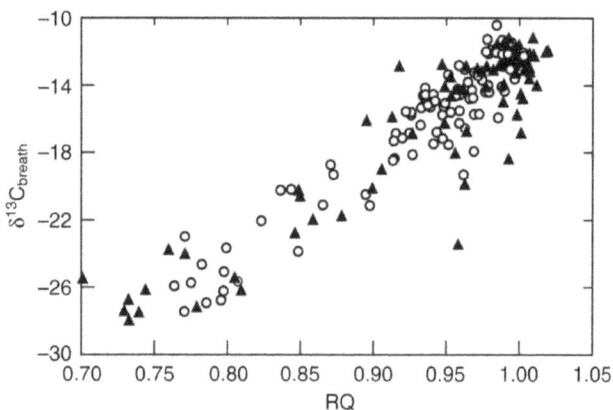

Figure 4. $\delta^{13}C$ of expired CO_2 as a function of RQ in hover-feeding rufous hummingbirds (*Selasphorus rufus*) (triangles) and nectar bats (*Glossophaga soricina*) (circles) (From [3]). More negative $\delta^{13}C$ values characteristic of maintenance beet sugar are observed when animals are hovering in the fasted state with RQ values close to 0.7. As RQ values rise to 1.0, indicating transition from fat oxidation to carbohydrate oxidation, $\delta^{13}C$ values also increase to approximate $\delta^{13}C$ of cane sugar provided in feeders during mask respirometry experiments.

The V_{max} values for hexokinase and carnitine palmitoly transferase in both hummingbird and nectar bat flight muscles (Table 1) indicate that catalytic capacities at these steps in both species are sufficient to account for the rates of glucose and fatty acid oxidation estimated during hovering flight (Table 2).

Table 2. Metabolic fluxes in hovering hummingbirds (*Selasphorus rufus*) and nectar bats (*Glossophaga soricina*). Glucose oxidation rates are estimated in animals performing aerial refueling, i.e., hover-feeding when RQ close to 1.0. Palmitate oxidation rates are estimated in animals hovering in the fasted state with RQ close to 0.7. Both glucose and palmitate oxidation rates are easily accommodated by V_{max} values for hexokinase and carnitine palmitoyl transferase, respectively (Table 1). Data from [3].

	Nectar Bat	Hummingbird
Whole-body V_{O_2} (mL O_2 g^{-1} h^{-1})	24.5	33.3
Flight muscle V_{O_2} (mL O_2 g^{-1} h^{-1})	84.7	119.8
Glucose oxidation rate (μmol g^{-1} min^{-1})	9.1	14.8
Palmitate oxidation rate (μmol g^{-1} min^{-1})	2.0	2.8

A mechanistic requirement for this process to work as hypothesized is a high enough rate of sugar uptake by the flight muscle fibers. In mammalian muscles, rates of glucose transport are increased when the glucose transporter, GLUT4, is translocated from intracellular vesicles to the cell membrane in response to exercise or insulin [44,59]. Nectar bat pectoralis muscles express remarkably high levels of GLUT4 (Figure 5), indicating high capacities for sarcolemmal glucose transport. Along with their high hexokinase V_{max} values, this makes nectar bats the natural analogues to mice engineered to express high levels of both GLUT4 and hexokinase [44]. In mouse muscles overexpressing GLUT4, transport is enhanced and glucose phosphorylation becomes limiting during exercise. Overexpression of both GLUT4 and hexokinase leads to higher rates of glucose metabolism during exercise than overexpression of GLUT4 or hexokinase alone. The results obtained using mice, through the elegant and powerful combination of genetic, physiological and biochemical approaches [44], were arrived at independently when nectar bats evolved millions of years ago [10].

NECTAR BAT PECTORALIS   MOUSE GASTROCNEMIUS

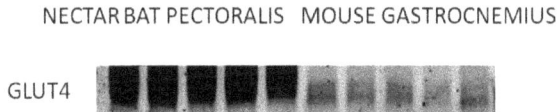

GLUT4

Figure 5. Western blot showing much higher GLUT4 expression in nectar bat (*Glossophaga soricina*) pectoralis muscles (lanes 1–5) than in mouse gastrocnemius (lanes 6–10). 40 μg protein was loaded into each lane. Staining intensity in nectar bat lanes was sixfold greater than in mouse gastrocnemius lanes. Generously provided by Robert Lee-Young and David Wasserman.

In a separate experiment of nature, birds evolved to not express GLUT4 and may not even possess the gene for it [60,61]. Consistent with these findings, the flight muscles of ruby-throated hummingbirds (*Archilochus colubris*) show no sign of GLUT4 expression, but do express GLUT1 and GLUT3 [62] (Figure 6).

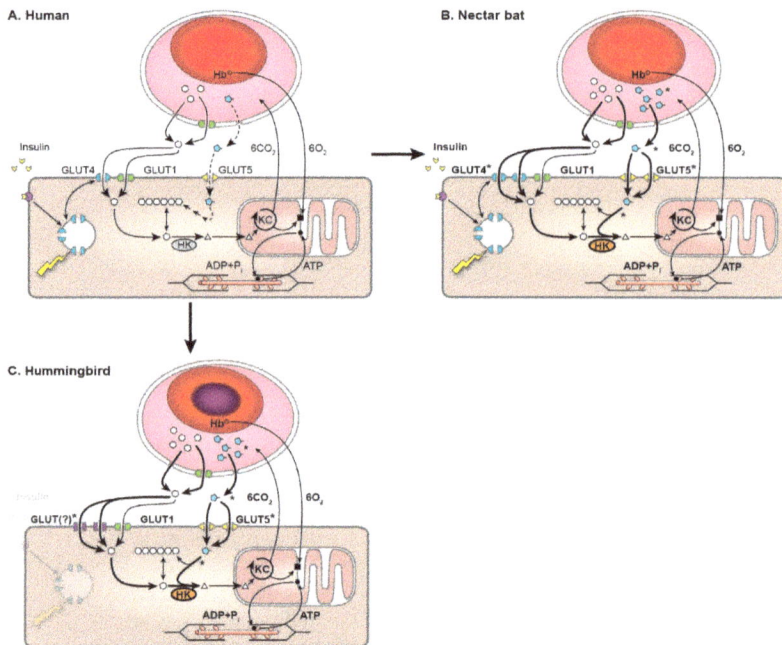

Figure 6. Comparison of mechanisms of muscle uptake and oxidation of circulating glucose and fructose in humans, nectar bats and hummingbirds. (**A**) Pathway for uptake and oxidation of mainly glucose into human skeletal muscle fibers, highlighting key regulatory steps (e.g., sarcollemal transport, regulation of transport capacity via insulin and contractile activity; (**B**) Glucose and fructose uptake and oxidation in nectar bats highlighting enhancements (in bold; those hypothesized are noted by asterisks) to various pathway elements; (**C**) Glucose and fructose uptake and oxidation in hummingbirds highlighting key upregulated steps (bold and asterisks used as in (**B**)). Details regarding functional enhancements are discussed in the main text and in Welch and Chen [63]. Figure from [63].

Experiments involving feeding of hummingbirds with ^{13}C-labeled glucose or fructose and determination of $\delta^{13}C$ of expired CO_2 reveal hovering flight can be fueled equally well by either sugar [64]. This contrasts with the skeletal muscles of rats and humans that transport and metabolize fructose at much lower rates than glucose [65,66] and, as noted previously, their more limited capacity to directly fuel exercise metabolism with dietary glucose and fructose [67].

Blood glucose concentrations in hummingbirds increase up to 40 mM during repeated bouts of hover-feeding on sucrose solutions and are maintained at 14 mM in the fasted state [63,68]. In contrast, blood glucose concentrations in fasted, resting nectar bats are maintained at about 3 mM. Values increase up to 30 mM after feeding on sucrose solutions and return close to fasted, resting values as a result of exercise after meals [69]. Because both hummingbirds and nectar bats make primary use of the paracellular route in transporting glucose and fructose across the intestinal wall [16,18], differences in flight muscle GLUT expression (Figure 6) offer a likely explanation for the differences in blood glucose kinetics. It appears likely that the ability to restore low concentrations of blood glucose in nectar bats is at least partly the consequence of GLUT4 recruitment and elevated rates of glucose uptake and phosphorylation in the flight muscles in response to insulin and exercise [44]. Birds are generally regarded as "hyperglycemic" relative to mammals and this appears to be due to the absence of GLUT4 and, therefore, the absence of insulin and exercise-stimulated GLUT4 responses in their muscles [61,63]. The ability to fuel muscle metabolism equally well with glucose or fructose [64] underscores the need for further study of sugar metabolism in nectarivorous vertebrates. The roles and mechanisms of regulation of sarcolemmal sugar transporters in hummingbirds during rest and flight, fasting and feeding await elucidation.

5. A New Concept: The "Sugar Oxidation Cascade"

We have named the process by which hummingbirds and nectar bats ingest sucrose, glucose and fructose from floral nectars, assimilate glucose and fructose through their intestinal walls, transport and oxidize them in exercising muscles the "sugar oxidation cascade" [3] (Figure 7). It operates in parallel with the oxygen transport cascade [70,71], the process by which animals take in O_2 from the environment and, via a series of convective and diffusive processes, transports it to exercising muscles where it serves as the terminal electron acceptor. The sugar oxidation and O_2 transport cascades converge as the carbon derived from recently-ingested sugars is oxidized in flight muscle mitochondria. Hummingbirds and nectar bats are unique among vertebrates in being able to fuel their locomotory muscles during exercise directly with recently-ingested sugar to the extent that their oxidation accounts for most of the V_{O_2} during hover-feeding. In contrast, ingested sugar can directly fuel only about 30%, at most, of the V_{O_2} during exercise in humans [57]. The operation of the sugar oxidation cascade is analogous to aerial refueling in aircraft, wherein fuel "ingested" from a flying tanker is directly combusted to fuel flight.

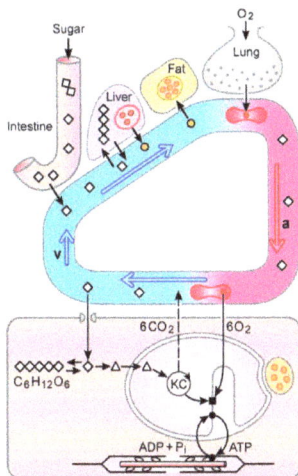

Figure 7. The sugar oxidation cascade provides most of the energy required for flight in hover-feeding hummingbirds and nectar bats. This diagram shows how the sugar oxidation and O_2 transport cascades operate in parallel in hover-feeding hummingbirds and nectar bats. During hovering flight, >90% of whole-body O_2 consumption rates are due to flight muscle mitochondrial respiration. In the O_2 transport cascade, O_2 travels from the external environment through the respiratory and cardiovascular systems and into muscle mitochondria through a series of convective and diffusive processes at rates determined by muscle energy demands. In the fasted state, mitochondrial respiration is fueled by fatty acid oxidation. During repeated hover-feeding, dietary sugars (twin diamond denotes sucrose; single diamonds denote glucose and fructose) are ingested. Sucrose is hydrolyzed; glucose and fructose cross the intestinal epithelium primarily through a paracellular pathway and enter the blood. Most of the ingested sugar is transported into the flight muscles and broken down. The sugar and O_2 transport cascades converge in the mitochondria where carbon compounds derived from dietary sugar (pyramids) are oxidized to provide reducing equivalents for respiration and oxidative phosphorylation. Ingested sugars in excess of energetic needs are converted to glycogen (strings of diamonds) and fat (yellow-filled circles). From [3].

In both hummingbirds and nectar bats, V_{max} values for glycogen phosphorylase (Table 1) are sufficient to account for the rates of carbohydrate oxidation required to fuel hovering flight [32,49]. However, metabolic rates during hovering are so high that, if on-board glycogen stores were to serve as the sole fuel for oxidative metabolism in the flight muscles, they would be totally depleted after only several minutes. Of course, this would be unlikely to occur. Instead, we suggest that glycogenolysis during repeated bouts of hover-feeding might function in the flight muscles as it does in mammalian hearts, i.e., glycogen "turns over", the relative rates of synthesis and breakdown change dynamically, and the process serves to buffer hexose phosphate concentrations [72,73]. Flight muscle power outputs vary as hummingbirds and nectar bats engage in different kinds of flight, e.g., level flight, hovering, aerobatic maneuvers or in response to changes in wing loading and altitude. It seems likely that glycogen resynthesis would occur at rest, between feeding bouts, and that the contribution of glycogenolysis to carbon flux through glycolysis becomes greater under certain circumstances, but only transiently, as in normoxic hearts operating within the range of their physiological power outputs [73]. At this time, the obvious difficulty of assessing rates of muscle glycogenolysis and resynthesis in hummingbirds and nectar bats precludes further discussion beyond the formulation of testable hypotheses.

What might be the advantages derived from direct oxidation of dietary sugar during hover-feeding? One benefit appears to be the direct consequence of the difference between carbohydrate and fatty acid oxidation in ATP yield. Expressed as the P/O ratio, i.e., the number of ATP molecules made per O atom consumed, the oxidation of glucose or glycogen yields a 15% higher P/O ratio than the oxidation of fatty acid [49,50]. This might be advantageous during foraging at high altitude, when hummingbirds must increase muscle power output while experiencing hypobaric hypoxia [49,74]. Another possible advantage is a consequence of the energetic cost incurred when dietary sugar is converted to fat. If this investment were to occur, followed by the oxidation of fat to fuel exercise, then the net energy yield would be 16% lower compared with the direct oxidation of ingested sugar [52]. Direct oxidation of dietary sugar allows more rapid accumulation of fat synthesized from sugar consumed in excess of daily energetic requirements. The rate of fat synthesis appears to be enhanced in nature by foraging behavior that keeps the sugar oxidation cascade turned on and muscle fatty acid oxidation turned off [52,75–77].

6. Premigratory Sugar Conversion to Fat in Hummingbirds

Certain species of hummingbirds fly long distances during seasonal migrations. Ruby-throated hummingbirds migrate non-stop across the Gulf of Mexico [78]. Rufous hummingbirds make multiple refueling stops as they migrate as far north as Alaska to breed in the summer and as far south as Mexico to escape the cold of winter [79]. As in all other species of flying migrants, hummingbirds make use of fat as the main oxidative fuel for long-term, steady-state flight. Given their high resting and active metabolic rates, the need to maintain daily energy balance (time averaged energy intake = time averaged energy expenditure) is, by itself, a significant challenge. Thus, making an energetic profit (energy intake > energy expenditure) and accumulating fat in preparation for migration is an even more impressive feat. Premigratory fattening becomes even more energetically challenging when higher energetic costs are imposed by low ambient temperature and high elevation [80,81]. Rufous hummingbirds stop to refuel in subalpine meadows during their late-summer, southward migration, where early morning temperatures can be near-freezing. Flight at high elevation requires higher muscle energy expenditure [21] while low temperature increases the energetic cost of thermoregulation [81]. Despite these challenges, hummingbirds have been known to gain about 10% of body mass per day and store up to 40% of body mass in the form of fat during refueling stops [82]. Laboratory experiments involving simulation of such conditions revealed that rufous hummingbirds allowed to perch and to hover-feed at 5 °C for 4 h are able to maintain or gain body mass when provided sucrose concentrations of at least 30%. At 5 °C, more dilute sucrose concentrations result in mass loss (energy intake < energy expenditure) even when the hummingbirds increase their feeding frequencies as they attempt to maintain energy balance [75,83]. At higher ambient temperatures, net fat accumulation can be achieved over a lower range of dietary sucrose concentrations. These experimental results lead to the hypothesis that the coevolution between hummingbirds and the flowering plants that they visit may have resulted in increased sucrose concentrations in floral nectars at higher elevation [83].

7. Metabolism in Nectarivorous Animals: Implications for Human Health

Basic research in comparative physiology and biochemistry is usually not done with human physiology or biomedical applications in mind. Instead, it is most often motivated by the desire to explore functional biodiversity across species or to investigate mechanisms of short-term (physiological) and long-term (evolutionary) adaptation. In addition, there is much interest among comparative physiologists in responses to environmental change and their ecological consequences. Nevertheless, studies such as those cited in this brief review illustrate how comparative approaches can benefit biomedical science by complementing traditional approaches, yielding new insights and inspiring new questions.

From an anthropocentric perspective, the idea that certain species of birds and mammals can fuel their extremely high rates of metabolism at rest and during exercise almost entirely with recently-ingested sugars is certainly cause for amazement. The mechanisms by which hummingbirds and nectar bats routinely hover at mass-specific V_{O_2} values about ten- and fivefold higher, respectively, than those of human athletes exercising at $V_{O_2 max}$ have been the subject of continuing investigation [2,63,84]. While the paracellular pathway plays a minor role in biomedical models, e.g., [85], it plays a dominant role, accounts for most of the intestinal glucose absorption in nectarivorous animals and operates at rates high enough to supply the fuel requirements of muscles during flight [16,18].

There is current debate concerning the possible roles played by dietary sugars in the development of obesity and diabetes [86,87]. However, what might be a toxic diet for humans serves as the main source of calories for nectarivorous animals. What might appear to be a persistent, severe and potentially harmful hyperglycemia is the natural state of blood glucose homeostasis in hummingbirds [68], animals that are extraordinarily long-lived [88,89] despite their high metabolic rates and small body size. In nectar bats, blood glucose concentrations increase to values high enough to be considered pathological in humans, and are restored to low, resting levels by exercise [69]. A large body of literature concerns how exercise contributes to disease prevention in humans [90,91]. Among the possible mechanisms underlying the beneficial effects of exercise is enhanced myokine production, which leads to autocrine, paracrine and endocrine effects [92,93]. This suggests that the persistent, night-time flight of foraging nectar bats [69] may counteract the negative effects of their sugary diets and hyperglycemia via similar mechanisms.

It has been suggested that honey accounted for a significant fraction of dietary energy intake early in human evolution [94]. Honey, with its high content of glucose (23–41%) and fructose (31–44%) [95], is highly prized and consumed in large quantities by forager societies in various parts of the world [94]. Studies have focused on the Hadza of northern Tanzania whose diet consists of 15% honey [96] but are thin, long-lived and do not suffer from chronic diseases common in Western societies [97]. A surprising finding, based on measurements using doubly labeled water, is that the average total daily energy expenditure of the Hadza hunter-gatherers is similar to that of Westerners. However, the Hadza walk about 6–11 km per day and thereby display higher levels of physical activity than Westerners [98]. Thus, rather than being the result of greater daily energy expenditure, the lack of obesity and metabolic disease among the Hadza may be due to their greater daily physical activity. This is supported by studies involving Western subjects whose walking was reduced to 1300–1500 steps per day for 2 weeks. The reduced activity was found to cause impaired glucose clearance, decreased insulin sensitivity, increased abdominal fat, loss of leg muscle mass and reduction in $V_{O_2 max}$ [99,100]. The high fructose content of honey in the Hadza diet is of special significance, given what is known concerning the harmful effects of excessive fructose ingestion [101]. Among Westerners, exercise has been shown to prevent the adverse metabolic effects of high fructose ingestion [102,103]. This is at least partly due to increased fructose oxidation and decreased storage resulting from exercise [104].

Taken together, these data lead to the suggestion that, just as in the case of nectar bats, exercise in humans counteracts the potentially harmful effects of ingestion of large quantities of sugar, particularly fructose. These findings call for further mechanistic studies of sugar metabolism in nectar bats as well as parallel studies on the GLUT4-lacking, chronically-hyperglycemic, nectarivorous hummingbirds. They call renewed attention to Nobel laureate August Krogh's dictum that "For many problems there is an animal on which it can be most conveniently studied" [105].

Acknowledgments: The work reviewed here was supported by a Natural Sciences and Engineering Research Council of Canada (NSERC) Discovery Grant (#386466) to KCW. RKS's work reviewed here was previously conducted in the Department of Ecology, Evolution and Marine Biology, University of California, Santa Barbara, with support from the US National Science Foundation and UC MEXUS-CONACYT. We thank Robert Lee-Young and David Wasserman for generously providing Figure 5.

Conflicts of Interest: The authors declare no conflicts of interest.

References

1. Heithaus, E.R. Coevolution between bats and plants. In *Ecology of Bats*; Kunz, T.H., Ed.; Springer: Boston, MA, USA, 1982; pp. 327–367.
2. Suarez, R.K. Hummingbird flight: Sustaining the highest mass-specific metabolic rates among vertebrates. *Experientia* **1992**, *48*, 565–570. [CrossRef] [PubMed]
3. Suarez, R.K. The sugar oxidation cascade: Aerial refueling in hummingbirds and nectar bats. *J. Exp. Biol.* **2011**, *214*, 172–178. [CrossRef] [PubMed]
4. Von Helversen, O.; Winter, Y. Glossophagine bats and their flowers: Costs and benefits for plants and pollinators. In *Bat Ecology*; Kunz, T.H., Fenton, B., Eds.; University of Chicago: Chicago, IL, USA, 2003; pp. 346–397.
5. Powers, D.R.; Nagy, K.A. Field metabolic rate and food consumption by free-living Anna's hummingbirds (*Calypte anna*). *Physiol. Zool.* **1988**, *61*, 500–506. [CrossRef]
6. Winter, Y.; Voigt, C.; von Helversen, O. Gas exchange during hovering flight in a nectar-feeding bat *Glossophaga soricina*. *J. Exp. Biol.* **1998**, *201*, 237–244. [PubMed]
7. Heinrich, B. Energetics of pollination. *Ann. Rev. Ecol. Syst.* **1975**, *6*, 139–170. [CrossRef]
8. Martinez del Rio, C.; Baker, H.G.; Baker, I. Ecological and evolutionary implications of digestive processes: Bird preferences and the sugar constituents of floral nectar and fruit pulp. *Experientia* **1992**, *48*, 544–551. [CrossRef]
9. Nicolson, S.W.; Fleming, P.A. Nectar as food for birds: The physiological consequences of drinking dilute sugar solutions. *Plant Syst. Evol.* **2003**, *238*, 139–153. [CrossRef]
10. Datzmann, T.; von Helversen, O.; Mayer, F. Evolution of nectarivory in phyllostomid bats (Phyllostomidae Gray, 1825, Chiroptera: Mammalia). *BMC Evol. Biol.* **2010**, *10*, 165. [CrossRef] [PubMed]
11. Baker, H.G.; Baker, I.; Hodges, S.A. Sugar composition of nectars and fruits consumed by birds and bats in the tropics and subtropics. *Biotropica* **1998**, *30*, 559–586. [CrossRef]
12. Kelm, D.H.; Schaer, J.; Ortmann, S.; Wibbelt, G.; Speakman, J.R.; Voigt, C.C. Efficiency of facultative frugivory in the nectar-feeding bat *Glossophaga commissarisi*: The quality of fruits as an alternative food source. *J. Comp. Physiol.* **2008**, *178*, 985–996. [CrossRef] [PubMed]
13. Martinez del Rio, C. Dietary, phylogenetic, and ecological correlates of intestinal sucrase and maltase activity in birds. *Physiol. Zool.* **1990**, *63*, 987–1011. [CrossRef]
14. Diamond, J.M.; Karasov, W.H.; Phan, D.; Carpenter, F.L. Digestive physiology is a determinant of foraging bout frequency in hummingbirds. *Nature* **1986**, *320*, 62–63. [CrossRef] [PubMed]
15. Karasov, W.H.; Phan, D.; Diamond, J.M.; Carpenter, F.L. Food passage and intestinal nutrient absorption in hummingbirds. *Auk* **1986**, *103*, 453–464.
16. McWhorter, T.J.; Bakken, B.H.; Karasov, W.H.; Martinez del Rio, C. Hummingbirds rely on both paracellular and carrier-mediated intestinal glucose absorption to fuel high metabolism. *Biol. Lett.* **2006**, *2*, 131–134. [CrossRef] [PubMed]

17. Hernandez, A.; Martinez del Rio, C. Intestinal disaccharidases in five species of phyllostomid bats. *Comp. Biochem. Physiol.* **1992**, *103*, 105–111.

18. Rodriguez-Pena, N.; Price, E.R.; Caviedes-Vidal, E.; Flores-Ortiz, C.M.; Karasov, W.H. Intestinal paracellular absorption is necessary to support the sugar oxidation cascade in nectarivorous bats. *J. Exp. Biol.* **2016**, *219*, 779–782. [CrossRef] [PubMed]

19. Price, E.R.; Brun, A.; Caviedes-Vidal, E.; Karasov, W.H. Digestive adaptations of aerial lifestyles. *Physiology* **2015**, *30*, 69–78. [CrossRef] [PubMed]

20. Welch, K.C. The power of feeder-mask respirometry as a method for examining hummingbird energetics. *Comp. Biochem. Physiol. A* **2011**, *158*, 276–286. [CrossRef] [PubMed]

21. Altshuler, D.L.; Dudley, R. Kinematics of hovering hummingbird flight along simulated and natural elevational gradients. *J. Exp. Biol.* **2003**, *206*, 3139–3147. [CrossRef] [PubMed]

22. Mahalingan, S.; Welch, K.C., Jr. Neuromuscular control of hovering wingbeat kinematics in response to distinct flight challenges in the ruby-throated hummingbird, *Archilochus colubris*. *J. Exp. Biol.* **2013**, *216*, 4161–4171. [CrossRef] [PubMed]

23. Norberg, U.M.L.; Winter, Y. Wing beat kinematics of a nectar-feeding bat, *Glossophaga soricina*, flying at different flight speeds and strouhal numbers. *J. Exp. Biol.* **2006**, *209*, 3887–3897. [CrossRef] [PubMed]

24. Voigt, C.C.; Winter, Y. Energetic cost of hovering flight in nectar-feeding bats (*Phyllostomidae: Glossophaginae*) and its scaling in moths, birds and bats. *J. Comp. Physiol.* **1999**, *169*, 38–48. [CrossRef]

25. Fons, R.; Sicart, R. Contribution a la connaissance du metabolisme energetique chez deux Crocidurinae: *Suncus etruscus* (savi, 1822) et *Crocidura russula* (Hermann, 1780) (insectivora, Soricidae). *Mammalia* **1976**, *40*, 299–311. [CrossRef] [PubMed]

26. Bartholomew, G.A.; Lighton, J.R.B. Oxygen consumption during hover-feeding in free-ranging Anna hummingbirds. *J. Exp. Biol.* **1986**, *123*, 191–199. [PubMed]

27. Taylor, C.R. Structural and functional limits to oxidative metabolism: Insights from scaling. *Ann. Rev. Physiol.* **1987**, *49*, 135–146. [CrossRef] [PubMed]

28. Blem, C.R. Patterns of lipid storage and utilization in birds. *Am. Zool.* **1976**, *16*, 671–684. [CrossRef]

29. Grinyer, I.; George, J.C. Some observations on the ultrastructure of the hummingbird pectoral muscles. *Can. J. Zool.* **1969**, *47*, 771–774. [CrossRef] [PubMed]

30. Suarez, R.K.; Lighton, J.R.B.; Brown, G.S.; Mathieu-Costello, O. Mitochondrial respiration in hummingbird flight muscles. *Proc. Natl. Acad. Sci. USA* **1991**, *88*, 4870–4873. [CrossRef] [PubMed]

31. Hermanson, J.W.; Ryan, J.M.; Cobb, M.A.; Bentley, J.; Schutt, W.A. Histochemical and electrophoretic analysis of the primary flight muscle of several Phyllostomid bats. *Can. J. Zool.* **1998**, *76*, 1983–1992. [CrossRef]

32. Suarez, R.K.; Welch, K.C., Jr.; Hanna, S.K.; Herrera, M.L.G. Flight muscle enzymes and metabolic flux rates during hovering flight of the nectar bat, *Glossophaga soricina*: Further evidence of convergence with hummingbirds. *Comp. Biochem. Physiol.* **2009**, *153*, 136–140. [CrossRef] [PubMed]

33. Dubach, M. Quantitative analysis of the respiratory system of the house sparrow, budgerigar and violet-eared hummingbird. *Respir. Physiol.* **1981**, *46*, 43–60. [CrossRef]

34. Maina, J.N. What it takes to fly: The structural and functional respiratory requirements in birds and bats. *J. Exp. Biol.* **2000**, *203*, 3045–3064. [PubMed]

35. Schmidt-Nielsen, K. *Scaling. Why Is Animal Size So Important?* Cambridge University Press: Cambridge, UK, 1984; 241p.

36. Canals, M.; Atala, C.; Rossi, B.G.; Iriarte-Diaz, J. Relative size of hearts and lungs of small bats. *Acta Chiropterol.* **2005**, *7*, 65–72. [CrossRef]

37. Mathieu-Costello, O.; Suarez, R.K.; Hochachka, P.W. Capillary-to-fiber geometry and mitochondrial density in hummingbird flight muscle. *Respir. Physiol.* **1992**, *89*, 113–132. [CrossRef]

38. Newsholme, E.A.; Crabtree, B. Maximum catalytic activity of some key enzymes in provision of physiologically useful information about metabolic fluxes. *J. Exp. Zool.* **1986**, *239*, 159–167. [CrossRef] [PubMed]

39. Suarez, R.K. Upper limits to mass-specific metabolic rates. *Annu. Rev. Physiol.* **1996**, *58*, 583–605. [CrossRef] [PubMed]

40. Suarez, R.K.; Staples, J.F.; Lighton, J.R.B.; West, T.G. Relationships between enzymatic flux capacities and metabolic flux rates in muscles: Nonequilibrium reactions in muscle glycolysis. *Proc. Natl. Acad. Sci. USA* **1997**, *94*, 7065–7069. [CrossRef] [PubMed]

41. Moyes, C.D. Controlling muscle mitochondrial content. *J. Exp. Biol.* **2003**, *206*, 4385–4391. [CrossRef] [PubMed]

42. Weber, J.M.; Roberts, T.J.; Vock, R.; Weibel, E.R.; Taylor, C.R. Design of the oxygen and substrate pathways. III. Partitioning energy provision from carbohydrates. *J. Exp. Biol.* **1996**, *199*, 1659–1666. [PubMed]

43. Crabtree, B.; Newsholme, E.A. The activities of phosphorylase, hexokinase, phosphofructokinase, lactate dehydrogenase and the glycerol 3-phosphate dehydrogenases in muscles from vertebrates and invertebrates. *Biochem. J.* **1972**, *126*, 49–58. [CrossRef] [PubMed]

44. Wasserman, D.H.; Kang, L.; Ayala, J.E.; Fueger, P.T.; Lee-Young, R.S. The physiological regulation of glucose flux into muscle in vivo. *J. Exp. Biol.* **2011**, *214*, 254–262. [CrossRef] [PubMed]

45. Fell, D.A. Signal transduction and the control of expression of enzyme activity. *Adv. Enzyme Regul.* **2000**, *40*, 35–46. [CrossRef]

46. Brooks, G.A. Mammalian fuel utilization during sustained exercise. *Comp. Biochem. Physiol.* **1998**, *120*, 89–107. [CrossRef]

47. Weber, J.-M.; Haman, F. Oxidative fuel selection: Adjusting mix and flux to stay alive. *Int. Congr. Ser.* **2004**, *1275*, 22–31. [CrossRef]

48. Johansen, K.; Berger, M.; Bicudo, J.E.P.W.; Ruschi, A.; De Almeida, P.J. Respiratory properties of blood and myoglobin in hummingbirds. *Physiol. Zool.* **1987**, *60*, 269–278. [CrossRef]

49. Suarez, R.K.; Brown, G.S.; Hochachka, P.W. Metabolic sources of energy for hummingbird flight. *Am. J. Physiol.* **1986**, *251*, R537–R542. [PubMed]

50. Brand, M.D. The efficiency and plasticity of mitochondrial energy transduction. *Biochem. Soc. Trans.* **2005**, *33*, 897–904. [CrossRef] [PubMed]

51. Welch, K.C.; Altshuler, D.L.; Suarez, R.K. Oxygen consumption rates in hovering hummingbirds reflect substrate-dependent differences in P/O ratios: Carbohydrate as a 'premium fuel'. *J. Exp. Biol.* **2007**, *210*, 2146–2153. [CrossRef] [PubMed]

52. Suarez, R.K.; Lighton, J.R.B.; Moyes, C.D.; Brown, G.S.; Gass, C.L.; Hochachka, P.W. Fuel selection in rufous hummingbirds: Ecological implications of metabolic biochemistry. *Proc. Natl. Acad. Sci. USA* **1990**, *87*, 9207–9210. [CrossRef] [PubMed]

53. Welch, K.C., Jr.; Herrera, M.L.G.; Suarez, R.K. Dietary sugar as a direct fuel for flight in the nectarivorous bat, *Glossophaga soricina*. *J. Exp. Biol.* **2008**, *211*, 310–316. [CrossRef] [PubMed]

54. Welch, K.C.; Bakken, B.H.; Martinez del Rio, C.; Suarez, R.K. Hummingbirds fuel hovering flight with newly-ingested sugar. *Physiol. Biochem. Zool.* **2006**, *79*, 1082–1087. [CrossRef] [PubMed]

55. McNevin, D.B.; Badger, M.R.; Whitney, S.M.; von Caemmerer, S.; Tcherkez, G.B.; Farquhar, G.D. Differences in carbon isotope discrimination of three variants of D-ribulose-1,5-bisphosphate carboxylase/oxygenase reflect differences in their catalytic mechanisms. *J. Biol. Chem.* **2007**, *282*, 36068–36076. [CrossRef] [PubMed]

56. Welch, K.C., Jr.; Peronnet, F.; Hatch, K.A.; Voigt, C.C.; McCue, M.D. Carbon stable-isotope tracking in breath for comparative studies of fuel use. *Ann. N. Y. Acad. Sci.* **2016**, *1365*, 15–32. [CrossRef] [PubMed]

57. Jentjens, R.L.P.G.; Venables, M.C.; Jeukendrup, A.E. Oxidation of exogenous glucose, sucrose, and maltose during prolonged cycling exercise. *J. Appl. Physiol.* **2004**, *96*, 1285–1291. [CrossRef] [PubMed]

58. Voigt, C.C.; Speakman, J.R. Nectar-feeding bats fuel their high metabolism directly with exogenous carbohydrates. *Funct. Ecol.* **2007**, *21*, 913–921. [CrossRef]

59. Huang, S.; Czech, M.P. The GLUT4 glucose transporter. *Cell Metab.* **2007**, *5*, 237–252. [CrossRef] [PubMed]

60. Seki, Y.; Sato, K.; Kono, T.; Abe, H.; Akiba, Y. Broiler chickens (Ross strain) lack insulin-responsive glucose transporter GLUT4 and have GLUT8 cDNA. *Gen. Comp. Endocrinol.* **2003**, *133*, 80–87. [CrossRef]

61. Sweazea, K.L.; Braun, E.J. Glucose transporter expression in English sparrows (*Passer domesticus*). *Comp. Biochem. Physiol. B* **2006**, *144*, 263–270. [CrossRef] [PubMed]

62. Welch, K.C., Jr.; Allalou, A.; Sehgal, P.; Cheng, J.; Ashok, A. Glucose transporter expression in an avian nectarivore: The ruby-throated hummingbird (*Archilochus colubris*). *PLoS ONE* **2013**, *8*, e7703. [CrossRef] [PubMed]

63. Welch, K.C., Jr.; Chen, C.C.W. Sugar flux through the flight muscles of hovering vertebrate nectarivores: A review. *J. Comp. Physiol.* **2014**, *184*, 945–959. [CrossRef] [PubMed]

64. Chen, C.C.W.; Welch, K.C., Jr. Hummingbirds can fuel expensive hovering flight completely with either exogenous glucose or fructose. *Funct. Ecol.* **2014**, *28*, 589–600. [CrossRef]

65. Kristiansen, S.; Darakhshan, F.; Richter, E.A.; Handal, H.S. Fructose transport and GLUT5 protein in human sarcolemmal vesicles. *Am. J. Physiol.* **1997**, *273*, E543–E548. [PubMed]

66. Zierath, J.R.; Nolte, L.A.; Wahlstrom, E.; Galuska, D.; Shepherd, P.R.; Kahn, B.B.; Wallberg-Henriksson, H. Carrier-mediated fructose uptake significantly contributes to carbohydrate metabolism in human skeletal muscle. *Biochem. J.* **1995**, *311*, 517–521. [CrossRef] [PubMed]

67. Jentjens, R.L.P.G.; Achten, J.; Jeukendrup, A.E. High oxidation rates from combined carbohydrates ingested during exercise. *Med. Sci. Sports Exerc.* **2004**, *36*, 1551–1558. [CrossRef] [PubMed]

68. Beuchat, C.A.; Chong, C.R. Hyperglycemia in hummingbirds and its consequences for hemoglobin glycation. *Comp. Biochem. Physiol.* **1998**, *120*, 409–416. [CrossRef]

69. Kelm, D.H.; Simon, R.; Kuhlow, D.; Voigt, C.C.; Ristow, M. High activity enables life on a high-sugar diet: Blood glucose regulation in nectar-feeding bats. *Proc. R. Soc.* **2011**, *278*, 3490–3496. [CrossRef] [PubMed]

70. Weibel, E.R. *The Pathway for Oxygen*; Harvard University Press: Cambridge, MA, USA, 1984.

71. Weibel, E.R.; Taylor, C.R.; Gehr, P.; Hoppeler, H.; Mathieu, O.; Maloiy, G.M.O. Design of the mammalian respiratory system. IX. Functional and structural limits for oxygen flow. *Respir. Physiol.* **1981**, *44*, 151–164. [CrossRef]

72. Goodwin, G.W.; Arteaga, J.R.; Taegtmeyer, H. Glycogen turnover in the isolated working rat heart. *J. Biol. Chem.* **1995**, *270*, 9234–9240. [CrossRef] [PubMed]

73. Goodwin, G.W.; Taylor, C.S.; Taegtmeyer, H. Regulation of energy metabolism of the heart during acute increase in heart work. *J. Biol. Chem.* **1998**, *273*, 29530–29539. [CrossRef] [PubMed]

74. Altshuler, D.L.; Dudley, R.; McGuire, J.A. Resolution of a paradox: Hummingbird flight at high elevation does not come without a cost. *Proc. Natl. Acad. Sci. USA* **2004**, *101*, 17731–17736. [CrossRef] [PubMed]

75. Suarez, R.K.; Gass, C.L. Hummingbird foraging and the relation between bioenergetics and behaviour. *Comp. Biochem. Physiol.* **2002**, *133*, 335–343. [CrossRef]

76. Gass, C.L.; Sutherland, G.D. Specialization by territorial hummingbirds on experimentally enriched patches of flowers: Energetic profitability and learning. *Can. J. Zool.* **1985**, *63*, 2125–2133. [CrossRef]

77. Hou, L.; Welch, K.C., Jr. Premigratory ruby-throated hummingbirds, *Archilochus colubris*, exhibit multiple strategies for fueling migration. *Anim. Behav.* **2016**, *121*, 87–99. [CrossRef]

78. Lasiewski, R.C. The energetics of migrating hummingbirds. *Condor* **1962**, *64*, 324. [CrossRef]

79. Calder, W. Southbound through Colorado: Migration of rufous hummingbirds. *Nat. Geogr. Res.* **1987**, *3*, 40–51.

80. Welch, K.C.; Suarez, R.K. Altitude and temperature effects on the energetic cost of hover-feeding in migratory rufous hummingbirds, *Selasphorus Rufus*. *Can. J. Zool.* **2008**, *86*, 161–169. [CrossRef]

81. López-Calleja, M.V.; Bozinovic, F. Maximum metabolic rate, thermal insulation and aerobic scope in a small-sized Chilean hummingbird (*Sephanoides sephanoides*). *Auk* **1995**, *112*, 1034–1036.

82. Carpenter, F.L.; Hixon, M.A.; Beuchat, C.A.; Russell, R.W.; Paton, D.C. Biphasic mass gain in migrant hummingbirds: Body composition changes, torpor, and ecological significance. *Ecology* **1993**, *74*, 1173–1182. [CrossRef]

83. Gass, C.L.; Romich, M.T.; Suarez, R.K. Energetics of hummingbird foraging at low ambient temperature. *Can. J. Zool.* **1999**, *77*, 314–320. [CrossRef]

84. Suarez, R.K. Oxygen and the upper limits to animal design and performance. *J. Exp. Biol.* **1998**, *201*, 1065–1072. [PubMed]

85. Lane, J.S.; Whang, E.E.; Rigberg, D.A.; Hines, O.J.; Kwan, D.; Zinner, M.J.; McFadden, D.W.; Diamond, J.M.; Ashley, S.W. Paracellular glucose transport plays a minor role in the unanesthetized dog. *Am. J. Physiol.* **1999**, *276*, G789–G794. [PubMed]

86. Basu, S.; Yoffe, P.; Hills, N.; Lustig, R.H. The relationship of sugar to population-level diabetes prevalence: An econometric analysis of repeated cross-sectional data. *PLoS ONE* **2013**, *8*, e57873. [CrossRef] [PubMed]

87. Tappy, L.; Mittendorfer, B. Fructose toxicity: Is the science ready for public heath actions? *Curr. Opin. Clin. Nutr. Metab. Care* **2012**, *15*, 357–361. [CrossRef] [PubMed]

88. Lutmerding, J.A. *Longevity Records of North American Birds*; USGS: Reston, VA, USA, 2016.

89. Calder, W.A. Avian longevity and aging. In *Genetic Effects on Aging II*; Harrison, D.E., Ed.; Telford Press: West Caldwell, NJ, USA, 1990; pp. 185–204.

90. Pedersen, B.K.; Fischer, C.P. Beneficial health effects of exercise—The role of IL-6 as a myokine. *Trends Pharmacol. Sci.* **2007**, *28*, 152–156. [CrossRef] [PubMed]

91. Bishop-Bailey, D. Mechanisms governing the health and performance benefits of exercise. *Br. J. Pharmacol.* **2013**, *170*, 1153–1166. [CrossRef] [PubMed]

92. Pedersen, B.K. Muscles and their myokines. *J. Exp. Biol.* **2011**, *214*, 337–346. [CrossRef] [PubMed]

93. Pedersen, B.K.; Febbraio, M.A. Muscles, exercise and obesity: Skeletal muscle as a secretory organ. *Nat. Rev. Endocrinol.* **2012**, *8*, 457–465. [CrossRef] [PubMed]

94. Crittenden, A.N. The importance of honey consumption in human evolution. *Food Foodways* **2011**, *19*, 257–273. [CrossRef]

95. Ball, D.W. The chemical composition of honey. *J. Chem. Educ.* **2007**, *84*, 1643–1646. [CrossRef]

96. Marlowe, F. Male contribution to diet and female reproductive success among foragers. *Curr. Anthropol.* **2001**, *42*, 755–760. [CrossRef]

97. Pontzer, H. Lessons from the Hadza: Poor diets wreck efforts to prevent obesity and diabetes. *Diabetes Voice* **2012**, *57*, 26–29.

98. Pontzer, H.; Raichlen, D.A.; Wood, B.M.; Mabulla, A.Z.P.; Racette, S.B.; Marlowe, F.W. Hunter-gatherer energetics and human obesity. *PLoS ONE* **2012**, *7*, e40503. [CrossRef] [PubMed]

99. Krogh-Madsen, R.; Thyfault, J.P.; Broholm, C.; Mortensen, O.H.; Olsen, R.H.; Mounier, R.; Plomgaard, P.; van Hall, G.; Booth, F.W.; Pedersen, B.K. A 2-wk reduction of ambulatory activity attenuates peripheral insulin sensitivity. *J. Appl. Physiol.* **2010**, *108*, 1034–1040. [CrossRef] [PubMed]

100. Olsen, R.H.; Krogh-Madsen, R.; Thomsen, C.; Booth, F.W.; Pedersen, B.K. Metabolic responses to reduced daily steps in healthy nonexercising men. *JAMA* **2008**, *299*, 1261–1263. [PubMed]

101. Tappy, L.; Lê, K.A. Metabolic effects of fructose and the worldwide increase in obesity. *Physiol. Rev.* **2010**, *90*, 23–46. [CrossRef] [PubMed]

102. Bidwell, A.J.; Fairchild, T.J.; Redmond, J.; Wang, L.; Keslacy, L.; Kanaley, J.A. Physical activity offsets the negative effects of a high-fructose diet. *Med. Sci. Sports Exerc.* **2014**, *46*, 2091–2098. [CrossRef] [PubMed]

103. Egli, L.; Lecoultre, V.; Theytaz, F.; Campos, V.; Hodson, L.; Schneiter, P.; Mittendorfer, B.; Patterson, B.W.; Fielding, B.A.; Gerber, P.A.; et al. Exercise prevents fructose-induced hypertriglyceridemia in healthy young subjects. *Diabetes* **2013**, *62*, 2259–2265. [CrossRef] [PubMed]

104. Egli, L.; Lecoultre, V.; Cros, J.; Rosset, R.; Marques, A.-S.; Schneiter, P.; Hodson, L.; Gabert, L.; Laville, M.; Tappy, L. Exercise performed immediately after fructose ingestion enhances fructose oxidation and suppresses fructose storage. *Am. J. Clin. Nutr.* **2016**, *103*, 348–355. [CrossRef] [PubMed]

105. Krebs, H.A. The August Krogh principle: "For many problems there is an animal on which it can be most conveniently studied". *J. Exp. Zool.* **1975**, *194*, 221–226. [CrossRef] [PubMed]

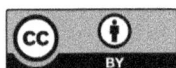

MDPI

St. Alban-Anlage 66

4052 Basel

Switzerland

Tel. +41 61 683 77 34

Fax +41 61 302 89 18

www.mdpi.com

Nutrients Editorial Office

E-mail: nutrients@mdpi.com

www.mdpi.com/journal/nutrients